Praise for THE PATIENT'S BOOK OF NATURAL HEALING

"A wealth of useful information about illnesses and their treatments with
a healthy dose of comfort, understanding, and knowledge."
—MICHAEL T. MURRAY, N.D., author of *The Encyclopedia of Natural Medicine,
The Encyclopedia of Nutritional Supplements,* and THE GETTING WELL NATURALLY series

❧

"Drs. Gaby and Wright have been effectively treating patients suffering from
a variety of chronic diseases for more than 25 years. This book powerfully
presents their wealth of wisdom and experience and makes it easily
accessible to the reader. It is an excellent reference for anyone with a
chronic condition willing to take responsibility for their own care."
—ROBERT S. IVKER, D.O., author of the bestselling *Sinus Survival* and
The Complete Self-Care Guide to Holistic Medicine

❧

"A perennial and devout believer in natural healing, I am delighted with
my copy of *The Patient's Book of Natural Healing* written by
a great pair of natural healers."
—JIM DUKE, author of *The Green Pharmacy*

JONATHAN V. WRIGHT, M.D. · ALAN R. GABY, M.D.

THE PATIENT'S BOOK OF NATURAL HEALING

PRIMA HEALTH

A Division of Prima Publishing

WARNING—DISCLAIMER

This book is for reference and informational purposes only and is in no way intended as medical counseling or medical advice. This information contained herein should not be used to treat, diagnose or prevent any disease or medical condition without the advice of a competent medical professional. The authors and Prima Publishing shall have neither liability nor responsibility to any person or entity with respect to any loss, damage, or injury caused or alleged to be caused directly or indirectly by the information contained in this book.

All products mentioned in this book are registered trademarks of their respective companies.

PRIMA HEALTH and colophon are registered trademarks of Prima Communications, Inc.

Library of Congress Cataloging-in-Publication Data

Wright, Jonathan V.
     The patient's book of natural healing / Jonathan Wright and Alan R. Gaby.
a cm.
          Includes bibliographical references and index.
          ISBN 0-7615-2018-X
1. Diet therapy. 2. Nutrition. 3. Health. I. Gaby, Alan R. II. Title
     RM216.W857 1999
     615.8'54—dc21   99-39232
                                                                        CIP

99 00 01 02 HH 10 9 8 7 6 5 4 3 2 1
Printed in the United States of America

HOW TO ORDER

Single copies may be ordered from Prima Publishing, P.O. Box 1260BK, Rocklin, CA 95677; telephone (916) 632-4400. Quantity discounts are also available. On your letterhead, include information concerning the intended use of the books and the number of books you wish to purchase.

Visit us online at www.primahealth.com

For Holly

—JONATHAN V. WRIGHT

❧

To my parents, for helping me to become what I am.
To Bonnie Raindrop and Pamela Snider, N.D., for teaching me the joy of service.

—ALAN R. GABY

CONTENTS

ACKNOWLEDGMENTS

The authors acknowledge and are grateful for the pioneering work of Roger Williams, Abram Hoffer, Linus Pauling, Carlton Fredericks, William Kaufman, John Yudkin, Broda Barnes, William Jefferies, John Ellis, Frederick Klenner, Emanuel Cheraskin, Robert McCarrison, Tom Spies, Weston Price, Francis Pottenger, Tom Brewer, James Duke, James Breneman, Wilfred and Evan Shute, and many, many others, whose innovative ideas have given us the tools to help thousands of patients and to make this book possible.

Dr. Wright is additionally grateful to Samuel Hahnemann, James Tyler Kent, Constantine Hering, C. von Boenninghausen, Albert Abrams, Ruth Drown, George Crile, Harold Saxton Burr, Reinhold Voll, William Tiller, the unknown originators of acupuncture, and many other pioneers in the field of "energy medicine."

INTRODUCTION

THIS BOOK EXPLAINS how natural medicine can be used to prevent and treat illness and promote optimal health. Although the term "natural medicine" has no universally accepted definition, to us it refers to the "medicinal" use of diet, nutritional supplements, natural hormones, herbs, and other naturally occurring substances.

We first became interested in natural medicine in the early 1970s, after we realized that the usual drug-and-surgery approach that we were taught in medical school was often dangerous, expensive, and ineffective. Seeking better ways to help our patients, each of us stumbled independently upon a vast, and largely ignored, body of scientific research that pointed to a promising alternative approach. As we tried these natural remedies in our practices, we quickly became convinced that the medical mainstream was overlooking something important. Patients with a wide range of both physical and mental medical conditions who had failed to respond to the best that modern medicine offered, or who suffered intolerable side effects, routinely showed improvements that ranged from gratifying to dramatic. We often heard a patient say, "I've been to 7 different doctors, and you're the first one who's helped me."

Hoping to unlock the full potential of natural medicine, we began a collaborative effort about 20 years ago to collect and review all the scientific research we could find in this field. Now, with more than 30,000 scientific papers in our files, and having between us more than 70,000 patient visits, we are firmly convinced that most chronic (and some acute) illnesses can be treated safely, effectively, and relatively inexpensively with natural medicines. In many cases, natural medicine alone can restore a patient to health. However, with some conditions (particularly more severe ones), natural treatments must be used in conjunction with conventional therapy.

In 1983, we began teaching natural medicine to health-care practitioners at an annual seminar. To date, more than 3,000 medical doctors, nurses, chiropractors, naturopaths, and other practitioners have taken our course. Those with whom we spoke at a later date all told us the same thing: Natural medicine really works for their patients.

The conventional medical community has for years either ignored or been openly hostile to natural medicine. In fact, some doctors practicing this type of medicine have been disciplined or had their medical licenses revoked on the grounds that they deviated from the professional "standard of care" (i.e., they dared to be different by choosing safer and more effective treatments). The pervasive bias against natural medicine was the topic of a recent commentary in a well-respected mainstream medical journal.[1] Part of this negative attitude may reflect the influence of the pharmaceutical industry (which spends heavily on both drug advertising and the funding of educational programs) on medical education. The negative bias of some government agencies, particularly the Food and Drug Administration (FDA), against natural medicine has also likely inhibited many doctors from taking a closer look at the natural approach. Another factor might be what psychologists call "cognitive dissonance:" Many doctors have a hard time considering the possibility that a simple and safe alternative exists, after they spent years learning to become experts at administering toxic drugs.

Fortunately, more and more doctors are beginning to look seriously at natural medicine, and the research supporting the effectiveness of this approach is stronger than ever. Of course, big changes usually come slowly, and there is still a great deal of resistance to using natural methods instead of drugs and surgery. We hope that this book will help to speed the transition of our health-care system from one that is too often ineffective and dangerous to one that is more humane and better meets the needs of the people it serves.

The first 4 chapters of this book provide general information about diet, digestion, allergies, and natural hormones. In Part 2, we discuss specific conditions and address how natural medicine—using both diet and nutrient supplements—can help. Overall, this book is designed to provide useful information related to the prevention and treatment of most of the common medical conditions that affect us.

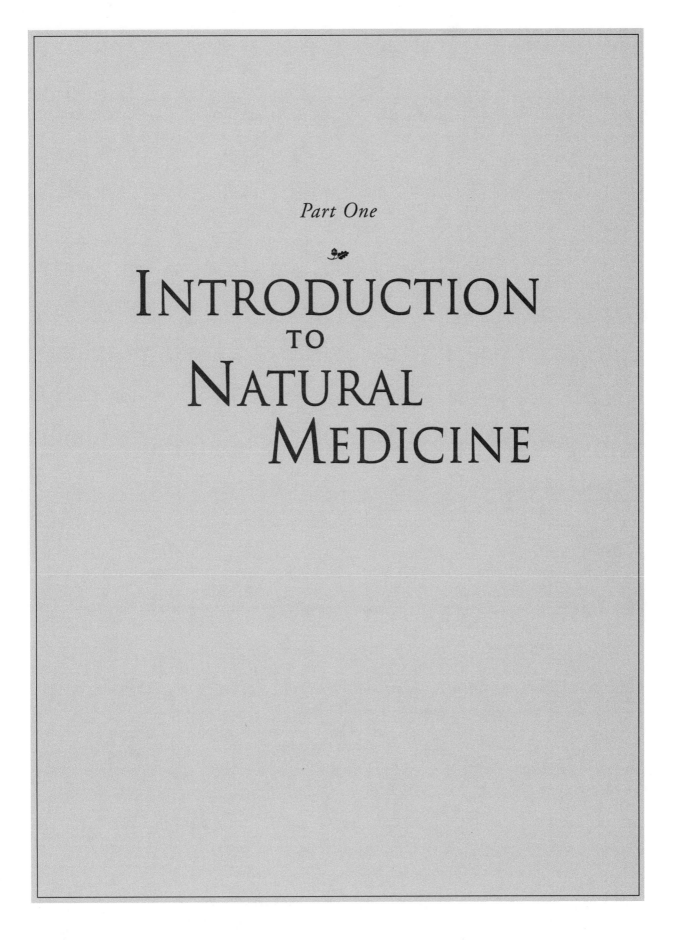

Part One

INTRODUCTION
TO
NATURAL
MEDICINE

CHAPTER ONE

FUNDAMENTALS
OF
NATURAL MEDICINE

For most people, a good natural-medicine program starts with their diet. The relationship between diet and health was recognized more than two thousand years ago by Hippocrates, the "Father of Medicine," who said, "Let your food be your medicine and let your medicine be your food." Additionally, in 1726, Jonathan Swift (*Gulliver's Travels*) wrote, "Kitchen, physic [medicine] is the best physic." More recently, Dr. Gaby's Uncle Ruben, remarked, "Health comes from the farm, not the pharmacy."

Many people come to our clinics looking for the magic vitamin or herb that will solve their problems, and they are not particularly interested in changing their diets. Some people who refuse to work on their diet do, in fact, see marked improvements when they take the right vitamins, minerals, amino acids, hormones, or herbs. However, most such individuals achieve less-than-optimal results. Those who are intolerant to refined sugar or have food sensitivities hardly improve at all until they make the necessary dietary changes. We recommend dietary improvement for two principal reasons: 1) a good diet may help prevent killer diseases such as cancer, heart disease, stroke, and diabetes from developing in the future, and 2) making appropriate dietary changes will often relieve today's symptoms and medical problems.

An Overview of Dietary Considerations

The most basic principle of nutrition is to consume a wide variety of health-promoting foods and to avoid (or reduce the intake of) foods that are known or suspected to cause adverse effects. Foods that are "good" for most people include whole grains, fresh fruits and vegetables, nuts and seeds, legumes, and moderate amounts of low-fat animal foods (beef, chicken, fish, and eggs). Potential "problem foods" include refined sugars, white flour, and foods that contain processed or modified fats, caffeine, or excessive amounts of salt. The relative merits and risks of consuming dairy products are still being debated. Consuming alcohol in moderation may be safe for many people, but drinking large amounts can be dangerous. Drinking pure, unpolluted water is also important. These issues are discussed in greater detail below.

Beneficial Foods

A health-promoting diet should consist of a wide variety of whole, unprocessed foods that are free of chemical additives and, if possible, grown without the use of pesticides. Such a diet generally includes liberal amounts of fresh fruits and vegetables, whole grains, nuts, seeds, and legumes. For most people, animal foods such as eggs, fish, chicken, and beef may be healthy in moderation. Of course, as most vegetarians have shown, good health can be maintained without eating animal foods. In fact, compared with meat-eaters, vegetarians may have a lower risk of heart disease, hypertension, gallbladder disease, kidney stones, and other disorders. However, if a vegetarian does not plan his diet carefully, he can develop deficiencies of protein, iron, zinc, vitamin D, vitamin B_{12}, and other nutrients.

A balanced, whole-foods diet provides the key nutrients—proteins, carbohydrates, fats, vitamins, and minerals—that are essential for life and good health. If those nutrients were all that whole foods provided, most of us could thrive on junk food, as long as we took nutritional supplements. That is not, however, the case. While many individuals do benefit, sometimes dramatically, from nutritional supplements, individuals who also work on their diet achieve the best results.

One reason whole foods are so important is that they contain many compounds that are not considered "essential nutrients," but that appear to play an important role in human health. For example, soybeans contain two molecules known as isoflavones—genistein and daidzein—that serve to modulate or balance the effects of estrogen.[1] In postmenopausal women who are deficient in estrogen, eating soy products has been shown to relieve hot flashes (apparently by exerting an estrogenic effect).[2] In women with too much estrogen, on the other hand, soy isoflavones compete with the stronger human estrogens, possibly reducing the risk of breast cancer and other hormone-dependent cancers.[3] Soybeans have also been shown to prevent atherosclerosis (hardening of the arteries) in experimental animals[4]—an effect that may be due at least in part to the isoflavones.

Many other foods contain "healthful" compounds. For example, broccoli, brussels sprouts, cabbage, and cauliflower contain indole-3-carbinol and several other compounds that appear to have anticancer activity.[5] Tomatoes, pink grapefruit, and watermelon contain another cancer-fighting substance called lycopene.[6, 7] Spinach, collard greens, and other dark-green leafy vegetables are rich sources of lutein, a carotenoid that may prevent the development of age-related macular degeneration.[8, 9] (See chapter on macular degeneration for more information.) Blueberries and grapes contain flavonoids called anthocyanosides, which may help prevent varicose veins and improve visual function.

Whole grains, fruits, vegetables, and other plant foods are good sources of dietary fiber. Most health-care practitioners accept that fiber promotes normal bowel function, prevents constipation, and helps prevent diverticular disease of the colon. In addition, evidence suggests that eating enough fiber may reduce the risk of heart disease, diabetes, hemorrhoids, and some types of cancer.

Refined Carbohydrates Cause Problems

IN addition to recommending health-promoting foods, we advise avoidance of those foods that promote illness. At the top of that list is refined sugar. By "refined sugar," we mean not just the table sugar that we put in our coffee and tea or on top of our cereal, but also the large amounts of sucrose, fructose, glucose, dextrose, high-fructose corn syrup, and other forms of sugar that are added by food processors to a wide variety of foods. "Refined sugar" does not include the sugar that occurs naturally in fruit, milk, and other whole foods. In the typical American diet, fully 19% of the calories come from added sugar. That translates to an average of 41 teaspoons of sugar per day. Most people find it difficult to believe they consume that much sugar. However, considering that a 12-ounce soft drink contains more than 8 teaspoons of sugar, and that pies, cookies, candies, doughnuts, pastries, cereals, applesauce, ketchup, and many other foods are heavily sweetened, 41 teaspoons per day becomes more believable.

Sugar is almost completely devoid of vitamins, minerals, and other essential nutrients. Thus, the typical American diet contains 19% fewer nutrients than it would if all of the sugar were eliminated. This across-the-board reduction of nutrient intake may have long-term consequences for our health, as well as affecting how we feel today. Studies described elsewhere in this book have shown that ingesting large amounts of sugar can cause adverse changes in risk factors for cardiovascular disease, impair the body's ability to fight infection, and possibly increase the risk of developing kidney stones and osteoporosis.

In our experience, sugar is also a major contributing factor to a wide range of symptoms, including fatigue, depression, anxiety, insomnia, premenstrual syndrome, headaches, joint pains, and abdominal complaints. Many of the negative effects of sugar may be due to the fact that it is absorbed very rapidly into the bloodstream, a phenomenon that the human body was apparently not programmed to handle efficiently. When blood-sugar levels rise abruptly, the body often overreacts and releases excessive amounts of insulin. This outpouring of insulin tends to push blood-sugar levels too low (hypoglycemia), resulting in a compensatory release of adrenaline and other blood-sugar-raising hormones. Thus, eating too much sugar can cause both wide swings in blood-sugar concentrations and elevated levels of various regulatory hormones. Some of the symptoms commonly attributed to "hypoglycemia" are indeed due to low blood sugar, but other symptoms appear to be caused by the high levels of adrenaline, insulin,[10] or other hormones that result from eating too much sugar. Whatever the biochemical explanation, we have found that for many individuals, removing sugar from the diet is extremely beneficial.

Refined grains, such as white bread and white rice, should also be avoided and replaced with whole-grain breads and brown rice, respectively. When whole grains are refined, the nutrient-rich germ portion and the nutrient- and fiber-rich bran portion are lost. Refined grains, which comprise approximately 30% of the calories in the American diet, contain substantially lower amounts of vitamins, minerals, and fiber than their unrefined counterparts. In addition, the carbohydrates in refined grains are absorbed relatively rapidly and may promote some of the same symptoms as eating sugar (albeit to a lesser degree).

Avoid "Bad" Fats

MOST doctors agree that our diets should be relatively low in fat. However, many people do not appreciate that the type of fats in the diet may be even more important than the amount of fat consumed. One potentially dangerous class of fats is the so-called *trans*-fatty acids that are produced during the processing of vegetable oils. *Trans*-fatty acids rarely (if ever) occur in natural foods. They are present in large amounts in most margarines and they are also found in foods that contain partially hydrogenated vegetable oil. Evidence shows that ingesting *trans*-fatty acids promotes the development of essential-fatty-acid deficiency.[11] Moreover, studies have suggested that consuming *trans*- fatty acids may increase the risk of heart disease.[12, 13] We therefore recommend that people avoid margarine and foods that contain partially hydrogenated vegetable oil.

Also potentially dangerous are vegetable oils that have been heated to high temperatures, as one would find in fried foods. The polyunsaturated fatty acids that are present in most vegetable oils are relatively unstable, and when they are heated in the presence of oxygen (from the air), some of these fatty acids are converted to toxic compounds called lipid peroxides. Consuming excessive amounts of lipid peroxides can lead to a chain reaction of chemical events known as free-radical damage. Free-radical damage is believed to accelerate the aging process and possibly contribute to heart disease, cancer, and other problems. Although the polyunsaturated fats found in vegetable oils have a number of positive effects on our health, the risks probably outweigh the benefits when these fats become oxidized.

Because of the chemical changes that occur in oils when they are heated to high temperatures, eating a lot of fried foods is not a good idea. Stir-frying is safer than deep-frying, because only a small amount of oil is heated and for just a short period of time. Also, if food must be fried, olive, coconut, or palm kernel oils are preferable, as they are less likely than other oils to form lipid peroxides during heating.

Cholesterol is also an unstable molecule. In the presence of heat and air, it can be converted into highly toxic cholesterol oxides. Animal studies show that eating pure cholesterol is not particularly harmful, but eating even small quantities of oxidized cholesterol causes considerable damage to the arteries.[14] High-temperature cooking with butter or lard is likely to produce significant amounts of oxidized cholesterol. In addition, broiling or baking beef or other cholesterol-containing foods at high temperatures probably produces more toxic byproducts than cooking at lower temperatures for longer periods of time. Poaching eggs or boiling them inside their shells presumably creates little or no oxidized cholesterol, because the cholesterol in the yolk is not exposed to oxygen during cooking. On the other hand, scrambling eggs or baking with eggs probably causes a significant amount of these toxic molecules to be produced. Other sources of cholesterol oxides include dried-egg products, powdered milk, grated cheeses, and processed meats.

The oxidation of unsaturated fats and cholesterol that occurs during cooking also takes place in the open air at room temperature, although at a much slower rate. For this reason, butter, nuts, vegetable oils, and other foods that contain unstable fats should be protected from exposure to air and kept refrigerated as much as possible.

In contrast to the "bad fats" described above, so-called "essential fatty acids" (EFAs) have a number of beneficial effects. EFAs are usually classified as either omega-6 or omega-3 fatty acids, depending on their chemical structure.

Sunflower oil, safflower oil, and soybean oil are good sources of omega-6 EFAs. The best sources of omega-3 fatty acids are flaxseed oil and fish oil. Increasing one's intake of EFAs can be helpful for a wide range of medical conditions, ranging from prostate enlargement to psoriasis to heart disease.

What About Dairy Products?

Cow's milk is heavily advertised by the dairy industry as a health-promoting food—one that "does a body good." However, while dairy products are a good source of protein, calcium, and some other nutrients, there are a number of important concerns about the safety of this food group. Research suggests that drinking milk may increase the risk of developing type 1 (juvenile onset) diabetes,[15] although not all of the studies agree. The mechanism by which milk might cause diabetes is as follows: First, certain proteins or partially digested fragments of proteins from milk are absorbed intact into the bloodstream. Next, the immune system recognizes these proteins as foreign and manufactures antibodies against them. Finally, in individuals who have a specific genetic makeup, these antibodies cross-react with cell-surface molecules in the pancreas, resulting in the destruction of the insulin-producing cells of the pancreas.[16]

Evidence also indicates that consuming cow's milk may be a cause of heart disease, independent of its saturated fat and cholesterol content. Cow's milk contains an enzyme called xanthine oxidase, which is said to be capable of damaging blood-vessel walls and promoting atherosclerosis (hardening of the arteries).[17] Normally, this enzyme would not cause any trouble, because it would be destroyed by digestive juices shortly after a person drinks the milk. However, the process of homogenization causes xanthine oxidase to become coated by fat molecules and effectively "walled off" from the digestive juices, possibly allowing it to be absorbed intact into the bloodstream. The absorption of xanthine oxidase from cow's milk has been demonstrated in animals.[18] Additionally, human atherosclerotic plaques have been found to contain xanthine oxidase.[19] Although these studies do not prove that milk causes atherosclerosis, it is noteworthy that the incidence of heart disease around the world correlates with consumption of homogenized milk, but not with consumption of butter or cheese (which are higher in fat, but which contain little or no absorbable xanthine oxidase).[20] Significant amounts of xanthine oxidase are presumably absorbed from whole milk, 2%-fat milk, and 1%-fat milk, whereas little or none of this enzyme would be absorbed from skim milk, cheese, butter, or yogurt.

Another problem with cow's milk is that many people lack the enzyme necessary to digest lactose—a sugar that is present in milk and most other dairy products (except some cheeses). Lactose intolerance is extremely common among persons of Asian or African descent (with an estimated 80 to 90 percent being affected), as well as among the population of southern Europe and India. Individuals with lactose intolerance often experience nausea, diarrhea, intestinal cramps, or bloating when they consume dairy products. Perhaps more important, the proteins in cow's milk are among the most common allergens in the human diet. We have seen hundreds of people whose problems (including nasal congestion, asthma, arthritis, ulcerative colitis, peptic ulcer, recurrent ear infections, manic-depressive psychosis, and various skin conditions) resolved after they removed dairy products from their diet.

For these reasons, we advise many individuals to restrict their intake of dairy products or to avoid them altogether, and to obtain their calcium from other sources, such as dark green vegetables (except spinach), whole grains, beans, and calcium supplements.

Caffeine

MOST American adults consume caffeine every day, primarily in coffee, tea, chocolate, or cola drinks. Because caffeine consumption is so widespread, many of us overlook the fact that it is an addictive and potentially toxic chemical that has profound effects on human physiology. While not all research agrees, caffeine consumption has been implicated as a contributing factor to anxiety, insomnia, hypertension, fibrocystic breast disease, impaired fertility, headaches, osteoporosis, heart-rhythm disturbances, and some gastrointestinal complaints. Although withdrawing from caffeine often causes fatigue and fairly severe headaches for a day or two, most people who make it through the withdrawal period feel considerably better than when they were consuming caffeine.

Alcohol

WHEN consumed in excessive amounts, alcohol can damage the liver, heart, brain, and other organs. Moderate alcohol consumption (such as one drink per day) does not appear to cause problems for most people, although some individuals (particularly those who are intolerant to refined carbohydrates), experience symptoms even from small amounts of alcohol. Drinking alcohol may aggravate hypertension, gout, psoriasis, and rosacea (a skin condition). There is some evidence (by no means conclusive), that drinking moderate amounts of red wine (or possibly other alcoholic beverages) may reduce the risk of developing heart disease. However, considering that heart disease can be prevented in many other ways, we are hesitant to recommend that a potentially toxic and addictive substance be used for that purpose.

Food Additives

MODERN processed foods contain so many chemical additives that it is impossible to determine all the effects they have on our bodies. Studies have implicated artificial colorings as a triggering factor for hyperactivity in children; tartrazine (Yellow Dye #5) and sulfites as factors in asthma; sodium benzoate as a cause of hives; and the artificial sweetener aspartame as a cause of a wide range of symptoms in susceptible individuals.[21, 22] Some farm animals are treated with hormones and antibiotics, and the residues of these substances may remain in the meat after the animals are slaughtered. Certain pesticides have estrogenic activity and could, in theory, increase the risk of reproductive problems and certain cancers. Although we still have a great deal to learn about the health effects of food additives, common sense suggests that we do our best to keep them out of our diet, by emphasizing fresh, unprocessed foods that are grown without the use of pesticides, antibiotics, and hormones.

Importance of Drinking Pure Water

MOST tap water in the United States contains two potentially toxic additives: chlorine (which is used as a disinfectant), and fluoride (which is put in the water to prevent dental cavities). Chlorine is a powerful oxidizing agent, and it has the potential to accelerate the aging process by inducing free-radical damage to cells. Evidence also suggests that ingesting chlorinated water may increase the risk of heart disease [23] and some types of cancer.[24]

Fluoride is a known poison that inhibits a number of essential biochemical processes. In addition, although fluoride has been reported to increase bone density, the quality of that bone seems to be impaired. This is demonstrated by an increase in the number of hip fractures in communities where fluoridated water is consumed.[25] While good evidence does show that drinking fluoridated water can reduce the incidence of cavities, an argument can be made that the risks of ingesting fluoride outweigh its benefits. Probably the most effective way to prevent cavities is to eliminate refined sugar from the diet.

Aluminum is another toxic metal that is commonly added to municipal water supplies in order to remove particulate matter. In addition, the drinking water in many cities, including Boston, New York, Philadelphia, Washington, Seattle, San Francisco, and Phoenix, contains excessive amounts of lead. According to one estimate, about 32 million Americans drink water that exceeds the federal safety limit for lead of 15 parts per billion.[26]

Because of these problems with tap water, we advise our patients to use bottled spring water, distilled water, or filtered water for drinking and cooking. Distilling water or filtering it by reverse osmosis or other powerful techniques removes not only toxic contaminants, but also essential minerals.

Individuals who consume demineralized water should therefore supplement their diet with a multimineral formula.

Living in a Polluted World

IN ADDITION TO concerns about the foods we eat, the modern world is contaminated with tens of thousands of chemicals, some of which have been shown to be allergens, carcinogens, or promoters of various diseases. The adverse effects of environmental chemicals may actually be greater than the research suggests. That is because most chemicals are tested individually for toxicity, but the combined effect of several chemicals is sometimes much greater than that of any single chemical by itself.[27] Although it is not possible to avoid pollution completely, you can take measures to reduce your exposure and possibly improve your health.

Lead

ONE of the most universal toxins is lead, which is widely used as an industrial metal. Low-level lead poisoning can cause muscle aches, fatigue, irritability, lethargy, joint pains, trouble concentrating, headaches, and weight loss. Lead may also contribute to heart disease, stroke, hypertension, and osteoporosis. As mentioned previously, some municipal water supplies contain excessive amounts of lead. In addition, approximately 200,000 tons of industrial lead aerosols are emitted annually into the atmosphere of the northern hemisphere. Some of this lead finds its way into our bodies through the lungs or by falling to the ground and entering the food chain through the soil. Other sources of lead include canned foods and some paints and cosmetics.

It is not known whether the amount of lead the average American is exposed to is a significant cause of symptoms or illness. However, it is noteworthy that the concentration of lead in the skeletons of modern Americans is about 500 times higher than the concentration in the bones of individuals living 1,800 years ago.[28] People can reduce their exposure to lead by avoiding canned foods and by drinking bottled water or water that is filtered in a way that removes heavy metals. In addition, animal studies and some research in humans suggest that people can reduce lead absorption and/or enhance its excretion by supplementing their diets with various nutrients, including vitamin C, zinc, calcium, and magnesium.

Aluminum

ALUMINUM is another potentially harmful metal that is widespread in the environment. Evidence shows that aluminum exposure may play a role in the development of osteoporosis and Alzheimer's disease.[29] As mentioned previously, aluminum is added to many municipal water supplies. Beverages stored in aluminum cans contain three to six times more aluminum than the same beverages stored in glass. Other sources of aluminum include food wrappings, aluminum cookware, sodium aluminum phosphate (a food additive), baking powder, processed cheese, pickles, and some antacids.

Mercury

MERCURY is perhaps the most toxic metal on the planet. Our two major sources of mercury exposure are fish and dental fillings. Fortunately, certain minerals or other molecules present in fish latch onto mercury and form a larger compound that, for some reason, is relatively harmless. However, the same is not true of the mercury in dental amalgams. The act of chewing has been shown to release measurable amounts of mercury vapor from these amalgams into the mouth. In animal studies, placing mercury amalgams in the mouth resulted in abnormalities of immune function, which returned to normal when the mercury was removed from the mouth.

The question of whether mercury fillings represent a health risk to humans has been heatedly debated. Although disagreements persist, we do not believe that the continued use of mercury fillings is justifiable, considering that many other materials are available in modern dentistry. Whether people should have their old mercury amalgams removed is another question. We have seen some patients in whom an autoimmune disease or other serious illness improved dramatically after their mercury fillings were replaced with other materials. However, only about 10% of those who have undergone amalgam removal have seen significant benefit. Changing one's fillings is expensive and traumatic to the teeth. When considering removing mercury fillings, the potential benefits should be weighed against the cost and the risk of damage to the teeth.

Many other environmental chemicals have been shown to affect human health. While space does not permit a discussion of every known pollutant, we recommend that you remain aware of when you are being exposed to toxic chemicals, and try to avoid unnecessary exposure as much as possible.

An Overview of Nutritional Supplements: Expensive Urine or Promising Therapy?

IN ADDITION TO improving one's diet and minimizing exposure to toxic chemicals, nutrient supplementation is often important for restoring and maintaining one's health. Numerous studies, described throughout this book, have shown that providing additional quantities of vitamins, minerals, amino acids, or other naturally occurring compounds can help relieve a wide range of symptoms and disorders.

Many doctors cling to the belief that the typical diet contains all the nutrients a person needs to stay healthy. We still occasionally hear that time-worn cliché that the only thing people obtain from taking supplements is "expensive urine." The beliefs that lead to such remarks reflect an incomplete understanding of human biochemistry and physiology. Perhaps if doctors better understood how nutrient supplements could work, they would be more inclined to pay attention to the research showing that they do work.

The rationale for using supplements extends beyond the rather obvious fact that refined, processed foods that are grown on depleted soil are low in vitamins and minerals. Even people who consume the most nutritious diets—particularly individuals suffering from illness—can often benefit from nutritional supplements. Some of the reasons that supplementation may be necessary or desirable are as follows:

- **To compensate for a weak digestive system.** Individuals who have difficulty digesting and assimilating nutrients may not be able to obtain what they need solely from their diet. Malabsorption may occur with advancing age, with the use of certain medications, and with a number of different diseases. In many cases, the effects of inefficient absorption can be overcome by providing higher-than-normal quantities of vitamins, minerals, and other nutrients.

- **To overcome a defect in the transport of nutrients into the tissues.** For example, in some individuals with heart failure, the capacity to transport magnesium into the heart muscle is impaired.[30] Some patients with dementia appear to have difficulty transporting vitamin B_{12} from the bloodstream into the brain.[31] In these patients injections of the respective nutrients resulted in clinical improvement.

- **To compensate for a genetically abnormal enzyme.** There are numerous examples of rare genetic disorders that result in unusually high requirements for a particular nutrient. We have only recently begun to discover that milder genetic variations are fairly common. For example, it is now well documented that many people are at risk of developing heart disease because they cannot metabolize homocysteine (a breakdown product of protein) efficiently. In these individuals, increasing the intake of vitamin B_6 and/or folic acid nearly always improves homocysteine metabolism.

- **To overcome the effects of pollution.** A number of environmental pollutants have been shown to interfere with specific nutrients. For example, a group of compounds called hydrazines and hydrazides, which are widely used in industry and agriculture, appear to interfere with vitamin B_6 utilization.[32] Carpal tunnel syndrome, a condition that causes problems in the hands, has been reported to respond to relatively large doses of vitamin B_6.[33] It is noteworthy that carpal tunnel syndrome, a fairly common problem today, was virtually unknown 50 years ago.[34] These observations suggest that the proliferation of hydrazines and hydrazides in our environment may have increased our requirement for vitamin B_6 by interfering with the way this vitamin works in the body.

- **To correct nutritional deficiencies induced by prescription drugs.** The list of drugs that can adversely affect nutritional status is long, and includes diuretics, antacids, acid-blockers, anticonvulsants, asthma medications, prednisone, and some cholesterol-lowering drugs. The most common ways in which drugs cause nutritional deficiencies are by 1) inhibiting nutrient absorption and 2) increasing the loss of nutrients through the urine. Certain drugs also block some of the normal biochemical functions of nutrients, resulting in an increased requirement for those nutrients. The interactions between drugs and nutrients can be rather complex, and working with these interactions usually requires the advice of a nutritionally oriented doctor. Unfortunately, drug-induced nutritional deficiencies are often overlooked by the average doctor.

- **To make use of direct chemical or pharmacological effects of some nutrients.** For example, vitamin C in high concentrations has been shown to kill viruses[35] and to inactivate histamine.[36] In addition, the presence of extra magnesium in the urine inhibits the formation of the calcium-oxalate crystals that cause kidney stones.[37] Vitamin B$_{12}$ has been shown to degrade sulfites,[38] an action that would be useful for individuals with sulfite sensitivity.

When nutrients are used in amounts greater than those normally present in the diet, it is not always clear whether the effects are "nutritional" or "pharmacological" (drug-like). Consequently, using nutrients therapeutically tends to blur the distinction between farm and pharmacy. But, considering how much people can benefit, and how little risk there is when nutrients are used with appropriate precautions, we believe that Hippocrates, Mr. Swift, and Uncle Ruben would understand.

CHAPTER TWO

DIGESTION
AND
ABSORPTION

EVERYONE HAS HEARD the saying, "You are what you eat." But from the standpoint of natural medicine, it would be more accurate to say, "You are what you assimilate." Even the best possible diet plan for a particular ailment might not produce the expected results if our capacity to digest and absorb food and nutrients is impaired. In addition, some individuals appear to absorb nutritional supplements poorly. They do not respond well to treatment unless the nutrients are given by injection or unless measures are taken to improve their gastrointestinal function.

Published research and/or our clinical experience have indicated that inadequate digestion or absorption of nutrients is a common problem among individuals with certain medical conditions, including: rheumatoid arthritis, osteoarthritis, hypothyroidism, hyperthyroidism, childhood asthma, rosacea, bursitis, chronic fatigue syndrome, depression, diabetes, gallbladder disease, lupus, age-related macular degeneration, multiple sclerosis, osteoporosis, "shingles" (herpes zoster), and cancer. In addition, as with many other bodily functions, digestion and absorption tend to become less efficient—even in healthy people—as they grow older. This impairment of gastrointestinal function may contribute to some of the infirmities of old age. Although not all causes of faulty digestion and absorption can be corrected, certain basic interventions are often helpful.

This chapter describes some of the important activities that occur in the body during the digestion and absorption of food and nutrients. It also explains some common problems that can occur during digestion and absorption and how these problems can be alleviated.

Digestion and absorption begin in the mouth, where food is partially broken down by chewing and by an enzyme in the saliva. In the stomach, food is further digested by the action of hydrochloric acid and pepsin. The food then passes into the small intestine, where it is acted upon by enzymes secreted by the pancreas, other enzymes produced by cells that line the intestine, and bile salts that are released from the liver and gallbladder. The vitamins, minerals, amino acids, carbohydrates and fats that are liberated by the process of digestion are absorbed through the small-intestinal wall into the bloodstream. The large intestine (colon) also contributes to the process of absorption, although its role is limited primarily to the absorption of water and certain minerals and electrolytes.

The Importance of Chewing

IN OUR ZEAL to provide the most up-to-date, sophisticated medical recommendations we sometimes forget to emphasize the obvious—like the importance of chewing our food thoroughly. One of the effects of chewing is to mix the food with saliva, which contains an enzyme that initiates the digestive process. Chewing also reduces the size of food particles, thereby increasing the surface area upon which digestive juices can act. The smaller the particles that come in contact with digestive juices, the more efficient the digestive process will be. Even the strongest digestive system would have difficulty dealing with a meal that has been gulped down. There is great truth in Upton Sinclair's statement that "Nature will castigate those who don't masticate."

Hydrochloric Acid

ONE OF THE functions of the stomach is to produce hydrochloric acid. The acid-secreting capacity of a healthy stomach is so great that at the end of its digestive process the pH (a measure of acidity) of the gastric contents is about 2.0 (highly acidic). The stomach also secretes pepsin, an enzyme that digests protein. Both the secretion of pepsin and its protein-digesting action are enhanced by the acidic environment provided by hydrochloric acid. Acting together, hydrochloric acid and pepsin represent a powerful first step in the digestion of protein. They can reduce even the toughest piece of meat to liquid. There is also evidence (occasionally conflicting) that hydrochloric acid enhances the absorption of iron, copper, folic acid, vitamin B_{12}, and calcium.

Impaired Secretion of Hydrochloric Acid and Pepsin

As we grow older, or with certain diseases, the stomach's capacity to secrete hydrochloric acid becomes impaired, resulting in decreased absorption of amino acids (the breakdown products of protein) and certain vitamins and minerals. This impaired secretion of hydrochloric acid and pepsin is called hypochlorhydria. Hypochlorhydria is probably the most common weakness in the digestive system, and it is frequently associated with the various medical conditions listed previously. Although conventional medicine minimizes the importance of hypochlorhydria, we have observed that some patients do not respond well to a nutritional program until hydrochloric acid and pepsin are added to their regimen.

Lack of stomach acid may also impair a person's response to some herbal remedies. A study was performed to determine why some patients respond well to a particular herb, whereas similar patients with the same medical condition fail to improve at all. Analysis of a number of medicinal herbs revealed that many were unable to exert their therapeutic effect until the "active ingredients" were released by the action of gastric juice. Individuals who responded well to herbal medications had more acid and pepsin in their gastric juice, compared with those who did not respond to the herbs.[1]

Symptoms of Low Hydrochloric Acid

INDIVIDUALS with hypochlorhydria may show signs of sub-optimal nutrition, such as broken fingernails or thinning hair (more commonly seen in women than in men, who have other major causes for hair loss). A wide range of other problems may also develop as a consequence of the nutritional deficiencies resulting from hypochlorhydria. Most (but not all) patients with hypochlorhydria experience gastrointestinal symptoms such as heartburn, bloating after meals, belching, or a feeling that food "just sits in the stomach" (particularly after eating meat). Most of us have been taught that these symptoms are caused by "excess acid," and we often treat the problem with antacids or acid-blocking drugs. However, when we actually measure the acid production of patients with these symptoms, we find that having too little acid is much more common than having too much.

Measuring Hydrochloric Acid

GASTRIC acid output has been measured traditionally by pumping out the stomach contents through a tube. A less invasive method is "radiotelemetry," using an instrument known as a Heidelberg machine. In this procedure, which is performed by some nutritionally oriented doctors, the patient swallows a device the size of a large vitamin tablet that contains a pH meter and a radio-transmitter. The device is tied to a string to prevent it from leaving the stomach. It transmits a radio signal to a machine that prints out a continuous recording of stomach pH. The patient then ingests a solution of baking soda, in order to make the gastric juice alkaline. As the stomach continues to secrete hydrochloric acid, its contents gradually return from alkaline back to acidic. The rate at which this change occurs provides a reasonable estimate of how well the stomach can produce hydrochloric acid.

Treating Hypochlorhydric Patients

FOR reasons that are not entirely clear, intestinal symptoms in hypochlorhydric patients can be relieved either by reducing the acidity further or by supplementing with hydrochloric acid (hydrochloric acid and antacids should never be taken at the same time). We prefer supplementing with hydrochloric acid, because replacing the missing acid often improves digestion and absorption, whereas reducing acidity further can make digestion and absorption worse. Indeed, we have observed that chronic use of antacids or acid-blocking drugs significantly contributes to malnutrition.

Individuals who are treated with hydrochloric acid are usually given capsules containing betaine hydrochloride or glutamic acid hydrochloride. Although the capacity to secrete pepsin is apparently preserved in many hypochlorhydric patients, there is no readily available test to measure pepsin secretion. Therefore, to "cover all of the bases," doctors often recommend products that contain both hydrochloric acid and pepsin. Patients usually take hydrochloric acid capsules during the early part of each meal, in order to maximize their digestive action. The number of capsules recommended depends on the severity of the hypochlorhydria, as well as the size and the protein content of the meal.

Individuals with a history of peptic ulcer and those taking medications that can cause ulcers (such as aspirin, ibuprofen, and other anti-inflammatory drugs) should not take hydrochloric acid, except in special circumstances. In addition, self-treating with hydrochloric acid is not a good idea. You should consult a nutritionally oriented doctor to help you determine whether you need to take hydrochloric acid and how much you might need.

Many individuals with low stomach acid, particularly those with the commonly occurring age-related decline in gastric function, need to supplement with hydrochloric acid indefinitely to maintain the best health possible. People with gastric atrophy due to chronic gastritis or autoimmune damage to the stomach lining may also fail to regain normal stomach function, even after their disease is effectively treated. On the other hand, acid production does return in some patients as they get well. Recent studies have shown that infection with *Helicobacter pylori,* an organism that is associated with chronic gastritis and peptic ulcer, can cause hypochlorhydria.[2] It is conceivable that if this infection is identified and treated before it causes chronic gastric atrophy, gastric acid secretion could be restored to normal.

Pancreatic Enzymes

IN A NORMAL stomach, after the "acid phase" of digestion is completed, the "food slurry" is dumped from the stomach into the upper small intestine (duodenum). The appearance of an acidic mixture in the duodenum causes the release of a hormone (secretin) that stimulates the pancreas to secrete bicarbonate and a group of enzymes that digest proteins, carbohydrates, and fats. All these enzymes function best in the more-alkaline environment provided by the bicarbonate.

Pancreatic Enzyme Deficiency

SYMPTOMS that might suggest pancreatic enzyme deficiency include indigestion beginning an hour or more after meals or excessive flatulence. The stools may be greasy and particularly malodorous. Signs of fat-soluble nutrient deficiency, such as dry, flaky skin, small, hard bumps on the back of the arms, or impaired dark adaptation (night blindness) may be present. Severe pancreatic enzyme deficiency can be diagnosed by stool analysis or by other tests; however, mild pancreatic insufficiency may be more difficult to identify with certainty.

One cause of reduced pancreatic activity is hypochlorhydria; i.e., there is not enough acid to stimulate the pancreatic secretions. This type of pancreatic problem is usually correctable by supplementing with hydrochloric acid. However, if the pancreas itself is weak, nutritional deficiencies could result. As is the case with low stomach function, the prevalence of pancreatic enzyme deficiency appears to increase with age.

Treating Pancreatic Enzyme Deficiency

THE most commonly used replacement therapy for pancreatic enzyme deficiency is an extract of pancreatic tissue from pigs or cows, known as pancreatin. In order to mimic the normal digestive process, pancreatin should be taken after meals—after the food has had adequate time to undergo the "acid phase" of digestion. Bromelain (from pineapple stem), papain (from papaya) or other enzymes derived from plant sources are often used as alternatives to pancreatin. It is not known whether plant-derived enzymes are equal in effectiveness to "animal" enzymes, which are much more similar in structure (and presumably activity) to human enzymes.

Bile Salts

BILE SALTS ARE secreted by the liver and stored in the gallbladder. They play an important role in the digestion and assimilation of fats. Individuals with weak liver function or those who have had their gallbladder removed sometimes benefit from taking a bile-salt supplement. One of us (J.W.) saw a woman in her late 30s who had a history of recurrent ulceration of the cornea of both eyes. She discovered that she needed to take 100,000 IU of vitamin A per day in order to prevent this problem from recurring. Despite taking such a large and potentially toxic amount of vitamin A, her blood level of the vitamin was at the low end of the normal range. This woman had had her gallbladder removed a number of years earlier. When she began taking bile salts after every meal, she was able to prevent her corneal problems with less than half of her previous vitamin A dose.

Bile Salts Deficiency and Treatment

THE clinical signs that might suggest a deficiency of bile salts include intolerance to fatty foods, indigestion, physical evidence of fat-soluble nutrient deficiency (described previously) and stools that are light in color or that float. Of course, each of these signs may be present for other reasons, so it is not always obvious when someone needs to supplement with bile salts. On the other hand, some patients have been able to determine that they need another course of bile-salt therapy by the reappearance of yellowish or floating stools. Certain herbs may be used to enhance the production or the flow of bile—including dandelion, artichoke, and Chelidonium. When these herbal treatments are insufficient, supplementing with bile salts is often helpful.

Only a small proportion of the bile salts secreted by the liver leave the body via the stool; the vast majority return to the liver to be re-used. Consequently, continuous supplementation with bile salts could lead to an excessive accumulation, resulting in diarrhea or green stools. Bile-salt supplements should therefore be used intermittently and only with professional supervision.

Allergic Malabsorption

WE ALL KNOW that certain foods do not "agree" with certain people. Preliminary evidence suggests that these food sensitivities or incompatibilities can result in disturbances of digestion or absorption.

Virtually any portion of the gastrointestinal tract can be a "target tissue" for allergic reactions. Studies have shown that ingesting allergenic foods can damage the lining of the stomach, small intestine, or colon. The classic example of food-induced intestinal damage is celiac disease (also called "gluten enteropathy"). With celiac disease, ingesting wheat or other gluten-containing grains results in severe damage to the small intestine. Individuals with celiac disease malabsorb a wide range of nutrients; however, when they remove the gluten from their diet, their intestinal function returns to normal or near-normal.

In addition to gluten, dairy is another food category that can cause allergic reactions that affect the gastrointestinal tract. One study in infants suggested that a cow's milk allergy can cause significant damage to the lining of the stomach. Fortunately, gastric function returns to normal within 6 months if cow's milk is removed from the diet.[3]

Although there has not been a great deal of research on the relationship between allergy and nutrient absorption, we have observed that patients with food sensitivities often require close attention to digestion and nutrient assimilation. Furthermore, when food allergies are effectively treated, nutritional status often improves.

Conclusion

IMPAIRED DIGESTION AND absorption are relatively common problems, particularly (but not exclusively) among individuals who experience gastrointestinal symptoms. In addition to relieving intestinal symptoms, appropriate use of hydrochloric acid, pepsin, pancreatic enzymes, and/or bile salts may improve nutritional status and increase the effectiveness of some herbal medications, thereby helping to relieve a wide range of medical conditions.

CHAPTER THREE

FOOD ALLERGY
AND
INTOLERANCE

I T IS WELL known that foods such as peanuts, shellfish, or strawberries, or additives such as tartrazine (Yellow Dye #5) or sulfites can trigger acute allergic reactions in susceptible individuals. These reactions may manifest as asthma, swelling, skin rashes, runny nose, or other symptoms. These types of allergic reactions are quite obvious and are easy to recognize.

Less obvious, and more controversial, are the hidden or "masked" allergies. These types of allergies are more difficult to identify because they are often delayed (sometimes for as long as several days after an individual eats an offending food) and because they do not necessarily occur every time the individual eats that food. Recognition of masked allergies is also hampered by the fact that many of the symptoms they cause are not generally perceived as being related to allergies. Nevertheless, doctors who have taken a serious look at hidden food allergy have found it to be a common cause of (or triggering factor for) a wide range of physical and emotional disorders. According to one estimate, as much as 60 percent of the population suffers from undetected food allergy.[1]

Symptoms of Food Allergy

SYMPTOMS AND DISORDERS that are commonly caused by food allergy include fatigue, migraines and other headaches, food cravings, obesity, fluid retention, irritable bowel syndrome, ulcerative colitis, Crohn's disease, gallbladder dis-

ease, arthritis, asthma, chronic bronchitis, chronic nasal congestion, recurrent infections, bedwetting, attention deficit-hyperactivity disorder, acne, eczema, and aphthous ulcers (canker sores). Obviously, food allergy is not the only cause of these problems, but it is one of the most common causes, and it is probably the one most frequently overlooked. Other conditions that are occasionally associated with food allergy include hypertension, heart-rhythm disturbances, angina, peptic ulcer, epilepsy, and psoriasis. Strictly speaking, food-induced symptoms should not be called allergies unless it can be shown that the immune system plays a role in the reaction. While many food reactions might be more appropriately labeled "sensitivities" or "intolerances," the term "allergy" will be used in this chapter to denote adverse reactions to foods.

Having treated thousands of allergic patients over the years, we are firmly convinced that working with food allergies is one of the most important components of natural medicine. We have seen hundreds of patients who had been sick for years and had spent thousands of dollars on ineffective medical treatments, who showed rapid and dramatic improvement with a simple change in diet.

Skeptical Doctors

FEW CONVENTIONAL doctors believe that hidden food allergy is a common problem, and some deny its existence altogether. These skeptics point out that many of the conditions that are said to be allergic in nature have a significant psychological component and fluctuate in severity. Consequently, it may be difficult to distinguish between a true food reaction and a conditioned (psychological) response or a spontaneous worsening of symptoms.

While food-allergic and psychosomatic illnesses do overlap, there is ample published research demonstrating that food allergy is a real clinical entity. At least three different disorders (rheumatoid arthritis,[2] attention deficit-hyperactivity disorder[3] and irritable bowel syndrome[4]) have been shown in well-designed, placebo-controlled studies to be triggered by reactions to foods. In these studies, patients experienced symptoms when challenged (in blinded fashion) with foods they had previously identified as offenders, whereas they did not react to "placebo" foods (those previously identified as safe). In addition to these carefully controlled studies, hundreds of observational studies implicate food allergy as a cause of one or more of the conditions listed previously. Readers interested in further information about food allergy are referred to various books and review articles on the subject.[5, 6, 7]

Diagnosing and Treating Allergies

FOOD ALLERGY SHOULD be suspected in individuals who have a childhood history of colic, recurrent ear infections, sore throats, runny nose, "growing pains," asthma, eczema, or "getting sick all the time." In addition, people with a family history of allergy are more likely to be allergic themselves. On physical examination, allergic individuals often have puffy dark circles under the eyes (known as "allergic shiners") and horizontal creases across the lower eyelids (Dennie's lines). Signs seen primarily in allergic children include a single horizontal crease across the lower portion of the nose (from repeatedly pushing the nose upward) and recurrent sudden redness of the ears.

Adults who notice a fluctuation in weight of more than two to three pounds per day (not related to menstrual cycles) frequently have food allergy.

Elimination Diets

SKIN tests are notoriously unreliable for detecting masked food allergy. Other diagnostic tools are used by some practitioners and will be discussed below. Probably the most reliable (and certainly the least expensive) method of identifying food allergies is to do an "elimination diet" for several weeks. A typical elimination diet (described in appendix A) is one that completely excludes the most common symptom-evoking foods: wheat, dairy products, sugar, corn, eggs, citrus fruits, chocolate, coffee, tea, alcohol, and food additives. For highly allergic patients, the initial diet may be even more restrictive, also eliminating soy products, yeast, all grains, and fish. During the elimination period, the patient, with the help of a nutritionist, consumes a balanced diet of nutritious "alternative" foods.

Eliminating all of the common allergenic foods at the same time often has two effects. First, the chronic symptoms from which the patient has been suffering may improve considerably or disappear completely; this typically occurs after 7 to 21 days on the diet. Second, by following a hypoallergenic diet for a few weeks, the body becomes "unwaterlogged" and the allergies become "unmasked." In this hyperalert state, the reintroduction of allergenic foods into the diet will provoke rapid and exaggerated reactions—usually reproducing the symptoms that had ceased with the elimination diet. In most cases, an elimination diet should be supervised by a nutritionally oriented health-care practitioner—both to prevent nutritional deficiencies and to aid in assessing the response to the elimination-and-challenge program.

The main advantage of the elimination-diet approach is that it is inexpensive and usually provides reliable information. Its major disadvantage is that many busy individuals have difficulty following it. For these individuals, one of the approaches that are described later may be satisfactory.

Long-Term Treatment After the Elimination Diet

MOST patients whose symptoms resolve on an elimination diet will remain symptom-free, as long as they avoid the foods that provoke their symptoms. Some patients are allergic to a large number of foods and their diet must be carefully planned—usually with professional help—in order to prevent nutritional deficiencies. Fortunately, food allergies often "settle down" within 3 to 12 months, if the offending foods are strictly avoided. Children tend to recover their tolerance to foods much faster than adults. After a period of avoidance, many allergenic foods can be safely returned to the diet, as long as they are not eaten more often than every three or four days. However, if the offending foods are consumed more often than that, the symptoms may gradually return. These observations suggest that the immune system can build up a tolerance to allergenic foods if it is given an adequate chance to rest, but that continual exposure to these foods will overwhelm the immune system.

In some cases, symptom-provoking foods can be safely returned to the diet right away (rather than having to avoid them for a number of months), as long as they are ingested no more often than every fourth day. The likelihood that an allergenic food will cause symptoms is also influenced by other factors, such as whether other allergens are being consumed at the same time, whether seasonal allergens are in the air, and the resistance level of the individual (which is influenced by infection, exposure to chemicals, emotional stress, etc.). A small minority of food allergies never resolve, even if the particular food has been avoided for years. These so-called "fixed allergens" will continue to evoke symptoms every time they are eaten.

Severely allergic people may eventually become sensitive to any food they eat every day. We therefore advise allergic patients to try to rotate their foods and diversify their diet as much as possible. Some individuals find that they must follow a four-day rotation plan, whereas others can maintain their health without being as strict.

Blood Tests

SEVERAL blood tests are available to measure antibodies to individual food extracts. Antibodies are protein molecules that are produced by the immune system when the body is exposed to allergens or other "foreign invaders" (such as microorganisms). Different antibodies are produced in response to different allergens, and it is possible to distinguish (through lab tests) one antibody from another. The antibodies most commonly measured in the lab are known as IgE and IgG_4 antibodies. Measuring IgE-antibody levels may be helpful for identifying classical allergic reactions (such as those that result in acute asthma or hives). However, IgE levels do not appear to be reliable indicators of hidden food allergy. Tests that measure IgG_4 antibodies to individual foods are also commercially available, and they are used by some doctors for diagnosing hidden allergies. However, while there is evidence that some IgG_4 antibodies can provoke symptoms, the IgG_4 fraction also appears to contain blocking antibodies, which might actually prevent allergic reactions.[8] Consequently, the theoretical basis for using this test to diagnose food allergies is open to question. Although at the present time, there are no studies demonstrating that measuring IgG_4 levels can reliably distinguish between allergenic and non-allergenic foods, many practitioners have found these tests to be useful clinically, especially for individuals who find an elimination diet too difficult to follow.

Another test, known as ALCAT, measures changes in blood platelets and white blood cells after mixing a sample of blood with various food extracts. ALCAT has been shown to be fairly reliable for identifying reactions to food additives.[9] However, in tests for allergy to foods, 18 (24.3%) of 74 positive results and 21 (30.9%) of 68 negative results were found to be incorrect.[10]

Skin Tests

WHILE "scratch testing" is considered by most conventional and natural physicians to be unreliable for identifying food allergy, other skin testing techniques called "provocation-neutralization" and "dilution-titration" are used by some practitioners to diagnose and desensitize food allergies. Nearly all of these practitioners are members of the American Academy of Environmental Medicine (AAEM), a 31-year-old professional association. The procedures involve administering carefully measured dilutions of food (and other) extracts intradermally (below the skin) or sublingually (under the tongue). Certain dilutions may provoke symptoms, whereas other dilutions may "neutralize" (relieve) the symptoms. After the testing is completed, the patient is treated with injections or sublingual drops of a mixture that contains various allergens in their respective neutralizing doses.

Although the efficacy of food-extract-injection therapy has been demonstrated in a small double-blind study,[11] other researchers have failed to find a beneficial effect,[12] and provocation-neutralization remains a controversial technique among many health-care professionals. However, it has been pointed out that the researchers who obtained negative results did not perform the procedures correctly. Having successfully treated hundreds of thousands of allergic and sensitive individuals, professional members of the AAEM and many of those with whom they have worked are firmly convinced of the effectiveness of this approach. Many point to "conventional" allergists' use of "allergy shots" for inhalant allergies as another successful allergy treatment used for decades without extensive "proof" by placebo-controlled, double-blind studies.

Meridian Stress Analysis

MERIDIAN Stress Analysis (MSA) is the most recent name for a rapidly evolving computerized testing/treatment system, previously known as "electrodermal testing," "EAV" (electroacupuncture according to Voll), "Vega" testing, "Interro" testing, and many other terms. Allergy and sensitivity testing may be done as part of an overall MSA testing and treatment program, or as an independent subset of tests, using the same equipment.

MSA evolved from the pioneering studies of a German physician, Reinhold Voll, M.D., who combined his knowledge of classical Chinese acupuncture with the electronics of the 1950s through 1970s. In the late 1990s, MSA uses the most recent computer equipment and programs to detect (without using needles) very small fluctuations in the flow of natural body electricity at acupuncture points and along acupuncture meridians. The treatment of allergies and sensitivities detected in this way is guided by observation of these fluctuations on the computer screen, and is done with homeopathic concentrations of the items to which each individual is allergic or sensitive.

The authors, doctors Wright and Gaby, have differing opinions on the usefulness of MSA. Our respective viewpoints follow.

Dr. Wright's Experience

Treatment of attention deficit-hyperactivity disorder (ADHD, see chapter on attention deficit-hyperactivity disorder) often involves allergy testing and treatment. In the mid-1980s, I had been working with children with ADHD following the procedures outlined in the books of Dr. Doris Rapp. These included the skin testing techniques of "provocation-neutralization" and "dilution-titration." While most of the children receiving these treatments improved considerably, they understandably did not like all the needles used. Our clinic obtained MSA equipment (then termed "Interro") and used it for allergy/sensitivity testing and as a guide to appropriate homeopathic treatment to desensitize allergies. The first few cases were children with ADHD, who were greatly relieved (as were their parents) that no needles were involved.

Nearly a year later, a physician who "couldn't believe" that either MSA testing or MSA-guided homeopathic desensitization "could possibly work" joined our clinic. He phoned one mother who "confirmed" that, indeed, MSA hadn't worked for her child. Instead, she reported that, "Tahoma Clinic must have replaced her child with another one without ADHD." Also in the early days of our "Interro" use, we saw a man in his mid-twenties who had been taking antihistamines/ decongestants for years, and had been through conventional testing and desensitization with no help for his intractable "year-round sinus allergies aggravated by seasonal hayfever." With MSA testing and homeopathic desensitization, his sinuses became entirely clear within a few months.

In 1998, a $1 billion Utah corporation, Icon Health and Fitness, Inc., reported the results of a pilot program using MSA techniques. The project was designed as an outcomes study—a type of study that monitors what a technique can achieve, rather than trying to explain how it works. The study had two objectives: 1) to see if company employees with long-term, unresolved health problems would find relief through MSA techniques; and, 2) to observe if the company's health-care costs could be cut by using MSA. ("Icon" has a self-funded medical plan.)

Each participating employee completed a symptom checklist (which weighted each symptom on a scale of 1 to 5) both before and after completing treatment. After approximately 7 months, an audit of results of the first 20 individuals was conducted by the testing/treating practitioner, the company's Director of Human Resources, and the company's independent medical-plan consultant. The involved employees provided considerable input through the "symptom checklists" and follow-up telephone calls. (The company supplying the MSA equipment did not participate in the testing, treatment, or audit, and did not financially underwrite the study.)

Results of the audit showed an overall 64% reduction in symptoms weighted for severity, and an estimated annual cost savings of $1,271 per participant. The cost savings did not include the cost of hospitalizations avoided, and didn't take into account the productivity improvement reported by individuals successfully treated for chronic fatigue syndrome or other conditions that had been interfering with job performance. Of the 20 employees in the outcomes study (which used MSA testing and MSA-guided homeopathic desensitization techniques as the only "intervention"), 6 had allergy symptoms. They reported the following results from MSA:

- Employee "Kim" reported a reduction in allergies and nasal congestion from 5 (severe) to 2.5 (moderate). She eliminated use of a "Nasonex" inhaler.

- "David" reported a reduction in asthma from 5 to 2, and other allergies from 3 to 0 (none). He discontinued his antihistamine (Claritin) and reduced his inhaler use by 99%.

- "Candi" wrote that her allergy symptoms decreased from 5 to 2, and that she had been able to discontinue Claritin altogether.

- "Layne's" allergy symptoms of many years were reduced from 5 (severe) to 1. Layne has needed no further allergy medication since completing the course of MSA-guided homeopathic desensitization.

- "Andrea" reported a reduction in asthma from 5 to 3, and a reduction in other allergies from 5 to 2.5, all in just 2 months.

- "Deborah" had the "worst" report, with a reduction in allergy symptoms only from 5 to 4. However, at the time of the audit, she had been in the study only 30 days.

- Icon's Director of Human Resources writes that, "the project is achieving the objectives hoped for." The involved employees agree.

MSA testing and treatment have not been "proven" by controlled clinical trials. However, none of the allergy treatment methods discussed in this chapter have been proven by controlled clinical trial. I have, at one time or another, used all of them and have found them all effective (although certainly not in all cases). I have presently settled on MSA techniques as most useful and convenient for the individuals with whom I work.

Dr. Gaby's Commentary

At present, no published studies support the concept that computers can reliably diagnose allergies. The few attempts I am aware of to investigate MSA showed that different technicians, testing the same individual on the same day, obtained widely divergent results. In addition, there is no scientific explanation for how drops of water, given an electromagnetic influence by a computer, could desensitize allergies.

In the Icon study described above, the reported improvements may have been due to a "participation effect" (i.e., people tend to report improvement when they participate in a study) and/or a placebo effect from the treatment they were given. Practitioners who use MSA also advise their patients to eliminate foods for a time, then to rotate them back into the diet. As mentioned previously, those dietary changes by themselves will frequently reduce sensitivities, so it may be difficult to determine exactly which component of the treatment is helping. In addition, patients who invest a significant amount of time and money in a procedure may experience a substantial placebo effect.

While clinical observations are often the starting point for advances in medicine, a properly conducted study is needed before the improvements described by Dr. Wright can be attributed to MSA, rather than to some other aspect of their medical treatment.

Conclusion

THERE IS STRONG evidence that food allergy is a contributing factor to a wide range of symptoms and medical conditions. In many cases, working with food allergies is the most important component of a natural-medicine program. Although there is some disagreement among practitioners as to the reliability and effectiveness of various testing and treatment methods, a number of different techniques are currently being used in clinical practice.

CHAPTER FOUR

NATURAL HORMONE THERAPY

THE WORD "HORMONE" is derived from a Greek word meaning "to set in motion" or "to spur on." Hormones are chemical substances produced in the body that regulate the function of various organs and tissues. While health problems can result from having either too much or too little of a hormone, deficiencies are much more common than excesses. One cause of inadequate hormone production is malnutrition. For example, a deficiency of zinc may reduce blood levels of testosterone and growth hormone, and may inhibit the conversion of thyroid hormone from the form that is transported in the bloodstream into the biologically active form. The levels of some hormones, such as estrogen, dehydroepiandrosterone (DHEA), and testosterone, tend to decline with age. In older individuals, these levels usually cannot be restored to normal by improving nutritional status. Certain diseases are also associated with hormone deficiencies, and drugs (such as prednisone) used to treat these diseases may make some of the deficiencies even worse. Genetic factors also play a role in determining hormonal status. In some cases, individuals have low levels of hormones for no apparent reason.

Conventional medicine recognizes the importance of hormone-replacement therapy (HRT) when a deficiency can be clearly demonstrated, as in laboratory-diagnosed hypothyroidism or adrenal failure. However, we believe that conventional endocrinology (the medical specialty that deals with hormonal problems) falls short in two important ways. First, it rejects the notion that subtle deficiencies of hormones (i.e., those that may not show up on standard laboratory tests) can cause illness and that these deficiencies can be safely corrected by gentle treatment with low doses of the appropriate hormones. For example, most doctors assume that if a person does not have Addison's disease (severe adrenal failure), then his adrenal glands are perfectly healthy. Doctors of natural medicine, on the other hand, understand that there are gradations between serious illness and total wellness. Many patients whose illness is due to sub-optimal glandular function can be helped by low-dose hormone therapy.

Second, some of the drugs that are used for HRT, such as Premarin, Provera, and methyltestosterone, have a different chemical structure than the estrogens, progesterone, and testosterone, respectively, that are produced in the human body. While these drug-company alternatives to human hormones are usually effective for the purposes for which they are intended, they also have a long list of side effects, some of which are quite serious.

In our experience, appropriate use of human hormones in physiologic doses (i.e., doses similar to what the body normally produces) often results in important clinical benefits, and causes fewer side effects than synthetic hormone-like drugs (or, in the case of Premarin, an extract of horse urine). Unfortunately, much of the research on humans has been done with synthetic or nonhuman hormones, particularly with respect to estrogen and progesterone. Consequently, some of our clinical observations regarding natural-hormone therapy have not been confirmed by scientific studies. However, the scarcity of research does not negate the intuitively obvious and logical idea that we should treat hormone deficiencies with the same molecules that the human body normally produces. In the absence of complete information, we usually prefer natural hormones (which appear to be effective and relatively safe) over some conventional hormone regimens (which the evidence indicates are effective but also potentially dangerous).

At the time of this writing, there is growing interest among research centers in studying natural hormones. In a few years, we will know a great deal more about this type of therapy than we do now. In the meantime, we will continue to look for subtle hormone deficiencies and try to correct them gently, carefully, and with gratitude that we possess such elegant tools. Following is a brief overview of the hormone therapies that we use most commonly in our practices.

Hypothyroidism

THE THYROID IS a gland located in the neck below the Adam's apple. It secretes two hormones—thyroxine (T4, approximately 90%) and triiodothyronine (T3, approximately 10%), both of which regulate the body's metabolism, as well as performing several other biological functions. The thyroid also secretes two other compounds, diiodotyrosine (DIT) and monoiodotyrosine (MIT). Conventional medicine views DIT and MIT as biologically inactive "slough off" products of thyroid-hormone synthesis. However, it is possible that these compounds have important functions that we have not yet discovered. DIT and MIT are not contained in synthetic thyroid-hormone preparations, but they are found in the whole thyroid extract prescribed by many doctors of natural medicine.

Diagnosing Hypothyroidism

HYPOTHYROIDISM (underactive thyroid) can cause any of a wide range of symptoms including fatigue, depression, difficulty concentrating, sensitivity to cold, hoarseness, dry skin, hair loss, constipation, fluid retention, menstrual abnormalities, infertility, reactive hypoglycemia, elevated serum cholesterol, and poor resistance to infection. On physical examination, people with hypothyroidism may have a sub-normal body temperature, dry skin, puffiness under the eyes or around the ankles, and yellowish palms.

Hypothyroidism is a well-recognized medical condition, and doctors frequently order blood tests for thyroid function as part of an overall medical evaluation. However, in our experience, these blood tests are unreliable, and they often fail to detect hypothyroidism. In his landmark 1976 book, *Hypothyroidism: the Unsuspected Illness* (Harper and Row, New York), Broda Barnes, M.D., argued that tens of millions of Americans suffer from undiagnosed hypothyroidism. While standard textbooks estimated that only about 3% of the general population is hypothyroid, Barnes believed the true figure to be much higher.

Treatment with Natural, Whole Thyroid Extract

OVER the years, we have seen thousands of patients who suffered from various combinations of the symptoms listed above. Although these symptoms can have many different causes, we have found hypothyroidism to be one of the most common causes. More than 2,000 of our patients have undergone a trial of a natural, whole thyroid extract (called desiccated thyroid) or, less often, synthetic T4. In the majority of these patients, chronic symptoms improved, often dramatically. Yet most of these individuals (perhaps 85%) had normal thyroid blood tests, including TSH (thyroid-stimulating hormone).

Thyroid-Hormone Resistance

ALTHOUGH our results in treating patients using thyroid-hormone preparations have been impressive, most conventional physicians are strongly opposed to (or even horrified by) the idea of giving a potent hormone to people whose blood tests are normal. However, that idea is not as farfetched as it might seem. By analogy, many diabetics require injections of insulin, even though the level of this hormone in the bloodstream may be normal or above normal. This phenomenon is known as insulin resistance. While there is plenty of insulin circulating in the blood, the cells of the body are inefficient at responding to insulin's message. As a result, some diabetics require higher-than-normal concentrations of insulin in their bloodstream in order to achieve a normal insulin effect.

A severe form of thyroid-hormone resistance is also known to occur, although it is a relatively rare disorder. However, it is possible that a more subtle form of thyroid-hormone resistance is present in a relatively large proportion of the population. If that is the case, then some individuals would need to maintain their thyroid-hormone level near the top of the normal range in order to feel well. While the existence of subtle thyroid-hormone resistance has not been proven, it could explain the dramatic results seen by innovative practitioners who diagnose and treat hypothyroidism on clinical grounds (i.e., the symptoms and physical exam suggest hypothyroidism, but the lab tests are normal).

Doctors who oppose this method of diagnosis, and rely instead on blood tests, point out that inappropriate use of thyroid hormones can put stress on the heart and promote the development of osteoporosis. While overtreatment can cause these problems, we argue that empirical use of thyroid extract, when done carefully, is neither inappropriate nor overtreatment. We have not seen any cardiac problems with thyroid therapy. A few patients developed chest pain, but it was alleviated by reducing their dosage. Our patients also have

not shown any evidence of accelerated osteoporosis. As a cautionary measure, we always recommend a bone-building nutritional supplement (see chapter on osteoporosis) for people taking thyroid-hormone preparations. In addition, bone density can be monitored directly by a type of X-ray (DEXA) or indirectly with a urine test. Most of our experience has been with desiccated thyroid, so we cannot be certain that synthetic preparations such as L-thyroxine have the same safety profile.

Conventional Treatment versus Natural Hormone Treatment

CONVENTIONAL treatment for hypothyroidism is L-thyroxine (Synthroid, Levothroid, and others). This provides replacement of the T4 hormone only. However, we agree with Barnes that some patients show a markedly better response to desiccated whole thyroid (extracts of thyroid tissue from pigs or cows, which includes brands such as Armour and Westhroid), than they do to L-thyroxine.[1] The superior effectiveness of desiccated thyroid may result in part from its T3 content. A recent study showed that the combination of T3 and T4 is more effective than T4 alone in improving mood and psychological functioning of hypothyroid patients.[2] In addition, the DIT and/or MIT contained in desiccated thyroid might enhance the effect of T3 and T4. Although such an effect has not been demonstrated scientifically, it could explain why a few patients have fared better with desiccated thyroid than with the combination of synthetic T3 and T4.

In our experience, somewhat more than half of patients with normal thyroid blood tests who benefit from desiccated thyroid are able to discontinue the treatment after one to two years without having a recurrence of their symptoms, whereas the remainder require continued treatment.

In a small minority of patients, synthetic T3 (Cytomel) is the most effective treatment. T3 appears to be the biologically active form of thyroid hormone, whereas T4 is thought to be the "storage and transportation" form. Normally, our cells convert T4 into T3 at a controlled rate. However, for some individuals (such as those with type 1 diabetes), this transformation is impaired. In those cases, treatment with T4 alone is relatively ineffective, and synthetic T3 achieves better results than even desiccated thyroid. Doctors can determine through blood tests whether T3 is the most appropriate treatment.

Treating Adrenal Gland Defects

THE ADRENALS ARE two small, almond-shaped glands—one gland sits on top of each kidney. Each adrenal gland can be divided into two major anatomical sections—like an almond "kernel" within a thick "shell." The "kernel" (termed the "medulla") produces adrenaline and adrenaline-like compounds. The thick "shell" (termed the "cortex") produces over 40 different steroid molecules. The precise function of most of these steroids is not known; some may be found to have hormonal activity, whereas others may be precursors to—or breakdown products of—active hormones. (From the 1930s through the 1970s, DHEA was thought to be one of these "unimportant" precursor molecules, but as we will see later, it has been shown to be an extremely important hormone.)

Adrenaline is the body's premier "emergency hormone"—it's often called the "fight or flight" hormone. Adrenaline is the substance that "energizes" the muscles and makes the heart pound during times of acute stress. In athletic terms, adrenaline might be compared to a sprinter—it's almost always reserved for short-term, high-intensity situations.

The major steroid hormones of the adrenal cortex are cortisol, DHEA, and aldosterone. Cortisol is the "medium and long range" stress hormone. In athletic terms, it might be compared to a middle-distance or marathon runner. Aldosterone regulates sodium, potassium, and water balance. DHEA has many functions. At present, DHEA and cortisol are the adrenal hormones used most widely by natural-medicine practitioners. We will discuss both cortisol and DHEA therapy in detail below.

Adrenal Failure

SEVERE adrenal failure was first identified by (and subsequently named after) Dr. Thomas Addison in the nineteenth century. Although Addison's disease is well recognized in conventional medicine, most doctors refuse to consider that milder degrees of adrenal weakness might also exist. Doctors of natural medicine, on the other hand, believe that there are many "shades of gray" between total adrenal failure and perfectly normal function. The majority of "weak adrenal" symptoms result from inadequate cortisol production.

"Whole Adrenal" Therapy

ADRENAL cortical extract (ACE) is a whole extract from the adrenal cortex of animals. It contains small amounts of every adrenal steroid—all in natural balance and proportion to each other. From the 1930s through the late 1940s, ACE (given by injection) was a major treatment for weak adrenals, used both by conventional and natural-medicine doctors.

In 1948, a pharmaceutical company marketed the first cortisol-only preparation. Although the cortisol was identical to the natural compound, it was not accompanied by the rest of the hormones found in normal healthy adrenal glands. It was often enthusiastically prescribed in amounts much larger than those produced by the human body. Unfortunately, such overdosing caused serious toxic effects, including hypertension, peptic ulcer, diabetes, cataract, and even psychosis. Even worse, pharmaceutical companies then introduced synthetic patentable drugs derived from cortisol (prednisone, dexamethasone, and others), which had even more severe toxic effects. People became quite nervous about the use of both cortisol and its synthetic counterparts (commonly called "cortisone").

Natural-medicine doctors continued to use

ACE, sometimes along with "adrenal support" herbals such as licorice and ginseng, and vitamins including vitamin C and pantothenic acid. The results were good, and patients reported no adverse effects from ACE. However, despite its track record of safety and effectiveness, in 1978 the Food and Drug Administration (FDA) tried to outlaw ACE. The FDA claimed this extract was ineffective, even though it had been perfectly effective when manufactured by Parke-Davis and other major drug companies in the 1930s through the 1950s. The FDA's attempted ban did not succeed, because pharmacies that were licensed, regulated, and supervised by individual states could still provide ACE on prescription. However, as part of a 1998–1999 attempt to take over the regulation of pharmacy compounding (i.e., mixing and compounding medicines on the premises), the FDA has again banned ACE. At present, it is difficult to obtain this "whole adrenal" preparation, and its future status is uncertain. While natural-medicine doctors are successfully using individual adrenal hormones such as cortisol and DHEA, one of us (J.W.) has found that certain patients do not respond as well to these individual hormones as they do to ACE.

Cortisol

CORTISOL (also known as hydrocortisone) is one of the major hormones produced by the adrenal glands. It has a wide range of physiological effects in the body, including regulation of blood glucose, blood pressure, fluid and electrolyte balance, and calcium metabolism. Cortisol is also required for normal functioning of skeletal muscle, the immune system, and the central nervous system. In addition, this hormone has a powerful anti-inflammatory action, and it is one of the main hormones the body secretes in response to stress.

Cortisol deficiency may result from a primary weakness of the adrenals, or less commonly from a failure of the pituitary gland to release sufficient amounts of ACTH (adrenocorticotrophic hormone, a hormone that stimulates the adrenals to secrete

cortisol). Individuals with mild degrees of cortisol deficiency may experience fatigue, weakness, recurrent episodes of "low blood sugar," heart palpitations, inability to gain weight or unexplained weight loss, and poor tolerance to stress. Some patients report that exercising makes them feel "wiped out." The blood pressure is frequently low, which can result in lightheadedness, particularly upon standing rapidly. With more pronounced adrenal weakness, patients may also experience nausea and vomiting, abdominal pain, loss of appetite, and salt cravings.

Severe adrenal insufficiency (Addison's disease) is a life-threatening condition. This disease is usually treated with a combination of cortisol and a synthetic steroid that has a more potent effect on fluid and electrolyte balance.

For reasons that are difficult to understand, few conventional doctors look for milder forms of adrenal weakness. Doctors of natural medicine, on the other hand, have found that cortisol has a definite role in treating some patients who have the various symptoms listed previously—including some who have been diagnosed with chronic fatigue syndrome. The effectiveness of low-dose cortisol in cases of chronic fatigue syndrome has been confirmed in a recent double-blind study.[3]

The need for cortisol therapy is usually determined by measuring the level of this hormone before and after an injection of ACTH. If the level is low initially, or if it fails to increase by a certain amount after stimulation with ACTH, then treatment with cortisol may be worthwhile.

As emphasized by William Jefferies, M.D., author of Safe Uses of Cortisol,[4] a deficiency of cortisol can be corrected with relatively small doses, as opposed to the larger amounts that are often used to treat inflammatory and autoimmune diseases. Jefferies also stressed the importance of administering cortisol in four divided doses each day, rather than the conventional twice-a-day regimen used by many endocrinologists. Spreading the treatment throughout the day minimizes the peaks (with their potential for toxic effects) and valleys (during which symptoms may not be controlled) of cortisol levels that would occur with less-frequent dosing.[5]

As noted previously, cortisol and its synthetic counterparts (such as prednisone) can be extremely dangerous in large amounts. But when cortisol is used carefully and according to the guidelines developed by Jefferies, it has not been found to cause diabetes, osteoporosis, cataracts, or any of the other side effects attributed to the synthetic drugs—even after many years or even decades of continuous treatment.

Dehydroepiandrosterone (DHEA)

DEHYDROEPIANDROSTERONE (DHEA) is a steroid hormone synthesized by the adrenal glands—and to a lesser extent by the testes and ovaries. DHEA is the most abundant adrenal steroid; blood levels of DHEA and its sister molecule DHEA-sulfate (DHEA-S) are 20 times higher than the levels of any other adrenal steroid. However, until recently, we did not know the function of DHEA in the body. Because it can be converted into other hormones, including estrogen and testosterone, scientists assumed that DHEA was merely a "buffer hormone"—a reservoir upon which the body could draw to produce the other hormones. However, in the 1980s, scientists found that DHEA has specific actions of its own.

Possible Benefits of DHEA

In recent years, there has been a great deal of interest in DHEA as a possible anti-aging hormone and as a treatment for various age-related medical conditions. This interest was sparked by the observation that DHEA levels decline progressively with age; the levels in 70-year-olds are only about 20% as high as the levels of people in their mid-twenties. In addition, population studies have suggested that higher levels of DHEA are associated with increased longevity and with a lower incidence of heart disease (in men only) and some types of cancer. Moreover, animals treated with

DHEA looked younger and had glossier coats and less gray hair, compared with animals not given the hormone.[6]

In a double-blind study, 30 individuals between the ages of 40 and 70 were given 50 mg of DHEA or a placebo for 3 months, then received the alternate treatment for an additional 3 months. During DHEA treatment, 67% of the men and 84% of the women reported a marked increase in physical and psychological well-being. No side effects were seen.[7] However, other studies have found that this hormone had little or no effect on well-being.

In our experience, some elderly individuals whose DHEA or DHEA-S levels are low experience dramatic benefits from this hormone. These improvements have included better appetite, energy level, memory and mood; an increase in muscle mass; and better skin tone and color. While not everyone responds, the results in those who do are often unmistakable.

A growing body of evidence suggests that DHEA may enhance immune function.[8] This hormone may also help prevent or reverse osteoporosis in postmenopausal women.[9] In a few of our patients, DHEA has been helpful in treating menopausal symptoms. It is not clear whether the benefit these patients experienced was due to DHEA specifically, or was the result of the production of additional amounts of estrogen and testosterone (which our bodies can make from DHEA). DHEA has also been used successfully to treat depression in individuals with initially low levels of DHEA-S,[10] as well as people with normal levels.[11] In a double-blind study of 20 women with lupus, treatment with 100 mg of DHEA per day resulted in improvements in energy levels and general well-being, and reduced the overall severity of the disease.[12] We have also found this hormone to be helpful for some patients with other autoimmune diseases, such as rheumatoid arthritis, dermatomyositis, ulcerative colitis, and Crohn's disease, although no studies have supported those observations.

Cautions in Using DHEA

Clearly, DHEA shows great promise for preventing and treating a wide range of health conditions. Furthermore, in contrast to the other major adrenal hormone, cortisol, DHEA appears to be relatively free of side effects—with the exception of acne or increased hair growth when large doses are administered. However, we must not forget that DHEA is a powerful steroid hormone, and that we know very little about the effects of long-term administration. Because DHEA is partially converted to estrogen and testosterone, there is a theoretical concern that it could promote the development of hormone-dependent cancers such as breast and prostate cancer. It has been observed that postmenopausal women with breast cancer tend to have elevated levels of DHEA. On the other hand, animal studies have demonstrated an anti-cancer effect of DHEA.

Until more is known about this hormone, individuals should use it with caution. People who are taking large amounts of DHEA because they heard that it boosts energy or builds muscle may be taking a significant risk with their health. Although DHEA is available without a prescription, we recommend that it be used only with medical supervision. In addition, some of the products sold over the counter have been found, when analyzed, to contain no DHEA at all. We advise our patients to obtain their DHEA from a compounding pharmacist or from other reputable sources.

The optimal "replacement dose" of DHEA is not known. Based on our experience with a few individuals whose lab tests showed extremely low levels of DHEA, it appears that the usual physiologic replacement dose is 5 to 15 mg per day for most women and 10 to 30 mg per day for most men. Larger amounts may be necessary in some cases, particularly for individuals with autoimmune disease. However, larger doses of DHEA, in addition to increasing the risk of toxicity, are not necessarily more effective. Some compounds have a so-called "therapeutic window," in which the optimal dose is more effective than either lower or higher amounts. Our clinical impression is that there may be such a therapeutic window with respect to DHEA.

Understanding the Ovaries, Testes, and Sex Hormones

NEARLY ALL OF us are aware of the location and relative size of our respective sex glands. Most of us also know that the glands' major hormonal products are estrogen and progesterone in women, and testosterone in men. (Both sexes also make small amounts of "opposite sex" hormones.) Estrogen and testosterone are not only responsible for the development of "secondary sexual characteristics," but they are also anabolic—that is, they promote tissue-building in "non-sexual" tissues (muscle, bone, connective tissue, and others).

With advancing age, the levels of sex hormones decline in both sexes—more abruptly for women around the time of menopause and more gradually for men. In women, the decline in hormone levels frequently causes "hot flashes," insomnia, mood swings, vaginal dryness, painful intercourse, and loss of libido. Estrogen-replacement therapy (ERT) has been clearly shown to reduce the risk of postmenopausal osteoporosis, and it may help prevent heart and blood-vessel disease and senility (including Alzheimer's disease).

Since testosterone levels typically decline very gradually in men, symptoms of deficiency aren't nearly as obvious as the symptoms of menopause. However, an accumulating body of research indicates that low testosterone levels in males may be an important factor in the development of heart and blood-vessel disease. Osteoporosis in men may also be due in part to low levels of testosterone. Many physicians who prescribe testosterone for men have observed a positive effect on mood, attitude, muscle mass, and memory.

Natural Hormone Replacement for Women

CONVENTIONAL medicine typically uses either Premarin (horse estrogens, concentrated from the urine of pregnant mares) or estradiol (one of the three estrogens made by humans), along with Provera (medroxyprogesterone acetate, a synthetic analogue of natural progesterone). Natural medicine uses the same estrogen and progesterone molecules that are present in women's bodies during the "cycling years."

Estrogen

There are actually three principal estrogens made by women: estrone, estradiol, and estriol. Estrone and estradiol are considered relatively strong estrogens, and they promote endometrial hyperplasia (a pre-cancerous change in the uterus) and possibly some forms of cancer. Estriol is a weaker estrogen which, according to some research, does not cause problems in the uterus or promote cancer. In fact, in a study of women with breast cancer that had metastasized (spread to other areas), treatment with estriol resulted in an arrest or remission of metastatic lesions in 37% of cases.[13] However, in another report, estriol did promote the growth of breast-cancer cells in a test tube. Several clinical studies have indicated that estriol, in doses that can relieve menopausal symptoms, does not cause uterine hyperplasia.[14] However, that observation has been challenged in some studies.[15] With regard to preventing osteoporosis, some studies have shown a beneficial effect of estriol, whereas others have not.[16]

These conflicting observations aside, it is clear that "being premenopausal" does not seem to promote cancer, whereas conventional ERT may. Therefore, logic suggests that the safest ERT regimen would be a combination of the three human estrogens given in the same proportions as those produced by premenopausal women. Unfortunately, no one is sure exactly what those proportions are.

Natural Replacement Estrogen. In 1982, in an effort to formulate an "identical to natural" replacement estrogen, one of us (J.W.) looked for data concerning the normal circulating levels of these three estrogens. Very little published research was available, so several clinical testing laboratories were asked what their "normal levels" (in blood tests) were for these three hormones. The "consensus" among the laboratories was 10% estrone, 10% estradiol, and 80% estriol. (More recent research shows a slightly different figure.[17]) However, estrogen levels in the bloodstream do not necessarily correspond to the optimal proportions for use in replacement therapy. That is because most of the body's estriol is manufactured in the liver from estrone and estradiol, and some of the estrone is produced by conversion from estradiol. Consequently, the amounts of these hormones circulating in the blood may be different than the amounts originally secreted. Despite these factors, using the 10%-10%-80% ratio, as suggested by the laboratories, would seem to err on the side of safety, possibly providing more estriol than the body actually secretes.

With the help of a compounding pharmacist, Dr. Wright put these proportions together into the first "triple-estrogen" or "Tri-Est" prescription. Triple-estrogen subsequently became widely used in natural medicine, and it is now available at most compounding pharmacies in the United States and Canada.

Expected Benefits and Side Effects of Estrogen. As mentioned previously, horse estrogens and other synthetic estrogens have been shown to reduce the risk of osteoporosis and possibly to reduce the risk of heart and blood-vessel disease as well as senility (including Alzheimer's disease). Although we do not yet have any "controlled studies" with triple-estrogen, logic and common sense give us reason to anticipate that it will do everything that horse hormones can do (if not more), and likely with less risk.

Occasionally, natural-hormone replacement

will cause "breakthrough" or other types of vaginal bleeding. In the early and mid-1980s, the few women who experienced this problem saw a gynecologist, and most had an endometrial biopsy. All of these biopsies were normal, suggesting that this hormone regimen (unlike conventional ERT) does not cause endometrial hyperplasia. Other practitioners who have used triple-estrogen have also found no evidence of endometrial hyperplasia. Now, our usual approach if vaginal bleeding occurs is to adjust the hormone dose first, and to refer for biopsy if bleeding persists. To date, neither of us has seen a case of endometrial hyperplasia resulting from the use of triple-estrogen. Of course, large-scale studies must be done before we can be sure of the long-term safety and effectiveness of natural-estrogen regimens.

Progesterone

In contrast to estrogen, progesterone is a single hormone. During a woman's "cycling years," progesterone levels increase dramatically after ovulation, and decline to their lowest levels just before and during the menses. Natural-hormone replacement attempts to mimic the natural cycle as closely as possible by using identical-to-natural progesterone (as well as triple-estrogen) on the same "timing schedule" as during the cycling years. The use of natural progesterone has been described in detail by a pioneer in the field, Dr. John Lee.[18]

Natural progesterone is considerably safer than Provera (the commonly used synthetic), which has been associated with a long list of side effects. In addition, according to a study published in the *Journal of the American Medical Association,* natural progesterone is as effective as Provera at preventing uterine hyperplasia in women taking conventional ERT.[19] However, although natural progesterone is available in over-the-counter creams, women should never change their hormone regimen without medical supervision. The required dosage of progesterone will vary, depending on the way it is taken and on which type of estrogen is being used.

Testosterone for Women

As previously noted, both sexes make small quantities of "opposite-sex" hormones. Although all sex hormones affect libido to some degree, testosterone appears to be the major "sex driver" in both sexes. Women who experience a decline in libido during or after menopause may have a deficiency of testosterone. This is especially true when menopause has been surgically induced by removal of the ovaries.

Because the human body can produce testosterone from DHEA, many natural-medicine doctors recommend DHEA for postmenopausal women before considering testosterone therapy. If testosterone levels are low after a few weeks of DHEA therapy, then a low dose of testosterone may be added. In addition to its effects on "sex drive," testosterone-replacement therapy may improve mood, increase strength, and prevent bone loss in postmenopausal women.

Natural Hormone Replacement for Men

THE first popular "hormone replacement" book was *The Male Hormone* by Paul de Kruif, published in 1945, some 20 years before the popularization of ERT. Unfortunately, the commonly prescribed "testosterone" was not testosterone at all, but methyltestosterone, an unnatural testosterone derivative that had the "advantage" of patentability. Methyltestosterone's unwanted effects (including angina and liver cancer) far outweighed its more desirable effects on libido, mood, and attitude. Male hormone replacement therefore fell into disrepute. It has been revived only in the last few years, aided both by Viagra and the aging of the "baby boom generation."

Since the late 1930s, we have slowly accumulated research showing that men with low testosterone levels tend to have a higher incidence of angina, more atherosclerosis, higher blood glucose, higher serum cholesterol and triglycerides, higher blood pressure, higher levels of blood clotting factors, and lower levels of blood clotting inhibitors. Researchers have shown that all of these problems, including angina and atherosclerosis, can be reversed with testosterone administration. While atherosclerosis has many other contributing causes (including poor diet, lack of key vitamins and minerals, and sedentary lifestyle), a relative deficiency of testosterone appears to be an important factor, as well.

Studies have also shown that men with osteoporosis have lower levels of testosterone than men with normal bone density. In one report, bone mineral density increased when otherwise healthy men with borderline-low testosterone levels were given testosterone. While osteoporosis is less common in men than in women, men who live into their mid-eighties have as much osteoporosis as do women of the same age.

A few studies have shown that men with lower levels of testosterone have more symptoms of depression, and other work has shown a lessening of depression when men with initially low levels took supplemental testosterone.

What About the Prostate?

There are two major beliefs concerning testosterone administration and the prostate. One theory (dominant among conventional physicians in the United States) is that administering testosterone may enlarge the prostate and possibly increase prostate-cancer risk. The other theory, more common in Europe, is that testosterone is necessary to maintain prostate health. Physicians who subscribe to the latter theory point out that men in their twenties (a time when testosterone levels are highest) have virtually no prostate enlargement or prostate cancer, whereas older men (who often have significantly lower levels of this hormone) commonly experience these problems.

There is insufficient research to determine which (if either) theory is correct. Many natural-medicine physicians are inclined to believe the latter, and they prescribe testosterone accordingly, making certain to recommend regular prostate examinations and PSA (prostate-specific antigen) tests to screen for prostate problems.

Other Side Effects

Because testosterone is a powerful hormone with the potential to cause adverse effects, testosterone treatment should be monitored by a physician experienced in its use. Reported side effects include breast enlargement (in men), acne, and an abnormal elevation of the hematocrit (blood count).[20]

Further Reading

FOR additional information and more research details about natural-hormone replacement for women and men, please see *Preventing and Reversing Osteoporosis* by Dr. Gaby,[21] and *Natural Hormone Replacement for Women Over 45* and *Maximize Your Vitality and Potency for Men Over 40*, by Dr. Wright.[17, 22]

Part Two

CONDITIONS

ACNE ROSACEA

🌿 ROSACEA IS A *condition in which the skin of the cheeks, nose, and forehead become reddened as a result of capillary dilation. Acne-like pustules often occur, as well. The cause of rosacea is unknown. It appears to be associated with a bacterial infection, since oral or topical antibiotics are sometimes beneficial. Individuals with rosacea should avoid substances that cause blood-vessel dilation, such as hot liquids and foods, spicy foods, alcohol, external irritants, and excessive heat or cold. Coffee, seafood, pork, or allergenic foods may also cause problems in some cases. Conventional therapy includes oral or topical (applied to skin) antibiotics or other topical medications.*

DR. WRIGHT'S CASE STUDY

One of David Flanagan's problems was obvious. His entire face was shiny and pinkish-red, —more pink around the edges and more red and shiny on and around his nose and the central areas of his face. There were a few small nodules scattered at random on his forehead, cheeks, and chin, and an unfortunately larger one on the end of his nose.

"I'm here from Chicago," he said. "And you can see why! I've had this 'rosacea' thing since I was 22 or 23, and I'm 41 now. I've had more tetracycline than I can remember, and it helps when I take it, but it's been helping less and less the last few years. I asked my dermatologist about cortisone ointment or cream, but she said if I kept using it for a chronic skin condition like this, my skin would just thin out. She's tried other antibiotics, but they don't even work as well as the tetracycline. So my face just keeps getting redder and redder, and now I just use the tetracy-cline when the pimples," he pointed to his nose, "get particularly bad."

"Like now?"

"Yeah, though I haven't gotten as many bad outbreaks as I've gotten older."

"Any other problems with your health?"

"Not really."

"Any heartburn, gas, indigestion?"

"Yeah, but no more than a lot of other guys my age. Besides, that happens more when I overeat."

"Tired?"

"I don't think so. 'Course I'm not as full of energy as when I was younger."

I asked other questions about possible symptoms; his answers were negative. After his physical exam, we returned to my office.

"So, what vitamins should I take? That's why I'm here from Chicago. My wife says your clinic does a lot with vitamins, and minerals, and herbs and all, and that's an approach I haven't tried. If I need to stay a few days, that's OK; I'm staying with my brother here in Seattle."

"You'll just need a day or two at most," I said. "You'll need to have your stomach tested. . . . "

"My stomach? The rosacea's on my face."

"I know. But your face is reflecting a gastrointestinal problem."

"Heck of a reflection. So if rosacea 'reflects' a gastrointestinal problem, how come no one told me that before? Besides, this gas and heartburn thing is minor, and just started. I've had this rosacea thing for years."

"I don't know why no one told you," I said. "An article published in 1948 said that '. . . every dermatologist knows about stomach malfunction—specifically low or no stomach acid—in cases of rosacea'."

"No stomach acid? What's that got to do with my face?"

"What's tetracycline got to do with your face?"

"Kills germs, I guess."

"Where are the germs?"

"In these pimple things."

"How about all the red skin in between the pimples—or when you don't even have pimples? The redness of your skin doesn't go away then, does it?"

"Not really, I guess. So where are the germs?"

"Don't know for certain, but I can guess. When you swallow the tetracycline, where does it go?"

"My stomach."

"And into the intestines after that. Biggest reservoir of bacteria in the whole body, the intestines, especially the colon. And if we don't have strong hydrochloric-acid production by our stomachs, the pH—the acid-alkaline balance—of the intestines and colon is made more alkaline. When that happens, . . . 'unfriendly' germs are more likely to grow. . . . "

"And maybe that's why tetracycline works—at least some?"

"That's my guess. It's also probably why several hydrochloric-acid and pepsin capsules taken with every meal help control rosacea as well as or better than tetracycline."

"Because the hydrochloric acid changes the pH—the acidity—back towards normal, and the 'unfriendly' germs can't grow as well?"

"Exactly right. And we get even better results when we add *Lactobacillus acidophilus*—those are 'normal' acid-loving bacteria—as well."

"That's certainly a different approach."

"Almost always works, though. Also, we add injections of vitamin B_{12}, which isn't absorbed as well when our stomachs aren't working, or when we have 'bacterial overgrowth' in the intestines. And as long as we're injecting vitamin B_{12}, we put the other B-vitamins in there, too."

Like nearly everyone with acne rosacea, Mr. Flanagan had very poor stomach function. After two years of replacement hydrochloric-acid/pepsin capsules with meals, *Lactobacillus acidophilus,* and B_{12} with B-complex injections, he flew back in from Chicago to visit his brother again, and came by to show us that his skin was almost normal, "for the first time in twenty years."

DR. GABY'S COMMENTARY

As you saw in David's story, conventional treatments may not work for everyone. Doctors have found that certain natural therapies might be helpful. You should discuss with your doctor which natural therapies might be useful for your condition.

The Role of Hydrochloric Acid

In studies performed during the early part of the twentieth century, 30% to 60% of patients with rosacea were found to have hypochlorhydria (low stomach acid). Treatment of these patients with hydrochloric acid during or after meals resulted in considerable improvement in their skin lesions.[1] Dr. Wright has found that as many as 80% of patients with rosacea have hypochlorhydria. This higher prevalence may be due to differences in methodology for measuring stomach acid. It is also possible that pollution and other aspects of modern-day living result in autoimmune damage to the stomach, which eventually leads to hypochlorhydria.

The effectiveness of hydrochloric acid against rosacea may be related to its capacity to kill unwanted organisms residing in the stomach or small intestine. In that respect, hydrochloric acid might be functioning as a natural antibiotic, without causing the usual antibiotic side effects. Hydrochloric acid also enhances the absorption of B-vitamins, iron, and many other nutrients. This effect may provide another explanation for why hydrochloric acid is helpful for patients with rosacea.

Hydrochloric-acid therapy is not advisable for all patients. Occasionally, a patient with rosacea will actually have too much, rather than too little, stomach acid. Gastric analysis (a test that measures stomach-acid production) can determine whether hydrochloric-acid therapy is appropriate for a particular individual.

Nutritional Supplements

In one study, 96 patients with rosacea received six tablets of brewer's yeast plus an iron formula daily. Most of these patients showed an improvement in their skin lesions.[2] In another study, oral administration of brewer's yeast, liver extract, and a B-complex vitamin formula, combined with injections of liver extract, was also found to be helpful.[3]

The authors of these studies attributed their good results to the B-vitamin component of the program. However, brewer's yeast and liver also contain a broad range of other nutrients, many of which promote healthy skin. Moreover, brewer's yeast is composed of living "friendly" organisms, which can compete effectively against certain harmful intestinal bacteria.[4] In studies in which synthetic B-vitamins alone were used to treat rosacea, the results have been conflicting.[5, 6] Thus, while B-vitamins may be useful for the treatment of rosacea, it seems that at least some of these B-vitamins should be obtained from brewer's yeast. Some products labeled "brewer's yeast" actually contain "nutritional yeast," which is a different organism that may not be effective against rosacea. Look for a product that states the yeast is a byproduct of the brewing of beer.

Another source of friendly bacteria is *Lactobacillus acidophilus,* which Dr. Wright has found to be helpful for patients with rosacea. Additional studies are needed to confirm the effectiveness of "probiotics" (friendly organisms) against rosacea, and to determine which organisms are the most beneficial.

Azelaic Acid

AZELAIC ACID IS a nine-carbon compound that occurs naturally in some foods. This compound has been shown to kill certain bacteria and to exert an anti-inflammatory effect on skin lesions. In a three-month double-blind study, 32 individuals with rosacea applied a 20% azelaic-acid cream to one side of their face and a placebo cream to the other side. There was a marked improvement or complete clearing of the lesions on 91% of the sides treated with azelaic acid, compared with only 34% of the sides treated with the placebo.[7] Azelaic acid is available as a 20% cream, either by prescription or (less expensively) from some distributors of natural products. The cream is usually applied twice daily to the affected areas. The incidence of skin irritation or other local side effects is lower with azelaic acid than with other commonly used topical treatments. However, on rare occasions, application of azelaic acid has been associated with a loss of skin pigmentation. Treatment with azelaic acid should therefore be monitored by a doctor.

Summary of Recommendations for Treating Rosacea:

- Hydrochloric acid (with pepsin) with meals, as directed by a doctor, if stomach acid is low.

- Brewer's yeast or *Lactobacillus acidophilus.*

- B-complex vitamins.

- Azelaic-acid cream; topical application twice daily, in selected cases. Discontinue after maximum improvement is seen.

ACNE VULGARIS

ACNE (ALSO CALLED ACNE VULGARIS) *occurs in most American teenagers and to a lesser extent in young adults. The severity of acne can vary from a few scattered lesions to severe inflamed pustules that result in permanent scarring. Acne results in part from excessive stimulation of the skin by androgens (male hormones). Bacterial infection of the skin also appears to be involved.*

Conventional treatment for acne includes topical application of benzoyl peroxide or retinoic acid (Retin-A, a vitamin A derivative), and topical or oral administration of antibiotics. In severe cases, the drug Accutane (another vitamin A derivative) is sometimes used. However, this drug can cause birth defects (if taken by pregnant women), as well as other significant side effects.

DR. WRIGHT'S CASE STUDY

Jason Jeffries didn't look happy, and didn't say much, so his mother spoke first.

"You can see Jason has a bad case of acne," she said. "It started when he was 12, and he's 15 now. We've been the antibiotic route—he's been using that antibiotic cream and taking oral antibiotics, and they just barely controlled it. And I know continuous antibiotics aren't good for anyone. He's tried Retin-A and benzoyl peroxide, but they both really irritated his skin. I've been reading more about health—not just for Jason, but for our whole family. My mother gave me a copy of your book—the one that told about the Eskimos and acne."

"I'm not an Eskimo, Mom."

"That's not the point, Jason. Those Eskimos didn't have any acne at all—they have picture proof for over fifty years—until they started eating refined food, especially all that sugar. Then all the teenagers got acne right away!"

"That sums it up," I said. "Not to mention an enormous and sudden increase in diabetes, heart and blood-vessel disease, gallbladder disease. . . ."

"And everyone in the family says Jason's acne has improved since we all switched to whole foods and no sugar about eight months ago. And I can tell when he's been eating sugar and junk food again away from home."

Jason looked uncomfortable, and wiggled in his chair. "It's tough, Mom."

"I know it is, Jason," I said, "but it's really better for our whole bodies—including for acne. There are some other things you can do, though, in addition to sticking with the natural, whole-food plan."

"I was hoping there were," Mrs. Jeffries said. "Jason's really tried, but unfortunately I didn't know enough to feed him the best food starting when he was very small. So he's not accustomed to it, and of course most of his friends tease him a lot."

"Are you taking any vitamins or minerals, Jason."

"Yeah."

"Which ones?"

"Don't know."

"For now, I'm just giving him vitamin C and a multiple vitamin. After I read your book, I was thinking about zinc, but then there's what you wrote about zinc and copper balance, so I thought I'd wait until I talked to you."

"Zinc is a good place to start. In small quantities for short periods of time, we usually don't need to worry about zinc-copper balance. But for acne, 30 milligrams of zinc three times a day for several months is usually necessary, so we'll make sure to check copper levels along the way."

"Your book mentioned food allergies, too. As far as I know, Jason doesn't have any, and they're not in the family as far as I know."

"In teenagers with acne, food allergies are sometimes important, sometimes not. Since you're not aware of them in your family, we'll postpone allergy testing for now."

"So we just add zinc to Jason's program?"

"Unless he eats much fish, unroasted nuts, or vegetable oils, it's wise to add a little 'essential fatty acid' such as flaxseed oil or perhaps cod-liver oil. Seems to help the zinc work better. Also, make sure there's vitamin A, not just beta-carotene, in Jason's multiple vitamin."

"Any special amounts?"

"For now, 15,000 to 25,000 IU of vitamin A. Years ago, a few dermatologists found that hundreds of thousands of units of vitamin A

worked against acne . . . but that's a lot, and now there are better alternatives, anyway."

"And those are . . . ?"

"In addition to zinc—and in some cases, selenium—there are two very useful natural skin creams. First, 4% niacinamide cream. Researchers compared the 4% niacinamide against the most popular antibiotic cream, and found the niacinamide worked better. And as far as anyone knows, there aren't any side effects."

"And it doesn't alter the normal skin bacteria unfavorably, either, does it?"

"No. Secondly, 20% azelaic acid . . ."

"What's azelaic acid?"

"It's a naturally occurring fatty acid found in some foods. It has an anti-inflammatory effect on the skin and kills some of the bacteria that cause acne. Researchers found azelaic acid is as effective as benzoyl peroxide or Retin-A, with many fewer side effects. It was just as effective as the antibiotic tetracycline, also."

"Which cream should Jason use?"

"Why not both? Perhaps one in the morning, and one at night."

"They won't interfere with each other if he uses them at the same time—in case he wants to use them more often?"

"Not as far as I know."

Jason stayed with what he called his "health food" most of the time, his mother later reported. He took the zinc (in addition to his multiple vitamin and vitamin C, along with added fatty acids) and used both the 4% niacinamide and the 20% azelaic-acid creams. After six months, his mother reported that his acne was "not totally gone, but much better."

DR. GABY'S COMMENTARY

Acne can be emotionally painful for already sensitive teenagers. As Jason learned, a healthy diet and limiting refined sugars can help control acne. In addition, a number of natural treatments for acne are frequently effective. Like Jason, teenagers (and adults with acne) can obtain a reasonable level of relief by using some or all of the natural treatments that Jason used.

Dietary Considerations

The importance of dietary factors in acne was illustrated by a study of Northern Canadian Eskimos. Prior to the 1950s, when their diet consisted of fish, game, and small amounts of fruits and vegetables, acne was unknown among this population. However, after refined foods—particularly refined sugar—were introduced into their diet, acne became epidemic among the teenage population.[1]

In our experience, a diet low in sugar and refined and processed foods is sometimes helpful for acne. Food allergy appears to be a major contributing factor in some cases of adult acne, but the effect of allergy on teenage acne is less pronounced. Although some individuals report that eating chocolate makes their acne worse, research has failed to confirm an association between acne and chocolate.

Nutritional Supplements
Zinc Therapy

One natural acne therapy involves zinc. In a double-blind study, 91 patients with moderately severe acne received either zinc (45 mg twice daily) or a placebo for 12 weeks. The skin lesions improved to a significantly greater extent in the zinc group than in the placebo group.[2] In another study, zinc was found to be as effective as oral antibiotics.[3]

Other studies have failed to show a beneficial effect of zinc. As a result, zinc therapy remains controversial and outside of the medical mainstream. However, the negative results were apparently due to inadequate duration of treatment (it takes about 12 weeks to see an effect) or to the use of a poorly absorbed form of zinc (zinc sulfate).

We prescribe one of the well-absorbed forms of zinc (such as zinc picolinate or zinc citrate) at a dosage of 30 mg, 2 to 3 times a day. Most patients notice improvement with this treatment. After 3 months, the dosage can often be reduced without causing a flare-up. Because large doses of zinc can promote copper deficiency, we recommend either a copper supplement (2 to 4 mg per day, depending on the dose of zinc) or periodic monitoring of copper status by a blood test.

Azelaic Acid

Azelaic acid[4,5] is a nine-carbon compound that occurs naturally in some foods. Azelaic acid has been shown to kill the bacteria that are associated with acne. However, unlike tetracycline, azelaic acid does not cause gastrointestinal problems, and it does not encourage the growth of fungus or resistant strains of bacteria. Azelaic acid also exerts an anti-inflammatory effect on skin lesions.

In a double-blind study, topically applied azelaic-acid cream was significantly more effective than a placebo. In other studies, azelaic-acid cream was about as effective as 0.05% Retin-A, erythromycin ointment, benzoyl peroxide, or oral tetracycline. However, the incidence of irritation and other local side effects was lower with azelaic acid than with Retin-A or other topical treatments. These studies demonstrate that azelaic acid is an effective alternative to antibiotics and topical agents in the treatment of mild to moderate acne.

Azelaic acid is not as effective as Accutane for

individuals with severe cystic acne, a type of acne that can lead to scarring. However, as many as one-third of such patients have achieved good to excellent results after 6 months of treatment with azelaic acid. The combination of azelaic-acid cream twice daily and 100 mg of oral minocycline (a tetracycline derivative) daily was even more effective, with 90% of patients achieving good or excellent results. Thus, azelaic acid, either alone or in combination with antibiotics, is an effective alternative to Accutane.

Azelaic acid is available as a 20% cream, either by prescription or (less expensively) from some distributors of natural products. The cream should be applied to the affected areas twice daily. Although azelaic acid is usually well tolerated, on rare occasions it has been associated with a loss of skin pigmentation. Treatment with azelaic acid should therefore be monitored by a doctor.

Topical Niacinamide

SEVENTY-SIX patients with inflamed acne lesions were randomly assigned to apply to their face twice daily a gel containing either 4% niacinamide or 1% clindamycin (a commonly used antibiotic). After 8 weeks, 82% of the patients receiving niacinamide were improved, compared with 69% of those treated with clindamycin.[6] The only side effect of the niacinamide gel was mild stinging or burning at the application site. However, that reaction was apparently caused by the gel used to carry the niacinamide, rather than by the niacinamide itself. The beneficial results obtained with niacinamide are thought to be due to an anti-inflammatory effect of the vitamin. Niacinamide for topical use can be obtained from compounding pharmacists, who should be able to identify a non-irritating gel or cream in which to mix the niacinamide.

Other Natural Treatments

SOME 106 teenage females who experienced premenstrual flare-ups of acne received 50 mg of vit-amin B_6 per day, beginning 1 week before and continuing through menstruation. A lessening of premenstrual acne was reported by 72% of the women.[7] Some individuals experience mild side effects from vitamin B_6, such as irritability or insomnia. These symptoms can usually be prevented by taking magnesium, 200 to 300 mg per day.

Very large doses of vitamin A are also effective in difficult-to-treat cases.[8] However, because of the potential for vitamin A toxicity, this treatment should be monitored by a physician knowledgeable in its use. In another study, selenium at a dose of 200 mcg twice a day for 6 to 12 weeks was reported to be helpful for individuals with acne.[9] However, there was no control group in that study, so a placebo effect cannot be ruled out. Long-term (greater than six weeks) use of more than 250 mcg of selenium per day should be monitored by a doctor.

Summary of Recommendations for Treating Acne

- Diet: Avoid refined sugar and other refined and processed foods. Work with food allergies in selected cases.

- Zinc (picolinate or citrate), 30 mg, 2 to 3 times per day for 2 to 3 months; then once or twice per day, depending on response. Balance with copper (2 to 4 mg per day, depending on zinc dose) or monitor copper status periodically.

- Azelaic-acid cream, topical application twice daily to affected areas, in selected cases. Discontinue after maximum improvement is obtained.

- Niacinamide 4% gel, topical application twice daily to affected areas, in selected cases.

- For premenstrual acne flare-ups: vitamin B_6, 50 to 100 mg per day premenstrually and during menstruation. Balance with magnesium, 200 to 300 mg per day.

ALCOHOLISM

> 🍂 ACCORDING TO ONE *point of view, alcoholism is caused primarily by a lack of willpower. Drinking to the point of self-destruction is a choice, and people who drink to excess could choose, if they wished, to remain sober. However, others consider alcoholism to be not a moral failing, but a disease. And, just like individuals with diabetes, heart disease, or arthritis, alcoholics need medical treatment.*
>
> *It is true that no one puts a gun to the head of an alcoholic and demands that he take a drink. However, physical and psychological addictions can be extremely powerful forces, and some people lack the tools needed to deal with these drives. Groups such as Alcoholics Anonymous help people get in touch with the emotional and spiritual aspects of their addiction. However, the candy, coffee, and cigarettes that permeate AA meetings are testament to how often the physical aspects of addiction are overlooked.*

DR. WRIGHT'S CASE STUDY

Mary Carter had been to Tahoma Clinic several times before, but not with her husband Tom. They sat down and looked at each other, appearing hesitant about who would talk first. I waited.

"Best to just say it, I guess," Tom started. "I'm alcoholic, probably always been alcoholic. Both my parents were, too. Started getting drunk when I was 11, and didn't even think of quitting until I met Mary here. Her father was alcoholic, she . . . you tell him, Mary."

"My father and grandfather were alcoholic, too," Mary said. "I made a promise to myself when I was eight years old—after watching my father beat my mother again—that I would never drink the first little bit of alcohol myself, and never, ever would my children be exposed to alcoholism. It's now 25 years since then, and I haven't had that first drink, and I never will."

Tom added, "For years, I hid my drinking from most all my friends and business acquaintances, but I never could fool Mary. She figured it out right away."

"Too bad I didn't promise myself never to fall in love with an alcoholic," Mary smiled. "That might be genetic, too, who knows? I've had plenty of other chances, but nobody ever 'clicked' with me until I met Tom. We met and got married all within seven months . . ."

"That was the first time I quit drinking," Tom broke in. "After Mary 'called me out' about alcohol, I decided it was time to stop. Lasted for nearly a year, but then the craving got too bad, and I started up again."

"I was almost expecting Tom to restart," Mary said. "I grew up with too many alcoholics around, I guess. That first time, Tom quit for me, not for himself, and he tried to do it almost alone. Of course he had my support, but he didn't get any counseling or go to AA."

"I was too proud," Tom said. "Here I was, a happily married, successful insurance salesman, and I just wasn't going to associate with all those drunks."

"So, anyway, he started again. Fortunately, Tom's such a nice guy, never has been a mean drunk. So I never thought of leaving him, but we had some rough times. The next time he was ready to quit, I persuaded him to go to AA meetings and see a counselor, too."

"I saw a specialist in alcoholism," Tom said. "Worked a lot better the second time. Three and a half 'dry' years. We were talking about having kids, and then I ran into serious business difficulties—only avoided bankruptcy by a tiny margin. The stress got to be too much, and I gave in again."

"I know it sounds weird, but in a way it's a good thing Tom had those business problems. It showed us his being sober wasn't solid, yet. Something inside told me not to let go of that promise I made to never expose my children to alcoholism. There was one other thing, too. I'd been here, told you my health history, and you suggested I try some things based just on my family history of alcoholism. I was skeptical, but went ahead, and I definitely felt better. I tried to get Tom to try, too, but he was 'on the wagon,' thought he was doing well, and didn't want to take any vitamins. Unfortunately, the counselor he was seeing then told him that diet and supplements have nothing to do with alcoholism."

"Fortunately, that's changing," I said. "But some still think that way."

"So we got through that, Tom's business is solid again, and he's quit drinking again . . ."

"For the third time," Tom said.

"This time, I've done enough reading to show Tom and to convince him that there's a biochemical side to behavior, as well as the psychological side. Now I hope it's OK with you, but I've already had Tom do that glucose-insulin tolerance test you had me do. When I was here, you told me it's often abnormal in alcoholics or their blood relatives. Here's the test report. I think it's abnormal."

"Thank you! Nothing like getting a head start." I looked at the report briefly, then turned to Tom. "Your test shows that your blood sugar drops too low—low blood sugar—a common problem for alcoholics and recovering alcoholics. Mary already knows what to do about this. Are you ready?"

"Yep. Mary's had me and alcohol figured right from the start, even if I'm too stubborn to go for it all at once."

"But I insisted he come in to talk to you," Mary said. "It's going to be hard enough getting Tom off the sugar—he's got quite a sweet tooth—without having to talk him into all the vitamins and things I think he needs."

"I'm glad you're trying. The diet helps reduce the craving for both sugar and alcohol.

"Let's go over supplements that can biochemically reduce craving for alcohol." I checked my notes. "Tom said he started drinking at age 11. There's been a recent publication noting that alcoholics who start at an early age may have a relative deficit in the amino acid tryptophan, which could cause a shortage of serotonin in the brain."

"What would that do?" Tom asked.

"In some people, it causes depression; in others aggressive behavior; and in some both."

"I've always been a little on the depressed side," Tom said. "Especially before I met Mary. And alcohol helps that somehow?"

"That's the thought. So, I'll start this list with tryptophan, 1,500 milligrams twice daily in between meals. That's especially important if you're going to be restricting carbohydrates in your diet to control low blood sugar."

"Why's that?" Mary asked. "I hadn't read about that anywhere."

"It's been found that dietary carbohydrates help tryptophan penetrate the brain and nervous system better. If we're cutting down carbohydrates for whatever reason, tryptophan may not penetrate the brain as well."

"And we have less serotonin, and get more depressed. Now I get it," Mary said.

"There are two other items that can reduce alcohol craving: one is based on research by the famous biochemist Roger Williams, and the other endorsed by Bill W."

"Bill W? The founder of AA?"

"Yes, that Bill W. Somewhere in our files is a copy of 'Letter to AA Physicians' by Bill W., very strongly endorsing the use of the niacin form of vitamin B3 to reduce alcohol craving. Many alcoholics have told me that Bill W. might not have been a biochemist or physician, but he knew what he was talking about when it related to alcohol. So, please get the time-release form of niacin and use 500 milligrams, twice daily. Bill W. advocated more, but if we use it in conjunction with good diet and other supplements, not as much appears to be necessary. Just in case it's still too much for you, we'll monitor liver enzymes to begin with, and then as necessary."

"What about the rest of the B-complex vitamins?" Mary asked.

"You're right. Whenever one B-vitamin such as niacin is used in relatively large quantities, it's best to 'back it up' with the rest of the B-complex. We'll get to that under general recommendations. First, let's cover the remaining alcohol-craving preventer. Dr. Roger Williams, a research scientist credited with the discovery of the B-vitamin pantothenic acid, did extensive animal research with glutamine, an amino acid. He found that supplemental glutamine noticeably reduced alcohol intake. It frequently does the same for humans, and reduces alcohol cravings, as well. Please use 1,000 milligrams of glutamine, twice daily."

"And all of that will cut down any craving for alcohol I have? I have to admit that it's been tough a lot of times even when I didn't give in."

"As Mary pointed out, fighting alcoholism is part psychological, and part biochemical. While these supplements won't do everything, they're an important part of the picture. Sticking strictly to a blood-sugar-control diet is very helpful. But before you think that's all—there's extensive evidence on other nutrients necessary to make up for what alcohol does to a person's nutritional status. You're . . ." I checked his record " . . . 35, and if I calculated correctly, you've been drinking alcohol steadily for 24 years, minus four and a half years 'on the wagon' since you met Mary. That's 19½ years. Just a short list of nutrients that may need some attention includes: vitamin A, the entire B-complex, vitamins C and E, zinc, magnesium, selenium, choline, gamma-linolenic acid, glutathione, pantetheine, and taurine . . . and I shouldn't forget some additional items very useful for blood-sugar control: chromium, manganese, essential fatty acids . . ."

"Hold on, you've already listed three supplements to cut down alcohol craving. That list must be another dozen or more."

"That's why there are multiple-vitamin combinations," Mary said. "Almost all of that stuff is in the multiple vitamin-mineral combination that I've been taking since I came here."

"You mean the ten-capsules-a-day formula you've been using?"

"That's the one," I said. "It's a lot of capsules, but all from the same bottle, which makes it easier. Actually, you're getting off easy—only four bottles, total, to work from."

"OK, I promised Mary I'd give it a try."

At his first return visit three months later, Mr. Carter observed that staying away from alcohol was "much easier this time," and that he felt better than he had in years. It's been eight years since that time. He and Mary have had two children who, according to both parents, "haven't been and won't be exposed to a (practicing) alcoholic parent."

As TOM LEARNED, when an alcoholic acknowledges his problem and is willing to accept both the psychological and biochemical factors that contribute to it, he can successfully stay dry. Tom's success came from understanding his own cravings and family history and using a combination of dietary approaches and natural medicine to reduce the craving for alcohol.

Biochemistry of Addiction

MANY HEALTH-CARE practitioners do not fully appreciate the biochemical component of alcoholism. For some alcoholics, the urge to drink may be as strong as a diabetic's need to eat sugar after overdosing on insulin. Thus, while some might disparage an individual who claims that "the spirit is willing but the flesh is weak," it would be more useful to seek ways of "strengthening the flesh," thereby increasing the person's willpower.

We know that alcohol addiction has a genetic component, although we have not defined the specific inherited biochemical abnormality. Despite the limits of our knowledge, there is evidence that we can use nutrition—both diet and supplements—to help alcoholics remain sober.

Dietary Considerations
The Hypoglycemia Connection

INDIVIDUALS who consume alcohol in excess frequently suffer from reactive hypoglycemia. When blood-sugar levels fall, people tend to develop anxiety attacks and to crave rapidly absorbable carbohydrates, including alcohol. Blood-sugar levels can often be controlled by avoiding refined sugar, other refined carbohydrates, and caffeine. Also helpful is consuming small, frequent meals and taking supplements including chromium, B-vitamins, magnesium, zinc, and other nutrients. When hypoglycemia is

kept under control, individuals with an alcohol problem sometimes find it easier to stay away from the bottle.[1]

The Role of Allergy

SOME doctors have observed that alcoholics tend to be allergic to the foods from which their "drink of choice" is derived. The so-called "allergy/addiction syndrome," which has been described for foods, also appears to extend in some instances to alcoholic beverages. Certain alcoholics have been able to resume controlled social drinking, as long as they consumed only drinks derived from non-allergenic food sources.[2] However, that approach is generally not recommended, because it does not work for everyone, and because it requires the strict limitation of only one or two drinks every 5 to 7 days.

Nutritional Treatments
Considering Nutritional Deficiencies

ALCOHOLICS are often deficient in a wide range of vitamins and minerals. These deficiencies can result from a dilution effect (calories from alcohol replace more nutritious foods) or from malabsorption (alcohol damages the gastrointestinal tract). One of the consequences of nutritional deficiency may be an increased desire to drink alcohol.

For example, when animals were fed a diet low in vitamins and minerals, their voluntary consumption of alcohol was three times higher than when the same diet was supplemented with vitamins and minerals.[3] In another study, thiamine-deficient rats had a 180% increase in voluntary alcohol consumption.[4] However, when the diet contained a higher-than-normal amount of thiamine, alcohol intake was reduced by 80%, compared with alcohol intake on a normal diet.[5] Deficiencies of riboflavin, niacin, pantothenic acid, or vitamin B$_6$ also caused some, but not all rats, to drink large amounts of alcohol. Of 10 mice fed a niacin-deficient diet, 3 exhibited an extreme drinking pattern—they drank the entire ration of alcohol offered them.[6, 7] If these findings are applicable to humans, they would suggest that nutritional deficiencies might increase the tendency to alcohol addiction, and that some individuals would be more susceptible than others to the effects of these deficiencies.

In human studies, six alcoholics were treated with a combination of vitamins A, B-complex, C, E, and essential fatty acids. All patients noted a decrease in their desire to drink alcohol, as well as a reduction in tension, hostility, and insomnia.[8] In a double-blind study using a similar treatment program, 56% of patients receiving nutritional support remained abstinent or engaged in controlled drinking, compared with only 14% of those receiving a placebo.[9]

Niacin

NIACIN has been effective in treating alcoholics. In one study, approximately 30% of previously treatment-resistant patients showed some degree of improvement while taking niacin, as evidenced by less insomnia, improved mood, enhanced social and emotional function, and reduced need for medication.[10] Of course, niacin should be used with caution in alcoholics, because large doses (particularly of the time-release form) can trigger or aggravate liver disease. Although the dosage of niacin used by Dr. Wright (500 mg twice a day) is lower than the amount that has been reported to cause liver damage, individuals with a history of alcoholism and/or liver disease should not take niacin without medical supervision.

Glutamine

IN a double-blind study, 10 alcoholics received 1 gram of the amino acid glutamine per day for approximately 6 weeks, and a placebo for an additional 6 weeks. In 9 of the 10 cases, glutamine appeared to diminish the desire to drink alcohol. Some patients reported that glutamine relieved nervousness and improved their ability to sleep.[11] Some doctors have observed that larger doses of glutamine may be effective when 1 gram per day is not. In my experience, glutamine has been helpful for some patients who, despite their best efforts, had difficulty staying away from alcohol. One patient told me that glutamine was the only treatment that actually reduced his desire to drink. Although it is not known how glutamine decreases alcohol craving, this amino acid is known to have beneficial effects on brain function.

Essential Fatty Acids (EFAs)

EVIDENCE shows that chronic alcohol consumption interferes with EFA metabolism, leading to a deficiency of prostaglandin E$_1$ (PGE$_1$, a hormone-like compound that is produced from EFAs). While short-term alcohol consumption may increase PGE$_1$ levels, resulting in an elevation of mood, chronic drinking eventually depletes PGE$_1$, leading to depression. It has been suggested that some alcoholics continue drinking in order to prevent their PGE$_1$ levels from declining. Studies in both humans and animals have shown that supplementing with EFAs, in the form of safflower oil, cod-liver oil, or evening primrose oil, reduced alcohol intake or inhibited signs of alcohol withdrawal.[12, 13]

L-Tryptophan

ALCOHOLICS often have low blood levels of the essential amino acid L-tryptophan.[14] Because L-tryptophan is the precursor to serotonin (a molecule that plays a role in mood and normal sleep), tryptophan deficiency might be responsible in part for the depression and/or insomnia that commonly occurs in alcoholics. Studies have shown that giving alcoholics L-tryptophan can relieve both of these symptoms.[15, 16]

Toxic reactions to L-tryptophan in 1989 resulted in the removal of this amino acid from health-food stores. It was later determined that the toxicity was due to a contaminant, not to the L-tryptophan itself. Currently, however, uncontaminated L-tryptophan is available only by prescription through compounding pharmacists.

Other Treatments
Lithium Therapy

THE trace mineral lithium has long been recognized as an effective treatment for manic-depression (bipolar disorder). Lithium also has been used to treat alcoholism, although the results have been conflicting. In one double-blind study, 73 patients hospitalized for alcohol detoxification were randomly assigned to receive a placebo or therapeutic doses of lithium for up to 96 weeks. During the treatment period, 64% of the patients in the placebo group had a drinking binge severe enough to require hospitalization, compared with only 25% of those receiving lithium (a statistically significant difference).[17] However, in a similar study, lithium was no more effective than a placebo.[18]

Gamma-hydroxybutyrate (GHB)

GHB is a normal constituent of the brain that is believed to function as a neurotransmitter (chemical messenger) and to play a role in regulating nervous-system activity. GHB has been shown to have a calming effect in both animals and humans. A derivative of GHB (its lactone form) suppressed voluntary alcohol consumption in a strain of rat that had been inbred for a high preference for alcohol. In addition, GHB itself prevented signs of withdrawal in rats that had been force-fed alcohol.

In a double-blind study, 82 alcoholics were randomly assigned to receive GHB (50 mg per kg of body weight per day, in 3 divided doses) or a placebo for 3 months. The average number of drinks per day declined by about 50% in the GHB

group, but did not change in the placebo group. Craving for alcohol was also significantly lower in the GHB group than in the placebo group. At the end of the study, only 28% of the patients receiving GHB were still drinking excessively, compared with 77% of those receiving the placebo. No serious side effects were seen, although a few patients reported minor adverse reactions.[19] In another study, approximately two-thirds of a group of 91 alcoholics achieved abstinence while using a higher dose of GHB (50 mg per kg of body weight 3 times a day). Of those who failed to respond to the prescribed regimen, all but one stopped drinking completely when the same daily amount of GHB was spread out over 6 doses.[20]

These studies suggest that GHB is one of the most promising treatments for alcoholism currently available. Unfortunately, this compound has achieved a bad reputation as a "date rape" drug, and has been reported to cause a number of toxic effects. For those reasons, GHB is currently illegal in the United States. However, the adverse effects that have been attributed to GHB were usually associated with overdoses, or with the use of GHB in conjunction with other legal or illegal drugs. There is no question that GHB has been abused, particularly by individuals with addictive personalities. However, the scientific evidence suggests that, if used properly (and that might mean having the doses doled out by a family member or "significant other"), GHB appears to be an extremely valuable and relatively safe weapon against alcoholism.

Conclusion

ALCOHOLISM IS A serious disease that requires attention to the body, mind, and spirit. Although more research needs to be done, effective nutritional interventions exist to help alcoholics abstain. Nutritional treatment of alcohol addiction should monitored by a health-care practitioner.

Summary of Recommendations for Treating Alcohol Addiction

- Diet: Avoid refined sugar, other refined carbohydrates, and caffeine. In cases of reactive hypoglycemia, eat small, frequent meals. Work with food allergies in selected cases.

- High-potency multiple vitamin/mineral (adjust doses of other nutrients as needed).

- High-potency B-complex vitamin.

- Glutamine, 500 to 1,000 mg, 2 to 3 times per day.

- Niacin, essential fatty acids, and/or lithium in selected cases (supervised by a doctor).

- L-tryptophan (by prescription), 1,000 to 1,500 mg twice per day between meals, for depression and/or insomnia associated with alcohol consumption.

ANGINA

❧ ANGINA PECTORIS IS *the medical term for a type of chest pain that occurs in people with heart and blood-vessel disease. The pain is often accompanied by a feeling of suffocation and impending death. Angina is usually triggered by exertion or stress, but some individuals develop angina even when at rest.*

A major cause of angina is a lack of adequate blood flow to the heart, resulting from atherosclerosis (hardening and blockage) of the coronary arteries. However, some individuals experience angina despite having completely normal coronary arteries. These people apparently suffer from periodic spasms of the coronary arteries, leading to a temporary restriction of blood flow. A minority of scientists believes that a primary weakness of the heart muscle is an important cause of angina and that blood-vessel spasm is often a consequence, rather than a cause, of impaired cardiac function.

Conventional therapy consists mainly of drugs that reduce the demands on the heart or that dilate blood vessels. These drugs often provide relief from symptoms, but they do not address the fundamental causes of heart and blood-vessel disease. Cardiac drugs can cause numerous side effects—from depression to fluid retention—and concerns have been raised that some of these medicines might cause cancer. Coronary-bypass surgery or balloon angioplasty are often performed when drug treatment is ineffective or when certain types of coronary blockages are found.

DR. WRIGHT'S CASE STUDY

Maya Kim had been to Tahoma Clinic for her own health problems, but this time she was here with her husband John. "I want you to fix John before he dies of heart attack!" she declared. "He's having chest pains three years now. He's taking 'nitro' under his tongue all the time, the heart doctor says maybe in a few years he needs bypass surgery. I say maybe in a few years he won't be here, like his father—died of heart attack, age 55! John is 53! Tell him please!"

I looked at John who smiled and said nothing,

so I turned back to Maya. "I can't 'fix' John for you," I said. "The most I can do is make recommendations. Any 'fixing' will need to be done by John himself—with your help, of course."

Maya stared at John. "John?"

He smiled again. "I'm not stupid. I read newspapers, see the TV about eating less fat, vitamin E preventing heart attacks—all that stuff. I just know from my work to wait—make sure it's real, not just a fad. Then unless it's my own knowledge area, I find an expert, maybe two experts, get information, then decide what to do."

"John's always this way—careful to study, to

analyze. That's why he's so successful in business," Maya said. "I stay home, raise the kids. But I worry maybe anytime now, no more time to study, to analyze. Tell him doctor!"

"Studying's done," John said. "Maya's health improved more in two years following natural-health methods from this clinic than in six years before with all the best doctors and drugs. So here I am, now what do I do?"

"Please tell me about the chest pains first, and then what you've done so far."

"Started having chest pain three years ago. At first, just if I exercised hard or had a lot of stress. Kept happening, got worse, so I saw the doctor, he sent me to a cardiologist. I've had cardiogram, treadmill, recently an angiogram. I'm told several arteries have some block—none really bad. I'm taking these . . ." He pulled two vials out of his pocket, and handed them to me.

"Nitroglycerin and one of the 'calcium-channel blockers,'" I observed. "No other medicines?"

Mr. Kim smiled, this time much more widely, and reached into his other pocket. "More research," he said. "When the cardiologist said he was taking these himself, and didn't know if it would help but it couldn't hurt, it was time to come here for sure." He handed me the bottle.

"Vitamin E, 400 IU," I read.

"John, you didn't tell me you have vitamin E!" Maya exclaimed.

"I didn't take any yet, I want to ask the expert, but that's when I asked Maya to make me an appointment here. I know from business that when the competition adopts your methods, you must be doing it right."

It was my turn to smile. "We find it's usually safer and more effective to start with natural means first," I said. "University researchers are starting to learn that too. But back to you—how often do you have chest pain?"

"Mild pains—several every day. More severe—when I walk up hills or try to work hard outdoors. Every so often, a bad one with no exercise or stress. I take maybe six or eight 'nitro' every week."

"Have you started to change your diet?"

"Maya did that for me at home . . ."

"But he eats out a lot, travels on business. I know he isn't careful then!" Maya declared.

"I promise, I start now. I've made up my mind. From now on, I only eat like at home wherever I am."

"Tell me what you do at home," I asked Maya.

"What I learned here and from books you ask me to read. Only whole food, whole grain—we eat only brown rice at home—no sugar, no chemicals in the food, less meat, more fish, many more vegetables. I do more old-style Korean cooking, John says like his mother did at home. Not just for myself and John, for the children, too, even if they complain their high-school friends eat pizza, Coca-Cola, and other junk!"

"Maya really means it. No other food at home for two years now—since she started coming here. I'm away on business a lot, but from now on, I only eat like at home. Now, about vitamins and anything else—what do I do?"

"In addition to your health history, we should do a physical exam, and there are some basic tests, too. Particularly when we're past 50 and have health problems, it's wisest to check the efficiency of digestion and assimilation. We'll also check levels of key minerals, serum levels of homocysteine, routine tests including cholesterol, HDL-cholesterol and triglycerides, kidney-function tests, and please check for allergies . . ."

"I understand minerals—like calcium and magnesium, right? And cholesterol and so on . . . but why kidney tests? And allergies? What have allergies to do with chest pain, with angina?"

"Angina due to allergy isn't common, but if it's there, it's certainly easy to relieve. A doctor I know told me his mother's angina finally went away when she quit eating onions."

"And kidney tests?"

"In addition to diet changes and supplements, chelation therapy is usually very helpful for relieving angina and improving the circulation. To make sure chelation therapy is safe, we need to monitor kidney function."

"I'll do all that—that's why I'm here today. Now how much vitamin E and other vitamins should I take?"

"Vitamin E, 800 IU daily, to start. Other supplements useful in relieving angina include L-carnitine, 500 milligrams; coenzyme Q_{10}, 100 milligrams; magnesium (aspartate), 125 milligrams; L-arginine, 1,000 milligrams; and vitamin C, 1,000 milligrams. All should be taken 3 times daily. Also, please obtain a high-potency vitamin-mineral supplement with at least 50 milligrams vitamin B_6, 800 micrograms folate, and 500 micrograms vitamin B_{12}." I wrote these items on a note for him.

"In addition to swallowing the magnesium supplement, please come in for a short series of magnesium injections intravenously. Once those are done, we'll have you switch over to periodic intramuscular injections at home. You can do them yourself, or Maya can do them for you."

"Why do I need injection if I swallow the magnesium?"

"In a way, life insurance, but the real kind. In the 1950s, Australian researchers found that the death rate among individuals hospitalized with heart disease could be cut from over 30% to less than 1%, simply with a series of magnesium injections."

"Sounds like valuable life insurance to me."

"Inexpensive, too—usually less than a dollar per injection, and injections are once weekly or less."

"And chelation therapy?"

"If your kidney-function tests are OK, chelation therapy can be started. At intervals, we also do mineral-replacement IVs, to replace any beneficial minerals that might have been lost during the chelation therapy. If you can, please read *The Chelation Answer* by Garry Gordon, M.D., and Morton Walker, D.P.M., or *Bypassing Bypass* by Elmer Cranton, M.D. Either of these books will provide an extremely good explanation of chelation therapy, but make sure to save any questions about it for next time."

"OK. Anything else?"

"Actually, I forgot one other test. Please have your testosterone level checked."

"I think John has enough testosterone," Maya said. "Just too much chest pain."

"Let's make certain. Testosterone can be extremely valuable in strengthening the heart muscle, lessening atherosclerosis, and even favorably affecting cholesterol, triglycerides, and blood sugar. It's true that testosterone is much more likely to be low in somewhat older individuals, but just in case, please check."

Like many individuals with angina, Mr. Kim had inefficient stomach function, with low production of hydrochloric acid and (presumably) pepsin (see chapter 2). He was advised to take supplemental hydrochloric acid and pepsin with meals, and to add vitamin B_{12} and folate to his at-home injections. His homocysteine level was normal and allergy tests were negative. His cholesterol and triglyceride tests were both slightly abnormal; his testosterone was OK. Since his kidney-function tests were normal, he went ahead with chelation therapy. He changed the rest of his diet, and took the vitamin E, L-carnitine, coenzyme Q_{10}, magnesium (both orally and by injection), and a "back-up" high-potency vitamin-mineral. He was also asked to take L-arginine by injection and orally. Even though there are no studies to date concerning L-arginine and angina, this amino acid is known to be an aid to blood-vessel dilation, which very likely will help with angina by helping deliver more blood to the heart.

His angina started to diminish just two weeks after starting his program. By six weeks, he was down to "only two nitros" per week, and after six months he was off all medications and free of chest pain unless he exerted himself excessively. He undertook a gradually increasing exercise program at four months, and by one year could run two miles without angina. Five years later he remains free of any chest pain.

DIETARY MODIFICATION AND nutritional supplements offer great promise for preventing and treating angina and related cardiovascular problems. Furthermore, nutritional therapy appears to have a favorable influence on the various factors that can cause cardiovascular problems, including atherosclerosis, blood-vessel spasm, and poor cardiac function.

Dietary Considerations
Effect of Diet

FOR some individuals, eliminating refined sugar from the diet will reduce the number of angina attacks. Some individuals suffer from reactive hypoglycemia or other related disorders of blood-sugar regulation. When the blood sugar falls too far, the body compensates by pumping out extra adrenaline, a "stress hormone" that can trigger angina in susceptible persons. In patients with reactive hypoglycemia and angina, normalizing the blood sugar will sometimes control the angina.[1]

Most physicians are not aware that allergy can be a triggering factor for angina. Allergic reactions result in the release of histamine, a compound that promotes blood-vessel spasm. Individuals with angina who also have allergy-related symptoms will sometimes experience an improvement in their angina if they avoid allergenic foods and chemicals.[2] I have seen several patients whose angina was completely controlled by avoiding a few specific foods. Another patient who was unwilling to change her diet was able to control her angina by taking an antihistamine. Alcohol is another triggering factor for some patients, particularly those who experience angina at rest.

Individuals who have followed the program developed by Dr. Dean Ornish, which includes a low-sugar, low-fat diet plus daily meditation and yoga, have, in many cases, reported rapid relief of angina. In addition, angiograms performed on these patients after one year of treatment demonstrated a significant reversal of coronary-artery blockage in some cases (see the chapter on atherosclerosis treatment for additional discussion of the Ornish program).[3]

Nutritional Supplements
Magnesium Therapy

MAGNESIUM is one of the most important nutrients for individuals suffering from angina. In addition to preventing atherosclerosis,[4] magnesium promotes dilation of blood vessels and improves the functioning of the heart muscle. While taking extra magnesium by mouth may help prevent heart disease from developing, magnesium injections are usually necessary once the disease is already established. Fortunately, intramuscular or intravenous magnesium therapy is of great benefit in many cases. As early as 1958, a South African physician reported that patients frequently responded to magnesium injections in a "dramatic and almost unbelievable manner . . . after all conventional and accepted methods of therapy had failed and sufferers had lost hope of ever obtaining relief."[5] In our experience, that doctor was not exaggerating. Many patients do, indeed, have their life turned around by magnesium injections. Although no double-blind studies have been done, the results are often quite obvious.

A typical treatment regimen is 1 gram of magnesium sulfate injected intramuscularly, once a week for 6 weeks, then less often, as needed. Magnesium can also be administered intravenously; the higher blood levels that can be attained with inravenous therapy may, in theory, increase the efficacy of the treatment. However, intravenous magnesium can cause low blood pressure and other side effects, if administered too rapidly. Therefore, intravenous magnesium should be given only by doctors experienced in its use. When magnesium is given in combination with B-vitamins and vitamin C, it appears to work somewhat better than when used alone (see appendix B).

L-Carnitine

L-CARNITINE is a vitamin-like compound that transports fatty acids into the mitochondria (the "energy-producing factories") of cells where they are "burned" to produce energy. Tissues that require a lot of energy, such as the heart, depend on an adequate supply of L-carnitine for normal function. In one study, 12 patients with angina received 900 mg of L-carnitine per day for 12 weeks. After L-carnitine treatment, the patients were able to exercise significantly longer before developing angina or electrocardiogram abnormalities.[6] In a double-blind study, 44 men with angina received 1 gram of L-carnitine twice daily or a placebo for 4 weeks, then the other treatment for an additional 4 weeks. Compared with placebo, L-carnitine significantly increased the amount of exertion required to induce angina. In addition, 22.7% of the patients were free of angina while taking L-carnitine, compared with only 9.1% during placebo treatment.[7]

Coenzyme Q10

COENZYME Q10 (CoQ10) also plays an important role in energy production within the heart muscle. In a double-blind study, 10 patients with angina were randomly assigned to receive 150 mg of CoQ10 per day or a placebo for 4 weeks. Each patient then received the other treatment for an additional 4 weeks. Compared with the placebo, CoQ10 reduced the frequency of anginal episodes by 53%. Although this improvement was not statistically significant, CoQ10 therapy did significantly increase exercise tolerance on a treadmill (as determined by the time before onset of chest pain).[8]

Vitamin E

FOR nearly 50 years, the relationship between vitamin E and heart disease has been debated repeatedly. Early claims by Dr. Wilfrid Shute that vitamin E relieves angina were not confirmed by controlled studies. However, one double-blind study did demonstrate a small beneficial effect of vitamin E in the treatment of angina.[9] Since vitamin E is safe and since there is evidence that it prevents both atherosclerosis[10] and heart attacks,[11] we recommend vitamin E supplements for nearly all patients with angina. The protective effect of vitamin E on the heart is probably related to its capacity to improve blood flow and to prevent the production of tissue-damaging free radicals.

Vitamin C

IN a 1954 study, 10 patients with atherosclerosis received 500 mg of vitamin C, 3 times a day for 2 to 6 months. Six similar patients did not receive vitamin C. Arteriograms performed on the femoral arteries (in the legs) demonstrated significant regression of atherosclerosis in 6 of the 10 patients receiving vitamin C, whereas none of the 6 untreated patients showed improvement.[12] Because reversing or inhibiting the progression of atherosclerosis is a desirable goal for individuals with angina, we include vitamin C (at least 2 to 3 grams per day) on the list of nutrients recommended for angina patients.

Chelation Therapy

IN the 1950s, a drug given intravenously to treat lead poisoning was serendipitously discovered to relieve the symptoms of angina. This compound, known as ethylenediaminetetraacetic acid (EDTA), has been the subject of considerable controversy ever since. More than half a million Americans have received chelation therapy with EDTA for cardiovascular disease. The term "chelation" is derived from the Greek word for "claw."

EDTA binds to lead and other metals in a way that resembles a claw. The vast majority of cardiovascular patients treated with chelation therapy have reported a reduction in symptoms, and more than 80% have shown improvement by objective testing.[13] Several studies have demonstrated that chelation therapy opens up blocked arteries; for that reason, this treatment is often likened to a chemical "Drano." Patients have provided numerous testimonials about how chelation therapy saved them from bypass surgery, gangrene, or amputation of limbs. Dr. Wright and I have both seen some dramatic improvements in patients who received chelation therapy.

Despite these glowing reports, there has never been a definitive, large-scale placebo-controlled study to determine whether chelation therapy is really effective (some doctors believe that the benefits are due to a placebo effect). Furthermore, it is not clear how EDTA therapy actually works, although a number of different theories have been put forth. Nevertheless, because chelation therapy is much safer than coronary-bypass surgery, costs about 90% less, and has the potential to "clean out" all of the body's arteries (rather than just the ones being surgically bypassed), a definitive study is urgently needed. If chelation therapy were proven to be effective, millions of Americans would be spared expensive and dangerous bypass surgery, and tens of billions of dollars would be saved.

Hormone Therapy

TESTOSTERONE DEFICIENCY HAS been implicated as a contributing factor in various types of heart and blood-vessel disease.[14, 15] In a 1946 study, 100 patients (92 men, 8 women) with angina were treated with testosterone (propionate) injections for 4 to 5 months. Fifty-one patients showed "marked improvement" (defined as the ability to increase physical activity without precipitating angina for up to 2 months after discontinuing treatment), and 40 had "moderate improvement"

(defined as a reduction in angina attacks by at least 50%). Of 5 patients who received a placebo, none improved.[16] The men in this study appeared to improve slightly more than the women, but the number of women treated was too small for a reliable comparison. The beneficial effect of testosterone on angina was confirmed in a 1993 study. Sixty-two patients with angina were randomly assigned to receive testosterone or a placebo for one month, after which each patient received the alternate treatment for an additional month. Some 77.4% of patients reported an improvement in their angina while receiving testosterone, compared with only 6.5% during placebo treatment.[17] Because of the potential to cause side effects, testosterone should be administered only by a physician experienced in its use.

Estrogen therapy has also been found to relieve angina in some women. In a double-blind study, 25 postmenopausal women with angina but normal coronary arteries were randomly assigned to receive estrogen patches (providing 100 mcg of 17-beta-estradiol per day) or a placebo for 8 weeks, then the alternate treatment for an additional 8 weeks. The number of angina attacks was significantly lower—by 49%—during estrogen treatment, compared with the placebo period.[18]

Conclusion

ALTHOUGH THE NUTRITIONAL treatment of angina has not yet entered the medical mainstream, it is safe, and in many cases it is an extremely effective alternative to conventional drugs and surgical procedures. Cardiovascular disease is the leading cause of death in the United States and is a major contributor to the high cost of medical care. There is good reason to believe that nutritional therapy (combined with chelation therapy in selected cases) could save millions of lives and greatly reduce the cost of health care. Because of the high stakes involved with heart disease, these alternative approaches deserve serious research funding.

Summary of Recommendations for Treating Angina Pectoris

- Diet: Avoid refined sugar, caffeine alcohol. Consume whole foods, emphasizing fruits, vegetables, whole grains, nuts, seeds, legumes. Consume fish and other low-fat animal foods in moderation.

- Magnesium injections in selected cases. Oral magnesium, 300 to 600 mg per day.

- Vitamin E, 400 to 800 IU per day.

- L-carnitine, 500 to 3,000 mg per day.

- Coenzyme Q_{10}, 60 to 300 mg per day.

- Vitamin C, 1,000 to 3,000 mg per day.

- High-potency multiple vitamin/mineral (adjust doses of other nutrients as needed).

- Chelation therapy, in selected cases.

- Testosterone and/or estrogen therapy in selected cases.

- Other recommendations, as discussed in the chapters on atherosclerosis (treatment and prevention), may also be considered.

ANXIETY IS A *problem that affects millions of Americans. In many instances, anxiety is a reaction to life stresses; however, in other cases no apparent emotional cause can be found. Conventional treatment of anxiety consists mainly of a class of drugs called benzodiazepines (Xanax, Valium, and others). While these medications are often helpful, they can cause significant side effects and may also become addictive. A number of nutritional factors are related to anxiety, and this disorder can often be controlled by dietary changes and nutritional supplements.*

DR. WRIGHT'S CASE STUDY

"My nerves are just shot," Victor Hamilton said. "I've always been high-strung, it runs in my family—my mother was even worse. But the last few years I've had so much stress, going through a divorce and financial troubles that won't quit. I've been smoking non-stop—over two packs a day. But even that doesn't seem to steady me enough. My regular doctor says to go on tranquilizers until it's over, but I went that route 20 years ago and damn near got permanently addicted. One addiction—the nicotine—is bad enough. I've been reading about alternative medicine, so I thought I'd try something besides drugs first; even though I know nicotine's a drug, why add another one? There must be some vitamins or herbs or something . . . "

"There might be, but it's best to start with basic diet and exercise and techniques like meditation and biofeedback. Have you done any of those?"

"I've prayed some, but that meditation thing just doesn't work for me. Maybe I just can't sit still for long enough—I've been restless all my life, and besides, I just start worrying harder about my divorce and money and things . . . maybe I'll try again sometime, but this isn't the right time for me."

"Have you counseled with a pastor or a psychologist?"

"Yeah, that's why I'm praying and also why I'm here. My pastor is Reverend Saunders—he sent me here and says 'hello'. He thinks I could get some help with vitamins and herbs and things, too."

"Give my regards to Reverend Saunders."

"I will."

Please tell me a little more about your family's health history."

"Like I said, my mother's even more high-strung than me."

"She's how old?"

"Sixty-seven. She's got a touch of high blood pressure, and that older-age diabetes. Its not bad—no insulin, just diet and pills. Her mother had that, too. Her husband—my grandfather—

was alcoholic and died young in a car wreck. My older sister she's 45, she's real nervous, too."

"Your father?"

"Don't know much about him. Mom and he divorced when I was three. I haven't stayed in touch. He smoked a lot, I hear."

"His parents?"

"Don't really know."

"Do you have children?"

"Two, their health is OK."

"Tell me what you're eating every day."

"Well, in the morning I have two or three cups of coffee and sometimes a doughnut or muffin. Lots of times I skip lunch or just pick something up like a hamburger. Since I started going through this divorce, I've been eating dinner out a lot—usually steak and potatoes and a salad. If I eat at home—it's a little apartment, now—can't afford a house any more—I get pizza or Chinese take-out or KFC chicken with coleslaw. Later in the evening I have popcorn or chips."

"I definitely want you to talk with our clinic's nutritionist. Even though you don't cook and you eat out a lot, she can help you put together a healthful diet that's easy to do. Definitely more vegetables—don't worry, there are many that need little or no cooking, and fruits, nuts, seeds are good when you're eating out; you can still do fairly well from restaurant menus if you know which selections to make. I'll leave the details to her."

"OK, that's what I'm here for. Reverend Saunders made me promise to give it all a good try."

"How many cups of coffee do you drink every day? And do you put sugar in it, or eat very much sugar otherwise?"

"I get some fierce sugar cravings sometimes, and I eat candy bars and drink quite a bit of pop. I put two spoons of sugar in my coffee, and right now I'm drinking a pot or two a day."

"Have you ever heard of 'caffeinism'"?

"Can't say I have, but from the sound of it, I'm in for some real headaches?"

"Why is that?"

"Every time I try to quit drinking coffee and cola drinks I get headaches for three or four days. When you said 'caffeinism' I figured that's what was coming."

"For some of us, caffeine can be a 'hidden' source of anxiety. I've noticed that caffeine-induced anxiety—caffeinism—occurs more often in individuals from families with blood-sugar problems. And speaking of families with blood-sugar problems—it'll likely reduce your anxiety if you stop all the refined sugar intake, too."

"I don't know. I'm getting anxious just thinking about stopping caffeine and sugar all at once!"

"I know it's tough, but do it if you can. Some of the vitamins will help you through the withdrawal symptoms. You're very likely to have less anxiety afterwards."

"I'll give it my best try. Now what about those vitamins and herbs?"

"First, niacinamide. It's ironic, but in 1979, shortly after the original patent for Valium expired, research scientists for Hoffmann-LaRoche, the company that made Valium, published an article entitled *'Nicotinamide is a brain constituent with benzodiazepine-like actions.'* That means niacinamide—nicotinamide is the British version of the name—acts like Valium and Valium-category drugs in the brain."

"Valium is the stuff I damn near got addicted to. Could I get hooked on niacinamide?"

"No. Niacinamide is one form of vitamin B_3. Without it for long enough, we'd literally drop dead. Most people say it helps them feel clearer mentally, instead of dulled as Valium and other patent-drug tranquilizers often do."

"You're pretty sure it'll help?"

"Niacinamide at the right quantity is likely to help any of us with anxiety, but it's especially helpful against anxiety—and to some degree, depression—for individuals from families with blood-sugar problems. Please take 1,000 milligrams three times daily. Make sure it's niacinamide, not niacin—that much niacin would likely give you a terrific 'flush'. It's usually very well tolerated, but there's a very small chance it could cause queasiness or nausea. If it does, it's too much."

"Then what?"

"Just stop, call, and we'll adjust the quantity downward. But remember, adverse effects are very unusual. Next, a high-potency B-complex. B-complex vitamins help settle anxiety on their own, especially if we haven't been eating as well as we might, but in this case, they're also important to 'back up' the extra amount of niacinamide."

"Next, calcium and magnesium. Both of these minerals can 'settle the nerves' for many of us. Magnesium is found particularly in green vegetables, and you haven't been doing very well in that category . . . please take 1,000 milligrams of calcium and 500 milligrams of magnesium at bedtime each night. Look for calcium in the citrate or lactate form, and magnesium as aspartate, citrate, or glycinate. These forms absorb a bit better."

"Gee, that's a lot of stuff to take. One thing about drugs, you just have to take one little pill two or three times a day. Aren't all those things going to add up or fight with each other and cause me trouble?"

"Not at all. That's actually likely to happen with drugs—the longer the list, the more likely there are to be drug interactions and progressively more serious adverse effects. But remember, there are literally dozens of nutrients in even the simplest of foods, and they all work positively together to nourish our bodies. In fact, nutrients always work together with others, some more closely—like individual B-vitamins with the rest of the B-complex vitamins, and some more 'at a distance.' The group of nutrients I've recommended to you so far will all work together to settle your anxiety."

"So far? You mean there's more?"

"You mentioned herbs, didn't you? A Polynesian botanical—kava—has an extremely long history of use for many things, including 'nerves'. It's recently become available in natural-food stores. Please use 100 milligrams, three times daily."

"What else?"

"A famous Chinese botanical—*Panax ginseng*—has traditionally been used to combat stress. And recent scientific studies have shown it can help improve mood, attitude, and mental performance for those under stress. There are other useful herbs, too—ashwaganda, valerian, and Siberian ginseng come to mind—but let's just start with kava and *Panax ginseng* for now. 100 mg, three times daily."

"I can definitely use some of that *Panax ginseng*. I've got plenty of stress, and I could use it to improve my performance in all areas." He got up to go.

"One more thing. If we're using individual nutrient supplements, it's wisest to also use a high-quality, comprehensive multiple vitamin-mineral. Please check with your natural food store—they have several."

"Let's see—niacinamide, B-complex, calcium, magnesium, kava, *Panax ginseng*, a multiple vitamin-mineral."

"Changing your diet and cutting out caffeine and sugar."

"I hope I can do all this."

"I'm sure you can. Make sure to stay in touch with Reverend Saunders, and keep up with those prayers you've started."

Mr. Hamilton later reported that with a few setbacks, he'd been able to implement the entire program within two to three months, and his anxiety was "unbelievably less." He had decided to make his diet changes and supplements permanent, since "I feel better all over, as well as being less anxious!"

DR. GABY'S COMMENTARY

As victor learned, diet can contribute to anxiety. Sometimes, simply eliminating certain foods from the diet can decrease anxiety. If anxiety is still high after such changes, nutritional supplements may offer some relief.

Dietary Considerations

Hypoglycemia

Reactive hypoglycemia appears to be a common trigger for anxiety.[1, 2] When the blood-sugar level falls, the body compensates by releasing adrenaline. Although adrenaline does help restore the blood-sugar level toward normal, it also induces the so-called "fight or flight" reaction, which can manifest as anxiety, heart palpitations, sweating, hunger, and irritability. Individuals who experience these symptoms (particularly during the late morning or late afternoon, when the blood-sugar level tends to fall), will often improve after eliminating refined sugar, caffeine, and alcohol from their diet and supplementing with blood-sugar-regulating nutrients, such as chromium, B-vitamins, and magnesium.

A psychologist colleague told me of a man he once treated for agoraphobia (fear of being in large, open spaces). During the course of psychotherapy, he learned that the man's fear attacks occurred only on Wednesday evenings, the night that he habitually went out to dinner with his wife. It also turned out that dinner at home was always served at 6:00 P.M., whereas on Wednesdays, the meal was not served until around 8:00 P.M. Suspecting hypoglycemia-induced anxiety attacks, the astute psychologist advised the patient to eat a small snack at around 6:00 P.M. on the nights that he ate out. This simple advice resulted in a prompt cure of what had previously been considered to be an emotional problem.

Effects of Caffeine

In addition to interfering with blood-sugar metabolism, caffeine can also be a direct cause of anxiety. While it is well known that an overdose of caffeine will trigger anxiety, it is not well appreciated that even "normal" amounts of caffeine may cause problems for some people. This difference in sensitivity is probably related to the fact that some people metabolize caffeine more slowly than others. For example, while the half-life of caffeine for most people is 3 to 6 hours, it can vary among healthy individuals by as much as 5-fold.[3] In a slow metabolizer, the effect of caffeine may be amplified considerably. Indeed, one study has shown that patients with anxiety disorders are more susceptible to the effects of caffeine than are healthy individuals.[4] In another study, patients suffering from panic attacks were also found to be unusually sensitive to caffeine.[5]

Role of Food Allergies

Allergic reactions to foods can also cause anxiety.[6] The possibility of food-induced anxiety should be considered when symptoms develop after eating, or if the anxiety is associated with other allergic manifestations (such as gastrointestinal symptoms, migraines, joint pains, or nasal congestion). Allergic anxiety typically resolves when the offending foods are removed from the diet.

Nutritional Supplements

Animal studies have shown that niacinamide (vitamin B$_3$) has actions that resemble those of the benzodiazepine drugs (such as Valium, Xanax, and Ativan), which are used to treat anxiety.[7] Although there are no controlled studies in humans, our observation is that niacinamide supplements often have a calming effect. It should be noted, however, that large doses of niacinamide (more than 1,000 mg per day) can occasionally stress or even damage the liver. It should therefore be taken only under medical supervision.

Anxiety can also be caused by a magnesium deficiency, which appears to be an extremely common problem among Americans.[8] Magnesium has a mild sedative effect[9] and, along with calcium, seems to be useful in the treatment of anxiety.

In our experience, vitamin B_{12} injections are also effective for some patients with unexplained anxiety. Although no one knows how vitamin B_{12} works, a double-blind study has confirmed that injections of this vitamin can increase happiness and feelings of well-being.[10]

Herbal Supplements

PANAX GINSENG (also known as Korean or Chinese ginseng) has been shown in animal studies[11] to reduce anxiety, and it is also used to increase tolerance to stress. Although ginseng is usually well tolerated, it has a mild estrogenic effect and can occasionally cause breast pain or a return of vaginal bleeding in postmenopausal women. Excessive doses of ginseng may also cause high blood pressure.

Kava (*Piper methysticum*) has also been shown to relieve anxiety. In a double-blind study, 58 patients received either kava extract (100 mg, three times per day) or a placebo for 4 weeks. There was a significant reduction in anxiety in the group receiving kava.[12] Although kava was well tolerated by participants in this study, there is one case report of a toxic reaction to kava in a patient who was also taking a prescription anti-anxiety drug, as well as several other medications.[13]

Summary of Recommendations for Treating Anxiety

- Diet: Avoid refined sugar, caffeine, and alcohol. In cases of "reactive hypoglycemia," eat small, frequent meals. Work with food allergies in selected cases.

- Niacinamide, 500 to 1,000 mg, 2 to 3 times per day. Doses greater than 1,000 mg per day should be supervised by a physician, with periodic monitoring of liver-function tests.

- High-potency B-complex vitamin.

- Calcium, 600 to 1,200 mg per day; magnesium, 300 to 600 mg per day.

- High-potency multiple vitamin/mineral (adjust doses of other nutrients as needed).

- Kava and/or *Panax ginseng* in selected cases.

ASTHMA

🌿 MOST OF US *take breathing for granted. But for the 10 million or more Americans with asthma, taking a breath of air is often a major effort and, at times, a desperate struggle. During the past 15 years, the number of asthmatics has increased sharply and the death rate from asthma has nearly doubled in the United States. Worsening air pollution probably contributes to these troubling statistics, although other unidentified factors may also be involved.*

Conventional medications are often helpful for treating acute asthma attacks and for preventing recurrences. However, despite the best that modern medicine has to offer, many patients continue to experience acute attacks and/or chronic, low-level breathing difficulties. Moreover, most of the medications used to treat asthma can cause side effects. New ideas are needed, if we are to win the battle against asthma.

DR. WRIGHT'S CASE STUDY: CHILDHOOD ASTHMA

"We're here to finish off Bobby's asthma," Rebecca Cutler declared. "He's lots better already, but we can't do it all ourselves. We've done everything you told the Pizzolis to do for their son, Vincent, and it's working! We're all members of the same church, Bobby and Vincent are classmates, and when Vincent's asthma disappeared in three months we couldn't believe it. So we decided to try . . . "

"And Bobby's asthma is more than half-way gone," his father, David, added. "I think we just need that injectable B_{12}, some allergy work, that test for his stomach, and maybe we can get it gone completely. At least we hope so. Bobby's had a tough time—we've had to rush him to the emergency room five times in just the last two years. Since we started as much of Vincent's program as we could, he's off the theophylline. That stuff made him 'hyper' all the time and made his heart race. He still needs to use his inhaler fairly often, but his wheezing is a lot less when it happens, and it goes away easier. And he's sleeping better at night, not waking up near as much."

I turned to Bobby. "What have Mom and Dad had you doing about your asthma lately, Bobby?"

"I can't have anymore milk or cheese or ice cream, and I hafta take a bunch of vitamins and stuff." He looked worried. "Do I hafta take shots every day like Vincent?"

"Is your asthma better since you stopped drinking milk and started taking your vitamins like Vincent?"

"Yeah."

"Then it's possible that shots might help you like Vincent, too, isn't it?"

Bobby looked dubious. "I guess."

"I can't tell you for sure they'll work, Bobby, but it sounds likely." I turned back to his parents. His mother handed me a list.

"Here's a summary of what we're doing so far," she said. "Bobby's seven, the same as Vincent, so we just gave him the same; as much as we could."

I read from the list. "Let's see. No milk or dairy products of any kind. All other foods, each one eaten only every four days or less."

"We did it that way 'cause we have no idea exactly what foods Bobby's allergic to yet," Rebecca said. "But Monica, Vincent's mother, told me you said no cow's milk or dairy under any circumstances. And you asked her to 'rotate' Vincent's less-allergic foods every four days. So we made everything every four days until we had him tested."

"Makes sense." I resumed reading the list. "Vitamin B_{12}, 1,000 micrograms, 3 times a day; magnesium, 125 milligrams, 3 times daily; vitamin B_6, 50 milligrams, 3 times daily."

"The Pizzolis said vitamin B_{12} should be injected, but since it's harmless, we thought we'd try having Bobby swallow it anyway until we could see you. They also said that building up tissue magnesium levels reduces the tendency to muscle spasm, including bronchial muscle," David remarked.

"Exactly. Let's see, vitamin C, 1,000 milligrams, 3 times daily; one tablespoon of cod-liver oil daily; and a high-potency multiple vitamin-mineral, one-third the adult quantity, in 3 divided doses. Everything in capsules, not tablets . . ."

"That's because most asthmatic children have poor digestion, and capsules usually digest better than some tablets, right?" Rebecca asked.

"Right on both, though it's not 100% on either."

"Also, we threw every bit of sugar, refined carbohydrate, hydrogenated vegetable oil, and food chemicals out of the house," Rebecca said. "Monica told me you recommend doing that no

matter what the problem is, and also just for staying as healthy as possible."

"Absolutely!" I replied. "None of those items have any place in healthful diets."

"Takes some getting used to, but since we did, I've felt less tired," David observed.

"Let's check Bobby over, and then have lab tests done, with your permission, of course," I said.

"That's what we brought Bobby here for," David replied. "Monica said that food allergies are more important than inhalant allergies in childhood asthma, and you'll check both. But I didn't understand what testing his stomach has to do with asthma. Could you explain?"

"Sure. In a 1931 publication, Dr. George Bray, an asthma specialist, noted that 80% of 200 asthmatic children had underproduction of acid and (presumably) pepsin in the stomach. This, of course, impairs digestion, lowering nutrient absorption, and gradually increasing allergies to foods. In 1979, other researchers published proof that food allergy, particularly to cow's milk, can cause the stomach problem in the first place."

"So it's sort of circular—food allergy causes the stomach to malfunction, which leads to more food allergy and worsening asthma."

"For approximately 80% of asthmatic children."

"And what's the reason for injecting vitamin B_{12} instead of just swallowing it?"

"In the late 1940s and early 1950s, extra vitamin B_{12} by injection was found to be very helpful in many cases of childhood asthma. I'm not sure how it helps eliminate asthmatic wheezing, but fortunately it's quite harmless. Some parents who've read articles I've written about B_{12} and asthma have tried having their children swallow it. Sometimes it helps, but often the injections are much more effective."

"How often does all of this work?"

"I can only give you approximations, but of those following this regimen about 50% eliminate their wheezing, about 30% have major improvement, about 10% see only minor improvement, and about 10% have no change."

"And I've read the death rate from asthma has been climbing the last few years," Rebecca remarked. "We want to do all we can to get Bobby healthy."

Six months later, Bobby's wheezing was gone. Although I recommended lifetime exclusion of cow's milk and dairy products, the large majority of his food and inhalant allergies had been desensitized, and his mother had liberalized his diet, while keeping all the "junk" out. His was taking capsules of hydrochloric acid and pepsin to aid his digestion, and his vitamin B_{12} injections were down to a maintenance level of one or two a month. He continued his other oral supplements. Several years later, he remains free of asthma.

CASE STUDY: SULFITE-SENSITIVE ADULT ASTHMA

Ted Koskovich was back to hear about his test results. "I been getting that allergy desensitization," he announced, "and it helps. Never thought I was allergic to so much stuff. No wonder I couldn't breathe so good. Taking those vitamins, too—B_6, magnesium, and so on. Find anything else?"

"One thing that could be very significant. You have 20 to 30 parts per million sulfite in your urine specimen."

"Sulfur in my urine? What's that mean?"

"Sulfite. It's a partially metabolized form of sulfur, and can cause spasm in the bronchial tubes—asthma."

"Where'd I get sulfite?"

"Normal metabolism generates sulfite, but usually it's turned into sulfate almost immediately. Sulfate doesn't cause bronchial trouble."

"How do I make sulfate outa sulfite?"

"With the trace element molybdenum.

Molybdenum stimulates an enzyme called sulfite oxidase that turns sulfite into sulfate."

"Molybdenum? Never heard of it. So do I take some?"

"Over the years, we've observed that swallowing molybdenum doesn't work nearly as well as injecting it." I wrote a recommendation. "Please have molybdenum injections, one twice a week for a month, 500 micrograms each time. To help the molybdenum work, we put in vitamin B_6, magnesium, and vitamin B_{12}, but molybdenum is the key element."

"You sure I hafta do shots? I'm already doing the B_6 and magnesium."

"You certainly can try capsules, but it usually doesn't work as fast or as well."

"Is there a better chance the asthma will be gone if I take the shots, too?"

"With your sulfite test high, yes."

"Anything else?"

"Sulfite is produced internally, but it's used as a food preservative, too. It's used in some less-expensive wines, and used by many salad bars to keep unsold food from turning brown. Read labels, and ask in restaurants."

Mr. Koskovich nodded knowingly. "I knew them wines was trouble. Every once in a while I'd get a really bad wheeze on after a toot. Stopped when I switched to that preservative-free beer."

After his series of molybdenum injections, Mr. Koskovich's wheezing was gone. He then started on 1 milligram of molybdenum by mouth, twice daily, while continuing allergy desensitization and his other supplements. However, 11 months later, his wheezing started to return. A retest of his urine at that time showed that sulfite levels were again elevated. We gave him another series of molybdenum injections, and his wheezing cleared again. Mr. Koskovich was simultaneously pleased and disgruntled.

"Glad my asthma's gone again, but do I hafta take shots every so often for the rest of my life?"

"You can take more molybdenum capsules. That might do the job, but we'll need to monitor your red-cell copper levels from time to time. Molybdenum can sometimes cause a deficiency of copper."

"So I'll just take copper, right?"

"If your levels go low. Eat a lot of unroasted nuts. They're high in copper. Liver's the best source of copper, but eat liver only from organically-raised animals, because pesticides and other agriculture chemicals can accumulate in the liver."

"How 'bout high molybdenum foods?"

"The way your sulfite tests have been, food won't do it. You'll need supplements, but as long as you take them and watch your copper

levels, your wheezing should be controlled."

It's been 4 years now, and Mr. Koskovich's wheezing hasn't returned.

Mr. Koskovich had an unusual form of asthma. Reacting to "environmental" sulfite (usually from food-preservative use) isn't unusual, but finding high levels of internally-produced sulfite is. However, testing the urine for sulfite is very inexpensive and may lead to a successful treatment approach, particularly in difficult cases of asthma. When excess sulfite is found, it's a definite guide to treatment, usually with a favorable outcome.

DR. GABY'S COMMENTARY

FOR BOTH CHILDREN and adults, asthma can often be controlled by avoiding allergenic foods and chemicals and taking nutritional supplements. In rare cases, patients also need to be treated for a defect in their ability to detoxify sulfites. Individuals who respond to a nutritional approach may be able to discontinue or greatly reduce their medications.

Dietary Considerations
Role of Food Allergy

UNRECOGNIZED food allergy is a contributing factor in at least 75% of childhood asthmatics and about 40% of adult asthmatics. As early as 1959, Albert H. Rowe, M.D., a pioneer in the field of food allergy, successfully treated 95 asthmatic patients with dietary changes alone.[1] Most of the patients who responded were unaware that they had food allergies. However, when they went on an elimination diet, symptoms typically disappeared or improved within 1 to 4 weeks. Eliminated foods were then added back one at a time, and the ones that provoked asthma were kept out of the diet. Nearly 20 years later, another study con-

firmed Rowe's observations. In that study of 198 children with allergic rhinitis and/or bronchial asthma, 90% experienced a significant improvement using the elimination-and-retesting approach.[2]

Foods most likely to provoke asthma include dairy products, eggs, chocolate, wheat, corn, citrus fruits (orange, grapefruit, lemon, and lime), and fish. In addition, tartrazine (Yellow Dye #5), a common food additive, is thought to trigger asthma in as many as 100,000 Americans. Ironically, before this association was discovered, some popular anti-asthma medications had been colored with tartrazine. Although this chemical is no longer used in asthma drugs, it is still added to many other prescription medications and processed foods.

Sulfites are another class of chemicals that can trigger asthma in susceptible individuals. Sulfites are found in many wines and other alcoholic beverages and are often used as a preservative at restaurant salad bars. Sulfites may also be present in a wide range of other foods, particularly processed foods. If someone is extremely sensitive to sulfites, avoiding them completely requires a good deal of detective work. Your doctor can help you determine whether you are sensitive to sulfites.

Allergy Testing

It should be noted that skin tests are notoriously unreliable for diagnosing food allergies. Skin testing frequently "detects" food allergies that do not really exist, while failing to identify the ones that are clinically significant. The unreliability of skin tests may explain in part why conventional allergists do not believe food allergy has much to do with asthma. On the other hand, conventional allergy testing is quite helpful for diagnosing allergies to inhalants such as molds, dust, pollen, and trees. When such allergies are found, environmental control and desensitization treatments are often helpful for asthmatics.

A more reliable method of identifying food allergies is to eliminate all of the common food allergens (and additives) simultaneously, then retest them one at a time (foods that are already known to trigger reactions should not be tested). Asthmatics who wish to try an elimination diet, particularly those who have had severe asthma attacks, must be supervised by a doctor. As explained in chapter 3, during an elimination diet the body becomes more sensitive than usual, and reactions to individual food challenges can be particularly severe. Although life-threatening reactions are rare, they have been known to occur in asthmatics who undergo an elimination-and-challenge procedure.

One of the elimination diets I have used in my practice is presented in appendix A. Some doctors use other tests for allergy and sensitivity, as well as desensitization techniques. The reliability and effectiveness of some of these methods is controversial (see chapter 3 for additional discussion).

Nutritional Supplements
Vitamin B$_6$

In addition to avoiding allergenic foods and chemicals, taking nutritional supplements such as vitamin B$_6$ can be helpful in treating asthma. In laboratory studies of 21 asthmatic children, 17 showed evidence of vitamin B$_6$ deficiency.[3] While asthma is itself associated with low vitamin B$_6$ levels, the deficiency may be aggravated by anti-asthma drugs. For example, theophylline and aminophylline have both been shown to reduce blood levels of vitamin B$_6$.[4]

In a double-blind study, 76 children with moderate or severe asthma received vitamin B$_6$ (200 mg per day) or a placebo for 5 months. Compared with children given the placebo, those receiving vitamin B$_6$ had significantly fewer symptoms and attacks and required significantly less cortisone. Children who improved, generally saw results by the second month of treatment.[5] In another study, 7 adult asthmatics experienced a dramatic decrease in the frequency and severity of asthma attacks while taking 50 mg of vitamin B$_6$, twice a day.[6]

Magnesium

Asthma is frequently associated with magnesium deficiency. In one study, serum magnesium levels were below normal in half of 26 asthmatics during an acute attack.[7] As with vitamin B$_6$, some of the drugs used to treat asthma could make magnesium deficiency even more pronounced.[8, 9] Since magnesium promotes relaxation of bronchial muscles, a deficiency of this mineral increases the likelihood that the bronchi will go into spasm and cause an asthma attack. Magnesium deficiency can also increase the release of histamine into the bloodstream, thereby increasing allergic reactivity in general.[10] For both of these reasons, asthmatics should make sure to obtain an adequate supply of magnesium.

Recent studies have confirmed what nutrition-oriented doctors have been saying for a long time: giving magnesium intravenously during an acute asthma attack can relieve symptoms rapidly and often eliminate the need for hospitalization.[11, 12] I have treated dozens of cases of acute asthma in my office, using an intravenous "cocktail" of nutrients that contained magnesium, calcium, vitamin C, and B-vitamins. In most cases, the asthma improved markedly or subsided completely within a few minutes, saving the patient a trip to the emergency room. In my experience, this treatment is not only a lot safer than the usual adrenaline/bronchodilator regimens, it also works faster and is often more effective. For details on this treatment, please see appendix B.

Vitamin B12

SEVERAL reports from the 1950s suggested that vitamin B12 injections could relieve the symptoms of asthma. These studies were reviewed by Dr. Wright, in a 1990 article in which he also described his own experiences with vitamin B12.[13] Although it is not known exactly how vitamin B12 relieves asthma, one of its effects is to detoxify sulfites through a direct chemical interaction with these compounds (see below).[14] However, vitamin B12 probably also acts in some other way against asthma, since Dr. Wright has found this vitamin to be helpful in asthmatics (especially childhood asthmatics) who test negative for sulfites.

Using Molybdenum and B12 to Detoxify Sulfites

THE body is constantly exposed to sulfites, even if care is taken to avoid all dietary sources of these chemicals. That is because sulfites are produced in the body during the normal metabolism of certain amino acids. It is conceivable that some asthmatics have a defect in the enzyme (sulfite oxidase) that is responsible for disposing of sulfites. In such cases, supplementing with vitamin B12 would presumably allow the body to bypass the biochemical block, although large doses of the vitamin might be necessary. In addition to vitamin B12, the trace mineral molybdenum also plays a role in detoxifying sulfites.[15]

The presence of sulfites in the body can be identified by a simple urine dipstick test. If the urine contains sulfites (it is not supposed to contain any), then taking vitamin B12 and/or molybdenum might help to get rid of them, thereby relieving the asthma. In some cases, taking these supplements orally is effective; however, in more severe cases, injections may be necessary.

Taking large amounts of molybdenum can result in a deficiency of copper. If you are taking molybdenum as a separate supplement, it is probably wise to take 2 to 3 mg of copper at a different time of the day.

Other Nutritional Treatments

VITAMIN C HAS been shown in test-tube studies to destroy histamine and to inhibit the enzyme phosphodiesterase[16] (the same action as that of certain anti-asthma drugs). If vitamin C functions the same way in the human body, then it would be expected to be helpful for asthmatics. In one study, 41 asthmatics received either 1 gram of vitamin C per day or a placebo for 14 weeks. Compared with individuals taking the placebo, those receiving vitamin C had 73% fewer asthma attacks; and the attacks that did occur tended to be less severe in the vitamin C group.[17] However, in other studies, vitamin C was not effective against asthma.

Fish oil may also be helpful for asthmatics, possibly by reducing inflammation in lung tissue.[18] In a double-blind study, 12 asthmatics received either fish oil (approximately 3 grams per day) or a placebo for 1 year. A measure of lung function (FEV$_1$) improved by 23% in the fish-oil group, but was unchanged in the placebo group.[19] This improvement was not seen until the ninth month of treatment. A few other studies failed to show a beneficial effect of fish oil; however, these negative results may have been due to the shorter duration of the studies.

Some individuals with asthma have a deficiency of stomach-acid production (hypochlorhydria). In those cases, taking hydrochloric-acid supplements with meals may relieve the asthma.[20] Because of the potential for adverse effects, treatment with hydrochloric acid should be supervised by a nutritionally oriented physician.

Conclusion

A LOT CAN be done for asthmatics besides taking prescription drugs. If health-care practitioners gave more attention to the nutritional approach, we might see a reversal in the recent alarming rise in asthma mortality. However, it is important to remember that asthma is a serious condition and that any nutritional program should be properly supervised by a medical practitioner.

Summary of Recommendations for Treating Asthma

PRIMARY RECOMMENDATIONS:
(NOTE: Dosages are for adults. For children, doses are lower and should be monitored by a doctor.)

- Diet: Work with food allergies.

- Magnesium, 300 to 600 mg per day.

- Vitamin B_6, 50 to 200 mg per day.

- Vitamin C, 500 to 1,000 mg, 2 to 3 times per day.

- Vitamin B_{12} by injection in selected cases, particularly for children.

OTHER RECOMMENDATIONS:

- Cod-liver oil, 1 to 2 teaspoons per day, or fish-oil concentrate, 3 to 6 grams per day. (Larger amounts may be needed in some cases. However, because of their vitamin A and D content, doses of cod-liver oil greater than 1 tablespoon per day should be supervised by a doctor.)

- Molybdenum, orally or intravenously, in selected cases (dosage as recommended by a doctor). With long-term use of molybdenum, balance with copper supplements.

- Identify and avoid/desensitize inhalant allergies (particularly for adults).

ATHEROSCLEROSIS *(prevention)*

THE TERM "ATHEROSCLEROSIS," *is derived from two Greek words that mean "gruel" ("porridge") and "hardening." As a disease, atherosclerosis refers to the buildup of yellowish plaques in the walls of arteries. Atherosclerotic plaques consist of cholesterol, fatty material, calcium, and other substances. When it becomes extensive, atherosclerosis restricts the flow of blood to the tissues and organs of the body, and it can potentially result in a heart attack, stroke, gangrene of the extremities, or other serious problems. In the following chapter we discuss ways of treating the disease once it is established. This chapter will focus on ways of preventing the disease from developing.*

DR. WRIGHT'S CASE STUDY

"My father had his first heart attack at 48," Mack MacArthur said. "His father died of a heart attack at age 60, and his brother—my great-uncle—at 63. My grandfather on the other side had his right leg amputated because of diabetes and poor circulation. Both of his sons—my mother's brothers, started having angina in their 40s, and are taking heart medication right now. Even my mother—she's 53 now—has circulation problems in her legs. So when I turned 30, I decided to try to prevent all of this. Of course, I had a little push from Cindy here. We've been married three years now, and as you can see our first is on the way. I promised Cindy to come in before he or she is born."

"When's baby due?"

"Six more weeks," Cindy answered.

"Congratulations. You're right, it's definitely time for Dad to get started on his health."

"I already had my cholesterol and triglycerides measured," Mack said. "I made sure they measured the HDL cholesterol, the good one, too. I'm told I'm a little off on cholesterol and triglycerides both." He handed me the report.

"Thank you. Before we get to specific tests, I have a few other questions, and some other basics to cover."

"OK, I'm ready."

"Thanks for the family history; I understand why you're so concerned. Is there any diabetes on either side of your family, particularly your mother's?"

"Sure . . . grandpa . . . the one who had the amputation . . . his wife, mother's mother, had 'a touch of diabetes' when she was 70 or so. And Mom's doctor told her she's at extra risk because her babies were over 9 pounds. As far as we know, there's no diabetes on Dad's side of the family."

"Do you get regular exercise?"

"I sure do, I'm a carpenter, I work construction. But then so was Dad, it didn't seem to help him, anyway."

"We do a lot of hiking," Cindy said. "Except lately, of course. But once the baby's born, we'll just add to the backpacks and start hiking again."

"Good. Please tell me what you're eating these days."

"These days is right. When Cindy and I first met, I was doing your typical single-guy stuff, burgers, fries, shakes, ribs, chips, ice cream . . . you know the routine. Cindy told me with my family history, I'd set the record for the quickest heart attack."

"But he's changed," Cindy said. "It's taken awhile, but Mack's really trying. We have oatmeal and orange juice and usually coffee for breakfast, mostly; on weekends we have eggs, but I'm cutting those back. We use margarine instead of butter when we have toast . . . and we've switched to entirely whole grains. I send two sandwiches and two thermoses with Mack for lunch—one with milk, one with coffee. I also put in a couple of apples or oranges. At dinner we have mostly chicken, turkey, fish sometimes, potatoes, and lots of vegetables—broccoli, spinach, carrots, lettuce, tomatoes, brussels sprouts. We've cut back on sugary desserts and have mostly fruit or ice cream."

"How about snacks?"

"Since I got pregnant, we've gone to the natural-food store more. We get yogurt, ice cream bars, 'energy' bars, and we have those along with fruit."

"Do you do any frying or other cooking with oils?"

"Sometimes. I use safflower oil."

I finished taking notes and turned to Mack. "Do you buy doughnuts, cookies, croissants, or other bakery items when you're on the job?"

"Yeah, I gotta 'fess up. All of the above . . . but not near as much as before I met Cindy. I really am cutting back."

"He is, too. He's actually lost a few pounds since we got married."

"Good. Let's see. Where does your water come from?"

Mack and Cindy looked at each other. "The faucet," Cindy said.

"No filter on the line?"

"No."

"Let's start with that. To prevent infections, most water districts add chlorine to the water supply, even though safer methods such as ozonation have been in use since the 1920s. Animal research suggests that chlorination is damaging to arteries, and there's suggestive evidence for people, too. There's definite research showing that water chlorination raises cancer risk, so it's generally wisest to avoid it. Fortunately, there are relatively inexpensive filters available in most hardware stores and elsewhere that remove almost all the chlorine. Unfortunately, the fluoride isn't removed. . . . "

"I thought that was good for our teeth."

"It may be, but it's bad for the rest of our bodies. Fluoride is much more hazard than help; the sooner we can get it out of our water, the better."

"What about bottled water?"

"If you can get a certificate of analysis from the company. Not all bottled waters are the best quality. Speaking of that . . . I'm glad you're visiting natural-food stores more. They have a greater percentage of healthful food than regular supermarkets, but it's not all good for us. Let me see . . . you mentioned yogurt, ice cream, and 'energy bars'. It's true that natural-food-store versions are safer . . . usually less chemicals, but cow's milk products of any sort aren't such a good idea. Decades ago, a Dr. Kurt Oster demonstrated that homogenized milk is particularly hazardous to our arteries. . . . "

"That's what I drink at lunch every day," Mack broke in.

" . . . and cow's milk products are best limited to calves for many other reasons. Look for yogurt made from soy; there are two or three very tasty brands. Ice cream can be replaced with rice or soy based products—some of those are so good children will eat any amount available.

"Also, please make sure to read the labels on those 'energy bars', as well as on any other packaged foods. Some 'energy bars' are quite good, but others contain refined sugar and partially hydrogenated vegetable oils. Those should both be eliminated entirely."

"Because of the diabetes in Mack's family?"

"Yes, especially the refined sugar, although actually it's bad for any of us in varying degrees. In families with diabetes, sugar and refined carbohydrates contribute to an over-active insulin response, called 'hyperinsulinism', which can contribute to artery damage. And those partially hydrogenated vegetable oils are likely worse for us than saturated fats."

I turned to Mack. "Doughnuts, cookies, croissants, and other bakery products are usually sources of a lot of partially hydrogenated vegetable oil. Phase those out completely, and only buy whole-grain bakery products without them."

"You're both doing well cutting down saturated fat, but eggs should be an exception. Eggs contain cholesterol, but they contain four to five times as much phospholipid, which more than offsets the cholesterol. Phospholipids are vital components of brain-cell membranes. The only other source of phospholipid in our entire food supply is soy lecithin. Most of us don't eat much of that. Lastly, research shows that only about one in five of us has our cholesterol numbers elevated by eating eggs."

Mack looked worried. "How about me?"

"Since your cholesterol and triglycerides are both a little high, and you have diabetes in your family, it's much more likely that sugar and refined carbohydrates are behind that problem.

"Excuse me a second. . . . " I checked my notes again. "We've gone over exercise, chlorine in the water, cow's milk, sugar and refined carbohydrates, partially hydrogenated vegetable oils, eggs . . . remember, more of those . . . oh yes, before we get to lab tests and supplements, I almost forgot: margarine, and safflower oil for cooking. Margarine's usually a significant source of partially hydrogenated oils, and far worse than butter. Olive oil is far and away best for frying or other cooking purposes. Heat oxidizes other oils much more than olive oil . . . and it's actually 'oxidized' oils, fats, and especially oxidized cholesterol that cause the worst arterial problems.

"Now, about lab tests. You've already checked your cholesterol and triglycerides . . . please have a hair mineral analysis done. Several mineral deficiencies contribute to atherosclerosis. Lastly, with the strong history of atherosclerosis in your family, please have your serum homocysteine checked."

"Serum homo-what?"

"Homocysteine. Researchers have found that as many as 33% of men with very early atherosclerosis—like your father and uncles—have a genetic problem leading to excess homocysteine in the bloodstream. Excess homocysteine is quite damaging to arteries, among other things. But homocysteine levels can be brought down to normal with supplemental vitamin B_6, folic acid, and vitamin B_{12}."

"Should I get those?"

"Among other items. I'll make a list . . . vitamin C, 1000 milligrams twice daily, vitamin E, 400 IU daily, flaxseed oil capsules, two of the 1,000 milligram size twice daily. . . ."

"I've heard about vitamin E helping prevent heart attacks, but flaxseed oil?" Cindy asked.

"It's an excellent source of both omega-3 and omega-6 fatty acids. It will help keep platelets in the bloodstream more 'slippery', and less likely to form clots. Omega-3 oils have been found to lessen the risk of heart attack. Then you'll need magnesium, chromium, copper, zinc, and selenium. . . . "

"I'll have dozens of bottles of vitamin pills!" Mack exclaimed.

"Not really. Unless your tests show particularly bad deficiencies, only vitamins C and E and flaxseed oil are separate. All the others—B_6, folic acid, B_{12}, all the minerals . . . can be found in several different high-potency multiple vitamin-mineral formulas. I'll write the name of one of them. . . . "

"Four supplement bottles. That's not so bad, Mack," Cindy said.

"I guess not. But I don't know about giving up those doughnuts . . . just kidding, but we still have a lot of diet changes to make."

"And baby here will have a healthy daddy," Cindy replied. "Let's go do it!"

DR. GABY'S COMMENTARY

TAKING STEPS TO reduce the risk of artherosclerosis is especially important for people with a history of heart trouble in their families. Fortunately, there are a number of simple dietary and nutritional steps people can take to reduce their own risk of heart disease and related health problems.

Dietary Consideration
Dietary Fats

IT is generally accepted that a diet low in fats and cholesterol may help prevent atherosclerosis. However, there are some populations around the world (such as the French and the Masai tribesmen in Africa) who consume a high-fat diet, yet have a low incidence of heart disease. Clearly other factors besides fat intake are involved.

Although the research is complicated and controversial, evidence shows that the type of fat consumed is more important than the total amount ingested. For example, the unnatural fatty acids that are produced in the manufacturing of margarine and "partially hydrogenated vegetable oils" (known as *trans*-fatty acids) have caused severe atherosclerosis in animal studies[1] and have been associated with an increased risk of heart disease in humans.[2] While butter may not be the perfect food, the evidence suggests that it may be safer than margarine.

Oxidized fatty acids can also cause significant damage to the heart and blood vessels. Fatty acids become oxidized when unsaturated oils (such as sunflower, safflower, corn, or fish oil) are heated to high temperatures in the presence of oxygen (air), as in frying or baking. Olive oil is a safer oil for cooking, because it is less prone to become oxidized at high temperatures. However, whatever oil is used, some toxic byproducts will be produced during frying; therefore, individuals should keep the consumption of fried foods to a minimum. Stir-frying is less dangerous, because it involves a relatively small amount of oil. Cooking at a lower temperature for a longer period of time appears to produce fewer oxidized fatty acids, compared with cooking at a higher temperature for a shorter period of time. Oxidation of unsaturated fatty acids also occurs at room temperature, albeit at a slower rate. To prevent oxidation of the fatty acids in nuts and vegetable oils, these foods should be stored in airtight containers and kept refrigerated.

Oxidized cholesterol is also considerably more dangerous than cholesterol itself. In animal studies, ingestion of pure cholesterol produced no significant adverse effects, whereas even tiny quantities of oxidized cholesterol caused serious damage to blood vessels.[3] Oxidized cholesterol forms during high-temperature cooking of foods such as meat, milk, eggs, and butter. Cooking these foods at lower temperatures is probably safer for the heart. In addition, eggs that are poached or boiled inside the shell are probably much safer than scrambled eggs. When the yolk remains intact during cooking, the cholesterol does not come in contact with air, and it is therefore protected from becoming oxidized.

Evidence also shows that consuming certain types of fish (such as mackerel, salmon, tuna, halibut, cod, and sardines) may help prevent heart disease. The omega-3 fatty acids present in these fish prevent blood platelets from sticking together (excessive platelet stickiness is believed to promote the development of atherosclerosis). Omega-3 fatty acids also lower triglyceride levels, reduce blood pressure, and improve blood flow. Heart disease is rare among populations in which people eat large amounts of these fish.

Effect of Sugar

WHILE the dangers of a high-fat diet are widely publicized, the risks of eating refined sugar have been largely ignored by the medical profession. However, population studies show that sucrose consumption is closely associated with heart-disease risk.[4] In addition, ingestion of sugar by susceptible individuals (approximately one-third of the population) can cause adverse changes in a number of cardiovascular risk factors, including HDL cholesterol, triglycerides, blood pressure, platelet stickiness, and blood levels of insulin.[5]

Chlorinated Water

THERE are few, if any, communities around the world with chlorinated drinking water that have a low incidence of atherosclerosis.[6] Chlorine is a powerful oxidizing agent (that's why it is used for bleaching), which is capable of causing severe damage to blood vessels. American servicemen fighting in Korea and Vietnam who were killed in battle were found to have advanced atherosclerosis in more than 75% of cases. The water given to these men was so heavily chlorinated that it was virtually undrinkable. In animal studies, chlorine has been found to promote the development of atherosclerosis. Chlorine can be removed from tap water by boiling it for 5 to 10 minutes, or by adding a pinch of vitamin C crystals to the water.

Other Dietary Factors

EATING whole grains, fruits, vegetables, nuts, seeds, and legumes may help protect against heart disease. The apparent protective effect of nuts,[7, 8] which are high in fat, may be due to their essential-fatty-acid content.

In addition to the items discussed above, a number of other components of our diet may promote or contribute to atherosclerosis. First, research on caffeine is conflicting, although some evidence shows that it can promote atherosclerosis. Alcohol in moderation is either protective or neutral, whereas heavy alcohol consumption can clearly damage the heart. Research suggests that an enzyme present in cow's milk, known as xanthine oxidase, is capable of damaging the blood-vessel wall and promoting atherosclerosis.[9] While this enzyme would normally be destroyed during the process of digestion, homogenization of milk protects xanthine oxidase from human digestive juices, allowing it to be absorbed intact into the bloodstream. The incidence of heart disease around the world correlates with the intake of homogenized milk, but not with intake of butter or cheese (which are higher in fat, but which contain little or no absorbable xanthine oxidase).[10] Significant amounts of xanthine oxidase are presumably absorbed from whole milk, 2%-fat milk, and 1%-fat milk, whereas little or no xanthine oxidase would be absorbed from skim milk, cheese, butter, or yogurt.

Nutritional Supplements
The Homocysteine Connection

A GROWING body of research shows that homocysteine (a normal breakdown product of the essential amino acid methionine) is a toxic molecule, which promotes the development of atherosclerosis. An elevated blood level of homocysteine is an important risk factor for atherosclerosis,[11, 12] perhaps even more important than elevated serum cholesterol. The normal biochemical pathways by which homocysteine is broken down require folic acid, vitamin B_6, and vitamin B_{12}. Individuals whose diets contain inadequate amounts of these vitamins may see their homocysteine levels go up. On the other hand, supplementing with these nutrients can reduce homocysteine levels.[13, 14, 15]

In most studies, relatively low daily doses (for example, 0.4 mg of folic acid, 10 mg of vitamin B_6, and 50 mcg of vitamin B_{12}) have been effective in lowering homocysteine levels. Some individuals (about 2% of the population) have a genetic defect in their ability to metabolize homocysteine. These people are at high risk of developing cardiovascular disease (indeed, more than one-quarter of patients with premature atherosclerosis have this genetic defect).[16] Fortunately, even inherited elevations of homocysteine can usually be corrected by supplementing with larger doses of folic acid (such as 5 mg per day) and/or vitamin B_6 (such as 50 to 100 mg per day). Now that blood tests for homocysteine are available, doctors can determine how much of these vitamins an individual needs in order to maintain homocysteine levels within the normal range.

Magnesium

WHEN rats were fed an experimental diet that normally induced atherosclerosis, the severity of the condition could be reduced by increasing the amount of dietary magnesium 4-fold.[17] Surprisingly, magnesium was protective even though it did not prevent the diet-induced elevation of serum cholesterol. Magnesium can raise levels of HDL cholesterol (the "good" kind), inhibit platelet aggregation, improve heart-muscle function, lower blood pressure, and dilate blood vessels.[18] All of these actions would be expected to improve cardiovascular health. Considering that the average American diet contains less than the RDA for magnesium, the importance of increasing the intake of this nutrient cannot be overemphasized.

Vitamin E

THE relationship between vitamin E and heart disease, for years a controversial topic, is now becoming increasingly accepted. Epidemiological studies have shown that individuals whose vitamin E intake is relatively high develop heart disease about one-third less often than do individuals with low vitamin E intake.[19, 20] In another study, 147 healthy volunteers received either 100 IU or 3 IU of vitamin E per day for 6 years. Of those receiving the lower dose, 10% developed cardiac disorders. In contrast, not a single person in the higher-dose group suffered a cardiac problem.[21] It is not known how much vitamin E is needed to protect a healthy person from developing atherosclerosis, but most studies suggest that as little as 100 IU per day can do the job.

Other Nutrients

SPACE does not permit a complete review of all of the nutritional factors related to atherosclerosis. However, research suggests that vitamin B_3, vitamin C, carotenoids, flavonoids, calcium, potassium, selenium, chromium, zinc, copper, silicon, iodine, and essential fatty acids all play a role in atherosclerosis prevention. More-detailed information is available for individuals interested in further study.[22]

Excessive intake of iron, on the other hand, may actually increase the risk of heart disease,[23] although not all studies agree on that point. Because iron is an oxidizing agent, iron overload might cause some of the same problems we are trying to prevent by taking antioxidants. A small proportion of the population has a genetic abnormality that causes them to accumulate iron. For those individuals, taking iron supplements can be dangerous. A simple blood test can identify "iron accumulators," as well as those who need to take supplemental iron.

Conclusion

As with many slowly developing degenerative diseases, there is no single cause of atherosclerosis. It appears that this disease is caused largely by the cumulative effect of years of poor diet and marginal deficiencies of a wide range of nutrients. Other likely contributing factors include environmental pollutants (such as lead and cadmium), stress, and lack of exercise.

Preventing atherosclerosis therefore requires more than just a "magic bullet" or two. An effective approach should include a diet that emphasizes whole grains, fruits, vegetables, nuts, seeds, legumes, and fish; a comprehensive nutritional-supplement program; and regular exercise. Higher doses of individual nutrients (such as vitamin B_6 or folic acid) may be necessary for particular individuals; this can be discussed with a nutrition-oriented physician.

Atherosclerosis is one of the most common and serious illnesses in industrialized countries. Although all the research is not yet in, a growing body of evidence suggests that this disease is preventable.

Summary of Recommendations for Preventing Atherosclerosis

Diet:

- Avoid chlorinated water, refined sugar and other refined carbohydrates, homogenized milk, margarine, partially hydrogenated vegetable oils, fried foods, and caffeine.

- Emphasize fruits, vegetables, whole grains, legumes, nuts, and seeds.

- Non-fat dairy products and oily fish may be consumed in moderation.

- Restrict high-fat foods.

Supplements:

- Vitamin C, 500 to 3,000 mg per day.

- Vitamin E, 100 to 800 IU per day.

- Magnesium, 300 to 500 mg per day.

- High-potency B-complex vitamin.

- High-potency multiple vitamin/mineral (adjust doses of other nutrients as needed). The need for supplemental iron should be determined by laboratory testing.

- Essential fatty acids, in selected cases.

For additional information, see the chapters on angina and atherosclerosis (treatment).

ATHEROSCLEROSIS *(treatment)*

❧ THE TERM "ATHEROSCLEROSIS" *is derived from two Greek words that mean "gruel" ("porridge") and "hardening." As a disease, atherosclerosis refers to the buildup of yellowish plaques in the walls of arteries. Atherosclerotic plaques consist of cholesterol, fatty material, calcium, and other substances. When it becomes extensive, atherosclerosis restricts the flow of blood to the tissues and organs of the body, and it can potentially result in a heart attack, stroke, gangrene of the extremities, or other serious problems.*

Conventional treatment includes bypass surgery, angioplasty (blasting an artery open by inflating a balloon), and various medications designed to minimize the effects of the disease or slow its progression. However, these treatments (particularly surgery) carry significant risks, and they are not always successful.

DR. WRIGHT'S CASE STUDY

Hernando Ferguson walked slowly into the office, leaning on his wife's arm. "It's about one hundred yards from where we parked to your front desk, and that's about as far as I can go anymore without sitting down," he said. "Too bad you weren't behind time, I could have rested out there." He sat down slowly.

"Sorry. We get behind time too often," I replied. "Usually, someone has more concerns than can be covered in their appointment time."

"We know," Mary Ferguson said. "He's not really complaining about that, he's just upset about not being able to get around like he used to."

"And by seeing a bunch of doctors who tell me there's nothing further to do about it besides taking this drug that doesn't do me much good anyway. I used to be able to run a hundred yards before I'd think of getting tired! I remember the

time I took the ball in our end zone and ran it the whole hundred yards and practically out of the stadium before they caught me! Now I'm just waiting around for things to get bad enough so I can have my legs amputated."

"That was in high school, Hern, and even if your legs were perfectly OK, they'd likely catch you at the ten-yard line today—unless everyone else was 63 years old, too, of course. And quit grumbling about waiting for amputation, that's why we're here."

She turned to me. "It's taken me over two years to drag him in here, doctor. Remember, I mentioned his condition to you last time I was here, and you said there's a good chance he can at least get some improvement? Well, I would have mentioned it sooner, but until he got this bad he wouldn't think of coming in."

"If there's anything that really works, how come my doctor and all those vascular specialists he sent me to don't know about it? They're supposed to be the best. Besides, I've been watching

Mary take 67 pills or so a day and I don't know if I can handle that."

"It's only 33 a day, Hern, and not a drug in the bunch. Sixteen are nutrients, food basically, just concentrated, and the other 17 are just to help my digestion. I think you need those, too—the way you get gassy and heartburn and all. Besides . . ." She crossed her arms, sat back, and smiled. "Aren't I much healthier than I was before I changed what I was eating and started taking those '67 pills'"?

"Basically that's the only reason I agreed to come," Hernando said. "I'm worse, you're better, here I am."

"What drug are you taking?"

"Trental, but it doesn't do much. The doctors said that's all there is. I suppose you're going to give a long list of vitamins?"

"Likely, but basics first. Have you heard of Nathan Pritikin?"

"No, but he's probably not heard of me, either."

"Hernando Ferguson? That's a fairly distinctive name."

"Mother's Spanish, father Scots . . . guess which one named me? 'Black Scots', my father called me, like the 'Black Irish' from the wreckage of the Armada on Irish shores."

"Public schools were teaching history in your times," I said. "But back to Nathan Pritikin. He was the first to demonstrate that diet alone could relieve the symptoms of atherosclerosis. At autopsy, Pritikin himself was found to have totally clear coronary arteries, even though he'd had rather severe symptoms of coronary atherosclerosis decades before. However, since he wasn't an M.D., his contribution is often ignored. Later, Dean Ornish, M.D., showed by means of arteriograms that atherosclerosis could actually be reversed, using a diet similar to Pritikin's. Pritikin isn't with us anymore, but his book and books by Ornish are available."

"And I know just where to get them," Mary said.

"Please plan your diet along the lines you'll find in those books," I said. "There's only one part I don't recommend, and that's Pritikin's almost total elimination of essential fatty acids. There are some that are very important, in fact, —essential—just as they're named. Our clinic nutritionist will help you with this and other details."

"There are a few tests that should be done, too. In addition to cholesterol, HDL-cholesterol, triglycerides—which you've already had done—it sounds like checking the digestion would be wise. Also, decades ago, a Danish cardiovascular surgeon, Jens Moller, demonstrated that testosterone treatment could reverse even severe cases of atherosclerosis. We'll check your testosterone levels, too." I marked a lab form for the appropriate tests.

"Testosterone? We'll ask Mary whether I need some of that."

Mary just smiled.

"So what about those vitamins? Can they really help?"

"Yes, in most cases—but supplements don't do as much good without basic diet change, and unless the nutrients are digested and assimilated as well as possible."

"You mean I might need 5 or 6 of those . . . those hydrochloric acid and pepsin capsules Mary takes at the beginning of every meal?"

"You might, and you could well need digestive enzymes after meals, too. Inefficient digestion is a very common problem when we get into our fifties, sixties, and beyond, and if we don't correct it as best we can, then even the best of diet and lots of supplements won't help as we know they can. But of course we'll run the proper tests to make sure."

"OK, OK, now what about those vitamins?"

"Start with vitamin C, 1 gram, 3 times daily. In 1954, vitamin C was shown to partially reverse atherosclerosis in some cases. . . . "

"1954? So why haven't those specialists heard of it by now?"

"Don't do their reading in the right places, I guess. Next, magnesium—but since I'm also going to recommend IV treatments, we'll put the magnesium in there."

Hernando sat up abruptly. "IV treatments? What's that about? I don't like the sound of that."

"Let me finish the supplements to swallow, first, then I'll get to the IV recommendations. Wouldn't recommend them if they didn't usually do the job, though. Now—after the magnesium, there's vitamin E. Please use 800 IU of the mixed tocopherol type daily." I added to his list.

"Next, inositol hexanicotinate, 1 gram, 3 times daily. Studies have shown that both vitamin E and inositol hexanicotinate can improve walking distance for individuals with blood-flow impairment in the legs. L-carnitine is helpful, too. Please use 250 milligrams, 3 times daily. L-carnitine has also been shown to increase walking distance. Then there's fish oil, 1 tablespoon daily or the equivalent in capsules. Fish oil makes platelets more 'slippery', reducing the risk of clotting, and as an omega-3 fatty acid source it reduces inflammation.

"Last on this list, a high-potency multiple vitamin-mineral. It's always wisest to add a multiple to 'back up' individual nutrients in higher amounts."

"Let's see—vitamin C, vitamin E, inositol whatever, L-carnitine, fish oil, a multiple vitamin-mineral, maybe hydrochloric acid-pepsin, maybe enzymes, maybe testosterone . . ."

"And we haven't even gotten to the 'good part' yet—the chelation therapy," Mary said.

"Is that the IV stuff? Why didn't you mention that to me?"

"It was hard enough getting you here without scaring you, too. I know how much you don't like needles."

"So what's this IV-chelation stuff?"

"Years ago, doctors were working with an intravenous treatment for lead poisoning using a synthetic amino acid called EDTA. They noticed an unexpected effect—circulation improved remarkably in some individuals. So they started treating people with atherosclerosis on purpose

with intravenous EDTA, and many of them improved. Since that time, literally hundreds of thousands of people with various forms of atherosclerosis have had chelation therapy with intravenous EDTA, and the large majority have improved significantly—well beyond what diet change and supplements can do alone."

"EDTA, EDTA—I've seen that somewhere else, too."

"It's in a lot of foods as a food preservative, Hern."

"So why can't I just swallow it?"

"Doesn't absorb well."

"So why haven't the specialists told me about chelation therapy?"

"Perhaps a bit of 'mainstream chauvinism'. Chelation's generally regarded as 'alternative' treatment. Also, it hasn't been under patent for years, so no giant drug firm is pushing it, and it competes with much more expensive 'mainstream' surgical procedures. Oddly enough, many of those 'mainstream' surgical procedures have never been subjected to controlled trials. But I've seen chelation therapy work over and over again in cases like yours, so I definitely recommend you think about it. There are books about chelation at your local library, and for sale in natural-food stores."

"What about this Trental stuff?"

"I think you already told me what that was doing for you."

Mr. Ferguson decided to take chelation therapy. He changed his diet, found he needed digestive aids, took all his supplements, and even a small quantity of testosterone. Two years after starting treatment, he was back to walking "at least 2 miles, 3 times every week, without sitting down once!"

Hormones and Atherosclerosis

AN INCREASING BODY of research appears to be confirming the work of Jens Moller[1] and other pioneers in the testosterone treatment of atherosclerotic disease. For further discussion with citations to the research, please see *Maximize Your Vitality and Potency for Men over 40: Natural Testosterone and Other Supplements,* by Jonathan V. Wright, M.D., and Lane Lenard, Ph.D., Smart Publications, 1999.

For women, estrogen may play the same role. Please see *Natural Hormone Replacement for Women Over 45,* by Jonathan V. Wright, M.D., and John Morgenthaler, Smart Publications, 1997.

DR. GABY'S COMMENTARY

SEVERAL SAFE AND effective alternatives are available to treat atherosclerosis. These include dietary modifications, nutritional supplements, and chelation therapy. Although the latter of these is a controversial approach, it is apparently an effective method of improving circulation.

Dietary Considerations
Pritikin/Ornish Diet

IN the 1970s, Nathan Pritikin promoted a diet that was low in fats, cholesterol, protein, and refined carbohydrates and high in complex carbohydrates and fiber.[2] According to Pritikin, when combined with an exercise program, this type of diet could produce marked improvements in individuals suffering from angina, heart failure, hypertension, and other diseases of the cardiovascular system. Although Pritikin's ideas were not accepted by the medical mainstream, his work was followed up by Dr. Dean Ornish and colleagues.

In their landmark study, 48 patients with coronary atherosclerosis were randomly assigned to receive standard care (control group) or a combination of diet, smoking cessation, stress management, and moderate exercise.[3] The diet emphasized fruits, vegetables, grains, legumes, and soybean products. No animal products were allowed, except egg white and one cup of nonfat milk or yogurt per day. Approximately 10% of calories were derived from fat, 15 to 20% from protein, and 70 to 75% from predominantly complex carbohydrates. Patients in the treatment group

experienced marked reductions in the frequency, duration, and severity of angina, whereas patients in the control group experienced a worsening of their angina. In addition, angiographic studies done on the patients' coronary arteries before and one year after the start of the study showed regression (i.e., improvement) of atherosclerosis in patients in the treatment group, and continued progression of the disease in patients in the control group. The difference in outcome between the two groups was highly statistically significant ($p = 0.001$).

This study showed that a comprehensive program consisting of diet, stress reduction, exercise, and other lifestyle changes can reverse atherosclerosis—a condition which most physicians had believed to be irreversible.

Nutritional Supplements
Vitamin C

ORNISH was not the first doctor to demonstrate that atherosclerosis can be reversed. That honor goes to Dr. G. C. Willis, a Canadian physician who published a little-known study in 1954. In that study,[4] 10 patients with atherosclerosis received 500 mg of vitamin C, 3 times a day for 2 to 6 months, while 6 similar patients did not receive vitamin C. Arteriograms of the lower extremities showed regression of atherosclerosis in 6 of the 10 patients treated with vitamin C, whereas no improvement was seen in any of the 6 untreated patients.

Magnesium

IN addition to improving blood flow by acting as a vasodilator (promoter of blood-vessel dilation), magnesium helps the tissues of the body make more efficient use of a limited supply of oxygen. Magnesium has been shown to be effective in the treatment of intermittent claudication, a condition caused by atherosclerosis in the lower extremities. Individuals with intermittent claudication develop severe pain in their calf muscles after walking short distances, because their arteries cannot supply adequate amounts of blood to the leg muscles. In one study, 19 patients with intermittent claudication received 250 mg of magnesium hydroxide twice a day. After 60 days, these patients were able to walk an average of 82% farther than they could before receiving magnesium.[5]

In individuals with more severe cases of atherosclerosis, intravenous or intramuscular injections of magnesium have been found to be helpful.[6] I once treated an elderly man who had such severe atherosclerosis of the extremities that he had developed gangrene of 6 toes. Angiograms had shown no detectable blood flow to his feet. The patient had been advised to undergo immediate amputation of both legs, in order to prevent the development of a potentially fatal blood infection. I began treating him with weekly magnesium injections, plus large oral doses of vitamin C, vitamin E, and other nutrients. He gradually improved and, after many months of treatment, the gangrenous lesions sloughed off, revealing pink, healthy tissue underneath. Because of the advanced stage of his illness, the gangrene would start to recur unless he continued to receive periodic injections of magnesium (usually twice monthly).

Vitamin E

IN one study, 47 patients with intermittent claudication were given either 300 IU of vitamin E per day or standard treatment (an anticoagulant or vasodilator). After 4 to 6 months, the maximum distance that patients could walk had increased to a significantly greater extent in the vitamin E group than in the standard-treatment group.[7] Vitamin E appears to function as a mild vasodilator. It is also thought to increase the flexibility of red blood cells, thereby allowing them to travel through tiny capillaries more smoothly. In addition, evidence shows that vitamin E enhances the efficiency of oxygen utilization by the tissues.[8]

Inositol Hexanicotinate

NIACIN (one of the forms of vitamin B$_3$) is a vasodilator, and it exerts other beneficial effects on the cardiovascular system. However, niacin often causes an uncomfortable skin flush, and in high doses it may occasionally damage the liver. A derivative of niacin known as inositol hexanicotinate has been used as an alternative to niacin. Inositol hexanicotinate consists of one molecule of the B-vitamin inositol and 6 molecules of niacin. It is preferred by many individuals, because it rarely causes a skin flush. In addition, this compound is said to put little or no strain on the liver, although there is not enough research to know whether that claim is true.

In a double-blind study, 86 patients with intermittent claudication received inositol hexanicotinate (1 g, 4 times a day) or a placebo. After 9 weeks of treatment, the inositol hexanicotinate group experienced a significantly greater increase in walking distance than the placebo group.[9]

L-Carnitine

IN a double-blind study, 20 patients with atherosclerosis of the lower extremities were randomly assigned to receive L-carnitine (2 g, twice a day) or a placebo for 3 weeks, then the alternate treatment for an additional 3 weeks. The average pain-free walking distance was significantly greater by 76% during the L-carnitine period than during the placebo period.[10] Since administering L-carnitine did not improve blood flow, its beneficial effects were probably due to an improvement in cellular metabolism.

Chelation Therapy

IN THE 1950s, the standard treatment for lead poisoning was a drug called EDTA (ethylenediaminetetraacetic acid). EDTA treatment is referred to as chelation therapy (pronounced "key-lay-shun"; the term "chelate" means "to grab like a claw"), because of the type of chemical bond that the drug forms with lead and other metals.

One doctor who was administering EDTA to a patient with both lead poisoning and atherosclerosis noticed that the patient's circulation improved markedly. This observation enticed that physician and several others to try EDTA therapy on patients with atherosclerosis who did not have lead toxicity. Some of these doctors reported that EDTA therapy was of great benefit for a large proportion of their patients, although they were not sure how the treatment worked.[11, 12]

Since that time, chelation therapy has been a popular (but extremely controversial) therapy. More than half a million Americans have received chelation therapy. Many of them are convinced that it saved them from amputation, bypass surgery, or even death. Hundreds of physicians are now using chelation therapy, and interest in this treatment continues to grow every year. At least one study has demonstrated that chelation therapy can, indeed, "open up" atherosclerotic arteries.[13]

However, the official position of the medical establishment is that chelation therapy is unproven and potentially dangerous. A number of physicians have even been harassed and threatened with license revocation by their state licensing boards for using this "unproven" treatment. One of the main arguments against chelation therapy is that the results are anecdotal—they are not supported by placebo-controlled, double-blind studies. Although one small double-blind study did show a beneficial effect of EDTA,[14] that argument is basically true. On the other hand, the clinical results with chelation therapy are so obvious in many cases that nearly every physician who has tried the treatment has been convinced of its effectiveness. In addition, the official position against chelation therapy appears to reflect a double standard, since the "accepted" technologies (bypass surgery and angioplasty) also have not been validated by double-blind studies.

Opponents of chelation therapy also argue that the treatment can damage the kidneys. That claim is based on observations from the 1940s, before the appropriate dosage and rate of administration for EDTA was known. Since then, doctors have become more knowledgeable about how to use EDTA, and problems with kidney damage have become virtually nonexistent. In fact, properly administered chelation therapy has actually been reported to improve kidney function, probably by enhancing blood flow to the kidneys.[15]

It should be noted that chelation therapy is far less expensive than coronary-bypass surgery (about $3,000 for a series of 30 chelation treatments, compared with $50,000 for bypass surgery). In addition, chelation can improve circulation throughout the entire body, whereas the effects of surgery are limited to the area being operated on. Furthermore, chelation therapy is extremely safe, when administered according to standard protocols. In contrast, as many as 1 to 2% of patients die as a direct result of coronary-bypass surgery.

We have seen chelation therapy work wonders for patients with atherosclerotic disease. However, we realize that a well-designed placebo-controlled study is needed before the medical mainstream will be convinced. Because atherosclerosis is one of the major diseases affecting Americans and because chelation therapy shows such great promise, the National Institutes of Health should im-mediately begin organizing a clinical trial. For less than one-fifth of one percent of the annual NIH budget, the question of whether chelation therapy works could be answered to everyone's satisfaction.

Physicians interested in learning about chelation therapy should contact the American College for Advancement in Medicine (ACAM) at 1-800-LEAD-OUT. ACAM can also provide prospective patients with a list of physicians in their geographic area who offer chelation therapy.

Conclusion

SCIENTIFIC RESEARCH AND clinical experience have demonstrated that safe and effective alternatives exist for individuals with atherosclerosis. A combination of dietary modification, nutritional supplements, and chelation therapy has helped hundreds of thousands of patients avoid dangerous surgical procedures and achieve better health. Please see the preceding chapter for additional information on preventing atherosclerosis.

Summary of Recommendations for Treating Atherosclerosis

DIET:

- Avoid chlorinated water, refined sugar and other refined carbohydrates, homogenized milk, margarine, partially hydrogenated vegetable oils, fried foods, and caffeine.

- Emphasize fruits, vegetables, whole grains, and legumes.

- Nuts, seeds, non-fat dairy products, and oily fish may be consumed in moderation.

- Restrict high-fat foods.

SUPPLEMENTS:

- Vitamin C, 1,000 to 2,000 mg, 2 to 3 times a day.

- Vitamin E, 400 to 1,200 IU per day.

- Magnesium, 300 to 500 mg per day.

- Inositol hexanicotinate, 500 to 1,000 mg, 3 to 4 times per day (treatment should be monitored by a doctor).

- L-carnitine, 500 to 1,500 mg per day.

- Fish-oil concentrate, 3 to 6 grams per day or cod-liver oil, 1 to 2 teaspoons per day, or other source of essential fatty acids.

- High-potency B-complex vitamin.

- High-potency multiple vitamin/mineral (iron-free, unless laboratory tests indicate the need for iron); adjust doses of other nutrients as needed.

OTHER RECOMMENDATIONS:

- Chelation therapy in selected cases.

- Testosterone therapy in selected cases.

- For additional information, see the chapters on angina and atherosclerosis (prevention).

ATTENTION DEFICIT-HYPERACTIVITY DISORDER

🌿 ATTENTION DEFICIT-HYPERACTIVITY DISORDER *(ADHD) was a rare condition 50 years ago. Today, it is extremely common, affecting an estimated 5 to 20% of all children in the United States. Previously known by a number of different names (including hyperactivity, hyperkinesis, and minimal brain dysfunction), ADHD is characterized by learning disabilities, short attention span, easy distractibility, impulsive behavior, hyperactivity, and lack of coordination. Although children with ADHD are not mentally retarded, they often do poorly in school and have difficulty making friends.*

Conventional medicine has discovered that methylphenidate (Ritalin—a chemical related to the amphetamines) is often effective for children with ADHD. For reasons that are not understood, stimulants like Ritalin produce a paradoxical response in these children: slowing them down and helping them concentrate, rather than speeding them up. However, despite its effectiveness, this powerful drug can cause numerous side effects, including loss of appetite, insomnia, rapid heart rate, headache, and possibly growth retardation. Furthermore, Ritalin does not address the cause of ADHD; it merely suppresses the symptoms. Unfortunately, both teachers and parents sometimes look at Ritalin as a quick fix, or as the simplest way to deal with a complicated problem. Indeed, in some parts of the United States, as many as 6% of grade-school children are on this drug.

DR. WRIGHT'S CASE STUDY

"Jeremy is NOT going on Ritalin!" Susannah Bernstein declared. "I don't care if we have to put him in a private school, even if we can't afford it. They're not drugging our son. We've been asking around, and we heard sometimes your clinic can help."

"We know Jeremy can be a handful," David added. "But we couldn't understand why the school was pushing so hard for that Ritalin, even hinting they might not let Jeremy come back

without it. How do they know it's exactly the right thing for him? They're teachers and administrators, not doctors. He just saw the school psychologist once, to 'confirm' that he needed the stuff. I got suspicious and started doing some digging. I found out the school district gets $1,000 or so in extra federal money for every student they put on Ritalin! No wonder the number of kids on that stuff has skyrocketed in the last few years."

"And I started doing some research in the library and on the Internet," Susannah said. "I decided that we could make some diet changes on our own and see what happened. So at the same time we got this appointment, about 3 months ago, we started Jeremy—the whole family actually—on the Feingold diet program. I got the book, we read all the labels, and we've eliminated all chemical flavors, colors, and preservatives. We stopped all the natural salicylate-containing foods, and while we were at it we got rid of all the refined sugar, too. It hasn't been easy, and it really complicates eating out. But Jeremy's been a real trooper, and we've gotten it done."

"Have you noticed a difference?"

Susannah glanced at Jeremy, who was playing on the floor. "A little improvement overall, but the biggest thing is that Jeremy is having very few 'anger spells' anymore."

"Anger spells?"

"Jeremy's always been excitable, but starting about age 4, when he was in pre-school, he started having sudden 'anger spells' at the other children—yelling and screaming at them. He'd always be sorry after, but he just couldn't control himself."

"Did he—or does he—get violent?"

Susannah looked at Jeremy again. By now he was on the other side of the room, playing with something else. David answered.

"Unfortunately, he did. He'd hit or kick, and once he even bit another boy. As Susannah says, he was always sorry after, but that didn't seem to stop the next one. At first it wasn't often, but this last year in the second grade he'd have a spell as often as every week or two. That's when we decided we really had to do something. We didn't disagree with the school about that, we just disagreed that Ritalin was the only answer."

"His anger spells were so unpredictable," Susannah said. "He had them at home, too, and often we couldn't find anything in particular that set them off."

"Or stopped them," David added. "He just seemed to wind down on his own. But we're hopeful about this diet plan, because he hasn't

had one 'anger spell' since the second week on this diet plan."

"Actually, it seems to be one of Jeremy's motivations to stay with the program," Susannah observed. "He's noticed he has a few more friends in the last month or so, now that the 'anger spells' have settled down."

"What about the rest of his behavior? How's he doing in school?"

"His teacher says his attention span might be a little improved, but he's still not doing as well as he should. He's especially behind in reading, and isn't doing so well in his other classes, either."

"He's had those tests, and they say it's not for lack of intelligence," David said. "In fact, he's brighter than average, but he just can't seem to 'catch on.'"

"Hyperactive children frequently test as higher in intelligence than others," I noted. "Let's see if we can help him use that intelligence."

Susannah reached into her bag and pulled out a book. "I've been reading Dr. Doris Rapp's books lately, too, and I'm convinced Jeremy has allergies. He has those dark circles under his eyes, and the horizontal creases in his lower eyelids. And he had ear infections starting at 18 months that didn't quit until he was about 4 years old."

I laughed. "You're making it easy for me," I said. "You've got Jeremy's problems diagnosed already. You're right, nearly all children diagnosed as 'hyperactive' have allergies and sensitivities, especially food allergies."

"We don't mean to diagnose . . ." Susannah started.

"We're not doctors . . ." David cut in.

"Please, I can use all the help I can get, anytime," I said. "After all, you live with Jeremy and observe him 24 hours a day. No way I can do that. I'm very happy you found Dr. Rapp's books; she's done more to inform parents of hyperactive children than all the rest of us doctors combined. Have you tried any of her suggestions?"

"Eliminating the food chemicals and refined sugar was hard enough," Susannah said. "I found

Dr. Feingold's book in the library first, and Dr. Rapp's books later. Also, we heard you do some fairly accurate allergy testing so we wouldn't have so much 'trial and error.' Dr. Rapp describes very careful skin testing techniques for allergies," Susannah said. "But then I read about blood testing for food allergies on the Internet. That only involves drawing blood once, rather than lots of separate tests with needles. It's called an ELISA test, I think. Do you do that one?"

"Sometimes, and I think it's quite a good test for food allergy, too. But in the last few years, I've found that electrodermal screening is much more helpful for allergy and sensitivity screening, especially for children. Electrodermal testing has a much broader range, and is somewhat less expensive, too. Lastly, it doesn't involve needles at all."

"Good," Jeremy said from yet another corner of the room.

"Jeremy agreed he'd do any test we needed to do," David said. "But of course he'd be happier with fewer."

"I can't guarantee we won't ever need to do tests that require needles, but we try to do other tests first. Sometimes blood tests for amino acids or essential fatty acids or serotonin can be very helpful."

"Serotonin? Isn't that a brain chemical?" Susannah asked.

"Yes, a neurotransmitter, a molecule that carries information from one nerve cell to another. Studies have shown that if blood serotonin is low in hyperactive children, extra vitamin B_6 can be quite helpful. However, since vitamin B_6 is also safe except in very large doses, often we just recommend trying it to see what happens. Vitamin B_6 is also important to essential-fatty-acid metabolism, and at least one study has found hyperactive boys to be low in certain essential fatty acids. We frequently recommend the use of essential fatty acids—especially omega-3 fatty acids—for children with a diagnosis of ADHD.

"Then there are amino acids, which are precursors of neurotransmitters. In some hyperactive children, amino-acid levels are low or imbalanced, which can lead to lower than usual levels of one or more neurotransmitters—or to imbalances of neurotransmitters. However, speaking of neurotransmitters, we've learned always to check hyperactive children for sensitivities to neurotransmitters, such as norepinephrine, dopamine, acetylcholine, GABA, serotonin, and so on."

"How can anyone be sensitive to their own natural molecules like neurotransmitters?" David asked.

"Don't know, but it's very analogous to progesterone sensitivity in women who have PMS. Desensitization to progesterone helps some women dramatically improve PMS, just as desensitization to neurotransmitters helps some hyperactive children."

Susannah smiled at David. "Sounds like I'm next after Jeremy."

"And maybe I'll check in about my hay fever," David replied.

"If I need any shots, maybe you can get some, too," Jeremy said, coming over to join his parents.

"I don't think you'll need any today," I said. "I will ask your parents to trim off a little of your hair, though—to screen for toxic minerals like lead and cadmium, as well as to check 'normal' elements like calcium, zinc, and copper."

"Haircut's OK," Jeremy replied.

Jeremy was found to be sensitive to milk and dairy products, wheat, soy, oranges, and 27 other foods. With the help of our clinic nutritionist, Susannah put a temporary diet plan together for Jeremy, while desensitization was done. Jeremy was also found to be sensitive to 6 neurotransmitters, as well as to several molds. Desensitization was done for those also.

After screening several multiple vitamin-mineral preparations, one was found that Jeremy could take. He was also asked to take 50 milligrams of vitamin B_6 twice daily along with 100 milligrams of magnesium, and capsules of omega-3 fatty acids high in EPA.

It took 7 months to complete Jeremy's desensitization. His parents noticed that the neurotransmitter desensitization seemed to "really impact Jeremy's behavior the most and quickest," and "the rest of the program helped over time." His screening for heavy-metal toxicity was negative, and blood testing for amino acids and essential fatty acids was unnecessary in his case.

By the third grade, Jeremy's behavior was described by his teacher as "not hyperactive at all, just normal and bright." His "anger spells" were gone entirely. He caught up in all of his subjects, and by the end of the year had started to excel. After some experimentation, his parents decided it was best to continue the entire family on a diet that is free of sugar and chemical additives, as well as avoiding milk and dairy and using wheat only occasionally. They continued his multiple vitamin-mineral, vitamin B_6, magnesium, and omega-3 fatty acids. Jeremy's in the fifth grade now, and has had no further hyperactivity problems.

DR. GABY'S COMMENTARY

A Consequence of Modern Living?

WHENEVER THE PREVALENCE of a disorder has been increasing rapidly, it is logical to look for the cause in our changing environment. Life in the late twentieth century is very different than it was 50 years ago. Many more children today grow up in broken homes or in families where neither parent is home during the day. Kids today also engage in less physical activity and watch far more television than did children in years past. They also consume dozens of previously unknown chemical food additives and are exposed to more fluorescent lighting and electromagnetic fields than before.

Evidence shows that some of these factors may be contributing to the epidemic of ADHD that we are now seeing. For example, time-lapse cinematography studies show that first-grade children sitting under fluorescent lights become hyperactive, compared with those exposed to standard lighting. The radiation emanating from television sets (not to mention the questionable programming) may also have an adverse effect on behavior. In one study, rats were placed in a cage in front of a television set. Although the sound was turned off and all visible light from the screen was shielded by a piece of black cardboard, the rats became hyperactive. This effect could be largely prevented by placing a lead shield over the black cardboard.[1]

Evidently, X-rays from the television set caused the rats to behave like children with ADHD. Because of the results of this study, I advise parents of children with ADHD to limit their child's time in front of the television set. If children do watch television or play video games, I recommend that they sit as far away from the screen as possible. The amount of radiation exposure is inversely related to the square of the distance from the television set. For example, there is 16 times as much radiation exposure at a distance of 1 foot from the set as there is 4 feet away, and 36 times as much radiation at a distance of 1 foot as there is at 6 feet.

Dietary Considerations

DIETARY FACTORS AND nutritional supplements also play an important role in the treatment of ADHD. Some children are exquisitely sensitive to refined sugars, and they improve greatly when all of the sugar is removed from their diet. Some children react to artificial colorings, particularly tartrazine (Yellow Dye #5) and other synthetic chemical additives. A substantial proportion of children are allergic to common foods, such as milk, wheat, egg, corn, or citrus. Others react to a group of naturally-occurring food-derived chemicals called salicylates.[2] Foods high in salicylates include tea; certain fruits, vegetables, and nuts; honey; and some spices. Planning a low-salicylate diet is rather complicated, and requires the help of a dietitian.

In my office, I teach parents how to put their child on an elimination diet. After about 3 weeks, if there has been a noticeable improvement, the foods and additives are reintroduced one at a time, while observing for reactions. Foods that provoke symptoms or behavioral changes are removed from the diet. Elimination-and-rechallenge diets should be medically supervised to ensure that they contain adequate amounts of protein, vitamins, and minerals and that the results are interpreted correctly. In my experience, about 50 to 75% of children with ADHD improve considerably if they exclude the offending foods and/or additives from their diet.

Some doctors use other tests for allergy and sensitivity, as well as desensitization techniques. The reliability and effectiveness of some of these methods is controversial (see chapter 3 for additional discussion).

Why the Controversy About Diet?

WHEN children with ADHD improve, the results are often dramatic. It is therefore surprising that most doctors do not believe diet has much to do with this condition. This skepticism arises in part from some bad research that appeared in popular medical journals and subsequently received widespread media exposure. For example, a study published in the prestigious *New England Journal of Medicine* concluded that dietary sugar does not affect behavior or cognitive function in hyperactive children.[3] In that study, which compared the effects of a high- and low-sugar diet, the so-called "low-sugar" diet actually contained 5.3 teaspoons of refined sugar per day. That amount of sugar is enough to cause symptoms in a sensitive child, rendering comparisons between the two diets meaningless.

Numerous studies have investigated the Feingold diet, which is based on Dr. Ben Feingold's observation that artificial colors and salicylates contribute to ADHD. A few of these studies found that the chemicals caused only minor problems, and other studies found no effect at all. However, much of the research was seriously flawed. For example, in one investigation of food dyes, the placebo was a chocolate cookie.[4] Since many hyperactive children react to chocolate, it is not surprising that the effect of food dyes was no worse than that of the "placebo." Another problem was that studies of food additives or allergens usually investigated only one food or one class of chemicals at a time. Since most children with ADHD are sensitive to more than one substance, they would not be expected to improve much if only one of these substances was removed from their diet.

In a properly designed study, all of the major additives and allergens would be removed at the same time. In one such study, of 26 children with ADHD who went on a comprehensive elimination diet, 19 (73%) improved. Upon retesting, all of the children who had improved reported reactions to 3 or more foods or additives. These reactions were repeatedly confirmed by double-blind food challenges, indicating that the results were not due to psychological factors.[5] A similar double-blind study done 9 years previously produced almost identical results.[6]

The bottom line is that diet modification works well if it is done properly. Although making major diet changes is not always easy, many parents and children find that the benefits are well worth the extra effort.

Nutritional Supplements

VITAMIN SUPPLEMENTS HAVE also been used successfully to treat children with ADHD. Some hyperactive children have a deficiency of the neurotransmitter molecule serotonin. Best known for its relationship to depression, serotonin deficiency also seems to play a role in ADHD. In hyperactive children who had sub-normal blood levels of serotonin, treatment with large doses of vitamin B_6 (15 to 30 mg per kg of body weight) was even more effective than Ritalin.[7] It should be pointed out that not all children with ADHD are low in serotonin. Furthermore, the doses of vitamin B_6 used in this study were extremely large, and use of such large doses of vitamin B_6 must be monitored by a physician. Fortunately, we have found that lower doses of vitamin B_6 are sometimes helpful when combined with appropriate dietary changes.

Other nutrients, including thiamine, niacinamide, zinc, and essential fatty acids are occasionally helpful for children with ADHD. However, it can be difficult to predict which nutrients will work for which children, so trial-and-error is sometimes necessary to achieve the best results.[8]

Conclusion

ADHD HAS BECOME an epidemic among American children. Stimulant drugs such as Ritalin, though effective, do not address the cause of the problem and can be toxic. A diet that is free of refined sugars, chemical additives, and allergens, combined with a medically supervised nutritional-supplement program, will often permit children with ADHD to lead perfectly normal lives.

Summary of Recommendations for Treating Attention Deficit-Hyperactivity Disorder

- DIET: Eliminate all refined sugar, caffeine, and chemical additives. Work with food allergies. Reduce intake of foods high in salicylates in selected cases.

- SUPPLEMENTS: Vitamin B_6, B-complex vitamins, magnesium, zinc, and/or essential fatty acids in selected cases (dosages should be determined by a doctor).

- LIFESTYLE: Obtain adequate exercise. Minimize exposure to color-television sets and increase the distance from the set. Minimize exposure to fluorescent lighting.

BENIGN PROSTATIC HYPERPLASIA
(enlarged prostate)

ENLARGEMENT OF THE *prostate gland is one of the most common conditions affecting men past the age of 50. Known to doctors as benign prostatic hyperplasia (BPH), this problem causes various urinary difficulties. Men with BPH tend to urinate frequently, often one or more times in the middle of the night. They also experience difficulty starting their urine flow and have reduced pressure behind their urinary stream. If BPH becomes severe, it can result in obstruction of urine flow, which is a medical emergency. More often, BPH is just a nuisance, interfering with the quality of life. With time, the condition usually either becomes gradually worse or stays the same; it rarely gets better on its own.*

Conventional doctors often prescribe a drug called finasteride (Proscar) for men with BPH. Finasteride works by preventing the buildup of dihydrotestosterone, a breakdown product of testosterone that is thought to promote prostate enlargement. Although a 4-year study did show that finasteride improves urinary symptoms and reduces the need for surgery, this drug is not without side effects. Approximately 5% of men who take finasteride develop impotence or other types of sexual dysfunction, and about 4 of every 1,000 men experience breast enlargement.[1] The blood pressure-lowering drug terazosin (Hytrin), is also frequently prescribed for BPH. While this drug does relieve symptoms in some cases, it does not prevent the condition from progressing.

Surgery to remove a portion of the prostate gland is still considered the "definitive treatment" by most urologists. However, there are risks associated with prostate surgery, including perforation of the bladder, hemorrhage, infection, and persistent urinary incontinence.

DR. WRIGHT'S CASE STUDY

"My urologist says I'll probably need surgery on my prostate gland soon, but in the meantime I should take this 'Proscar' stuff," Aaron Spiegel said. He pulled a prescription from his pocket, and showed it to me. "Ann here wouldn't let me get it filled, at least not until I came to talk to you."

"Of course not!" Ann Spiegel exclaimed. "One hundred seventy-three dollars a bottle of 100 my pharmacist says it costs! And he says it has to be taken for a year at least! For years, Aaron hasn't listened to me about eating right and taking vitamins, but finally I put my foot down! One hundred seventy-three dollars!"

Aaron reached over and patted his wife's shoulder. "Now, Annie, I'm here, aren't I?" He turned to me. "I've been healthy most of my life, never been in the hospital, feeling pretty good, so I haven't worried. Besides, I'm a big city guy—we retired here from New York a few years back . . . never understood the herbs, nuts and berries thing. New York, you get sick, you see the doctor, get surgery, take a regular medicine—not a root or something."

Annie snorted. "In New York we had health food stores, too. And how many times have you told me about your grandmother's chicken soup when you got sick?"

"She was from the old country, times change. But we're here, so let's talk to the doctor. What can you tell us?"

"Before I can tell you anything, I should know more about what's going on. When did you first start having prostate symptoms?"

"Maybe 4, 5 years ago. At night, I was getting up more often, 2 or 3 times instead of just once. Waiting longer before anything would come—that sort of thing. I saw the urologist, he said a little enlargement, nothing to do, surgery if it got bad."

"In 1986 this urologist says 'nothing to do!'" Ann exclaimed. "I read to you from Dr. Wright's book, published 1979, where he quotes from research back to 1941! Take zinc, take flaxseed oil, eat pumpkin seeds. Did you do any of that?"

"The pumpkin seeds I ate, but nothing happened. The urologist said it wouldn't help anyway, surgery was the only thing, so I quit."

"So it got worse . . ."

"And every year I see the urologist. Last time, he says it's not bad enough for surgery, but there is this new drug I should take."

"Have you had the PSA test done?"

"The blood test for cancer? Several times. Ann insisted. It's always been OK—the last time it was 3 or so, very good the doctor says."

"Anyone else in your family have cancer, especially prostate?"

"No cancer, but in his time my father had prostate surgery, and a few years ago, my older brother."

"You said you've been healthy otherwise?"

"No problems I know about, except if you count a few less teeth, and a whole lot less hair than I started with."

We went over the rest of his health history, then to the exam room for a check-up. Since we planned no prostate check ("once this month is enough," he said), Mrs. Spiegel came along. Aside from a minor problem with dry skin, everything else appeared OK. Especially since we'd not done a prostate check, I asked him to have copies of his tests and records sent over from his urologist's office.

"No problem, I'll do that. Now what do I do, eat pumpkin seeds?"

"Wouldn't hurt. But they're not at the top of the list. There's an extract of the saw palmetto . . ."

"The 'saw' what?"

"The 'what' I've been trying to tell you about, Aaron. The saw palmetto plant, it grows in South Carolina, Georgia, Florida. It was used by American Indians centuries ago . . ."

"Exactly! Centuries ago. Annie, now we have modern drugs."

"Modern, shmodern . . . you think prostate glands are a new invention? If it worked on prostate glands in 1692, it'll work on prostate glands in 1992!"

"But modern drugs are extremely well tested, compared to folk remedies."

I laughed. "Excuse me. Modern drugs are frequently not as well tested as their manufacturers would like us to think. But to get back to your specific problem—saw palmetto has several placebo-controlled, double-blind studies behind it which show that it works as well as 'Proscar', and with none of the side effects. And saw palmetto isn't the only thing. It's near the top of the list, but zinc and flaxseed oil are extremely helpful, too." I wrote him a list:

- zinc (picolinate)—30 mg, 1 tablet, 3 times a day
- flaxseed oil—1,000 mg, 3 capsules, 3 times a day (or flaxseed oil liquid, 1 tablespoon per day)

- saw palmetto (standardized extract)—80 mg, 2 tablets, twice a day
- vitamin E (mixed tocopherols)—400 IU per day
- copper (sebacate)—4 mg, 1 tablet, once a day

Mr. Spiegel studied it. "What'll this all do? Maybe I should just have the surgery and get it over with. Isn't this just postponing the inevitable?"

"Surgery? Aaron Spiegel, haven't you heard enough from your brother about what surgery does? A good thing he's a widower, bless her soul."

"What this all will do for most men is reverse the symptoms and shrink the prostate gland! Now, hardly anything works every single time, but your chances are very good," I said.

"How long does it take? That's . . ." he paused. "Eighteen pills every day I'm supposed to swallow!"

Annie looked over his shoulder. "So? Even all 5 bottles won't cost anything close to $173! And I'm sure you take less as things get better."

"That's true," I said. "Usually symptoms begin to diminish in 3 to 4 months. When you check back after 6 months, we can cut back somewhat. In 1 or 2 years, only 1 or 2 of each item will be recommended for maintenance. Also, remember that if your prostate gland could use more zinc or flaxseed oil or whatever, it's likely that other areas in your body could use more, too. After all, these are nutrients, not drugs. For example, I expect you won't have much dry skin left at all in 6 months. The flaxseed oil should take care of that, also."

"OK. OK. I'll give it a try. If it doesn't work, then I can think about surgery. If I understand this correctly, though, the saw palmetto, zinc, and flaxseed oil are what actually do the job. So what are the vitamin E and copper for?"

"Vitamin E should always accompany essential fatty acids, such as flaxseed oil, as is the case in nature. Vitamin E prevents the unsaturated fats in flaxseed oil from undergoing potentially

dangerous oxidation in your body. Taking therapeutic amounts of zinc can lead to copper deficiency, which can adversely affect cholesterol levels or cause other problems. It's always wisest to 'balance' these two when they're used therapeutically."

"Remember, though, that these are supplements for an enlarged prostate—very necessary supplements to a good diet. It's likely that if your diet had included enough of these and other nutrients for the last 50 years or so, very little if any supplementation would be needed now. I noticed when we went over your diet . . ."

"You don't need to tell me again, Annie's been doing that for years. Now she's got our daughters doing it."

"It's because they love you too, Aaron."

"They're probably right," I observed.

Aaron groaned, "I know. If this works, I'll never hear the end. It'll be 'eat your vegetables, Aaron.' 'Eat your pumpkin seeds, father.'"

"Glad you reminded me about the pumpkin seeds again. Unroasted, they're an excellent source of essential fatty acids and zinc."

"Figures. Anything else?"

"Just one other item. It's likely a good idea to take one other supplement, too; one I suspect your wife already has—a good multiple vitamin and mineral. That will help make up for other things missing from your diet the last few years."

"I know just the thing," Ann said.

Three months later, the Spiegels were back. Aaron reported his symptoms were "at least 30 to 40% better." By 8 months, he reported the symptoms "mostly gone," and his urologist had found his prostate definitely smaller. At one year, he felt "like I don't have a problem anymore." We cut his supplements down to a maintenance level, and Ann told me he was ordering unroasted pumpkin seeds wholesale!

Before You Reach for the Saw Palmetto

SAW PALMETTO HAS a well-deserved reputation for reducing (and in many cases eliminating) the symptoms of benign protastic hyperplasia that are so common in men over age 50. Health-care practitioners have observed by direct examination that saw palmetto therapy reduces the size of enlarged prostate glands, as well as decreasing symptoms. Moreover, there appear to be no side effects from using this botanical preparation. So, why any caution at all?

In 1941, researchers at the Lee Foundation for Nutritional Research (founded by Royal Lee, one of the pioneers and innovators in nutritional research in the United States) reported research concerning 19 men with enlarged prostate glands. All had the expected symptoms of increased urinary frequency, decreased force of urinary stream, urinary "dribbling," and repeated night-time urination. The men took "vitamin F complex," a flaxseed oil-based concentrate containing essential fatty acids. All 19 had a reduction in the size of their prostates. Of the 19 men, 18 had no further "dribbling;" excess night-time urination was eliminated in 13 of 19 men; and 12 of the 19 had no further "residual urine" after urination. Most of the men also reported an increase in libido.

In 1974, Professor Irwin Bush, head of the Division of Urology at Cook County Hospital (Chicago), reported his results with the use of zinc by 19 men with symptoms of an enlarged prostate. After using zinc for 2 months, 14 of the 19 men had shrinkage of the prostate as determined by rectal palpation, X-ray, and endoscopy (internal examination with a "scope").

For years after reading about this research, one of your authors (J.W.) advised men with benign prostatic enlargement to supplement both zinc and flaxseed oil (as a source of essential fatty acids), along with extra vitamin E and copper, which should always be used when essential fatty acids and zinc, respectively, are supplemented. Occasionally digestive enzymes were also needed to facilitate the absorption of these nutrients. Although dozens of men were treated over the years, your author at one time kept track of 19 consecutive treatments, and observed that 18 of

19 men in this group experienced significant reductions in both symptoms and gland size.

So what's the difference between treatment with zinc and essential fatty acids on one gland, and saw palmetto and other herbs on another? The difference is simple: both zinc and essential fatty acids are essential nutrients, while saw palmetto and other herbs are not. Carrying this example to its extreme, we can die of either zinc or essential-fatty-acid deficiencies, but we wouldn't die if we never swallowed a microgram of saw palmetto. Obviously, we should correct deficiencies of essential nutrients first, even if the deficiency appears to be "only local" in the prostate gland.

Additionally, it's likely that if one body tissue is deficient in an essential nutrient, other tissues, glands, or organs are deficient, too, even if the deficiency isn't immediately apparent. So, if the prostate is "hurting" for lack of zinc and essential fatty acids, these nutrients should be supplemented, regardless of whether or not herbs are being used. These supplements can help the rest of the body, too, wherever they're needed. By contrast, taking saw palmetto will help the prostate, but it won't correct the possibly hidden deficiencies of essential nutrients elsewhere in the body. (As far as we know, saw palmetto doesn't work by supplying zinc and/or essential fatty acids.)

One might ask: "So, why not use all 3, or even more?" In fact, this might be the best solution—"covering all the bases." Several widely available "prostate supplements" follow exactly this pattern, adding in other nutrients (glycine, alanine, and glutamic acid are often used) and botanicals such as *Pygeum africanum, Urtica dioica,* flower pollen, uva ursi, and beta-sitosterol—all of which are known to be helpful for the prostate. Using a combination supplement that contains all the useful ingredients also saves space on the kitchen shelf. It's what I often recommend. Whatever you do, if you have an enlarged prostate along with the usual symptoms, don't reach for that saw palmetto without picking up the zinc and essential fatty acids, too!

DR. GABY'S COMMENTARY

CONVENTIONAL TREATMENTS FOR enlarged prostate are expensive, and they can have unpleasant side effects. Fortunately, natural medicine offers a number of safe, effective, and inexpensive options for men with enlarged prostates.

Nutritional Supplements
Zinc and Essential Fatty Acids

SUPPLEMENTING with zinc and essential fatty acids has been helpful for many men with BPH. EFAs are found in large amounts in sunflower oil, safflower oil, flaxseed oil, and to a lesser extent in soybean and other oils. In a 1941 study, men who supplemented their diets with EFAs experienced an improvement in urinary symptoms and a reduction in the size of their prostate.[2] Zinc supplements have been shown to produce a similar effect in men with BPH.[3]

EFAs and zinc act on a group of hormone-like molecules known as prostaglandins—so named because they are found in abundance in the prostate gland. Certain prostaglandins are believed to help prevent the prostate gland from enlarging. However, with advancing age, the prostate appears to lose its ability to manufacture prostaglandins.[4] EFAs are the raw materials from which prostaglandins are produced, and zinc influences the formation of these compounds. Supplementing with these nutrients might be expected to help reverse the age-related decline in prostaglandin production, and thereby improve the health of the prostate gland.

Admittedly, the two studies supporting the use of EFAs and zinc are fairly weak. Neither of these studies included a control group, so the possibility of a placebo effect cannot be ruled out. In addition, neither of the studies was ever published in a medical journal. Nevertheless, our clinical observation supports the fact that men with BPH frequently improve when they take these nutrients, so we continue to recommend them.

The usual dosage of EFAs that we recommend is 1 tablespoon per day for the first 3 to 6 months, with a possible reduction in dosage as symptoms improve. To enhance absorption, EFAs should be taken with a meal that contains some fat. Flaxseed oil is an excellent source of omega-3 EFAs, whereas sunflower oil (cold-pressed) is a good source of omega-6 EFAs. To provide balance, it might be wise to alternate these two oils: flaxseed oil one day, sunflower oil the next. However, since the American diet is usually deficient in omega-3 EFAs relative to omega-6 EFAs, we often recommend flaxseed oil alone for the first several months.

EFA deficiency may be caused in part by excessive consumption of certain types of fat. For example, ingestion of *trans*-fatty acids (modified fats that are present in margarine and in foods containing partially hydrogenated vegetable oil) has been shown to promote EFA deficiency in animals.[5] In another study, when animals were fed an EFA-deficient diet, the signs of deficiency appeared sooner if the animals were also fed large amounts of cholesterol.[6] We also suspect that eating too many fried foods might contribute to EFA deficiency. When oils are heated to a high temperature during frying, some of the EFAs are destroyed, and some of the by-products that are created might conceivably interfere with EFA metabolism. Therefore, we advise most of our patients (and particularly those with BPH) to avoid margarine, partially hydrogenated vegetable oil, and fried foods and to keep high-cholesterol foods to a minimum.

With zinc, we usually start with a relatively large amount, such as 30 mg, 2 or 3 times per day. After several months, the dose is typically reduced to 30 mg, once or twice per day, depending on the patient's response. Well-absorbed forms of zinc include zinc picolinate and zinc citrate, whereas zinc sulfate and zinc oxide are not as well absorbed.

EFAs and zinc increase the body's need for vitamin E and copper, respectively. If you are taking extra EFAs and zinc, be sure to supplement your diet with vitamin E and copper. In general, 400 IU of vitamin E per day should be adequate to balance an EFA supplement. With a daily dose of 30 mg of zinc, we usually add 2 mg of copper. With 60 to 90 mg of zinc, we typically include 3 to 4 mg of copper. Both zinc and copper can cause nausea in some individuals. All of these nutrients work best and are most easily tolerated when taken with meals.

Amino-Acid Therapy

ANOTHER effective natural remedy for BPH is a combination of three amino acids: glycine, alanine, and glutamic acid. This group of amino acids is sold in health-food stores under the name Prostex. In a placebo-controlled study done more than 35 years ago, treatment with Prostex relieved urinary symptoms in as many as two-thirds of patients.[7] The dosage used in the study was 2 tablets 3 times per day initially, and 1 tablet 3 times per day for maintenance. Each tablet contains about 375 mg of the amino-acid mixture. These amino acids appear to work by reducing the amount of swelling in the prostate gland.

Herbal Supplements
Saw Palmetto

PROBABLY the most effective treatment for enlarged prostate is an extract of saw palmetto berries (*Serenoa repens*). This extract has an action similar to that of finasteride—it inhibits the build-up of dihydrotestosterone. In addition, saw palmetto exerts other effects on the metabolism of steroids (such as estrogen) that may be beneficial for prostate health. Researchers are not exactly sure how saw palmetto works. However, clinical studies suggest that this herbal remedy is a strong (and effective) medicine for men with an enlarged prostate. In one placebo-controlled study, as many as 89% of men taking saw palmetto improved

after 1 month of treatment.[8] These improvements included less need to get up at night to urinate and a more powerful urinary stream.

A review article published recently in the *Journal of the American Medical Association* concluded that saw palmetto works about as well as finasteride, but causes fewer side effects.[9] Unlike finasteride, saw palmetto does not cause impotence. On the contrary, this herb has a reputation for being somewhat of an aphrodisiac. Saw palmetto was listed in the *United States Pharmacopoeia* as early as 1905, and it has been used safely for many decades. In addition, saw palmetto is less expensive than finasteride—approximately $20 per month for the herb, compared with $60 per month for the prescription medication.

The dosage used in most of the clinical studies was 320 mg per day of a saw palmetto extract standardized to contain 85% fatty acids (a single daily dosage of 320 mg has been found to work as well as 160 mg twice a day). However, some of our patients have found that lower doses are effective for them (either initially or for maintenance). We usually advise our patients to start with 320 mg per day. After a few months, when symptoms have improved, the dosage can be reduced (perhaps by half), as long as the symptoms do not begin to return.

Other Herbal Remedies

SEVERAL other herbals have been shown to be effective for men suffering from BPH. *Pygeum africanum* is an evergreen tree indigenous to Africa. An extract from the bark of this tree has been used for more than 25 years in Europe and for about a decade in the United States. Numerous controlled studies have demonstrated that pygeum is effective in treating mild to moderate BPH.[10, 11] Published data on more than 2,200 patients have shown this extract to be almost entirely free of side effects. The usual dosage of pygeum is 100 to 200 mg per day of an extract standardized to contain 14% triterpenes.

A chemically defined mixture of phytosterols

(plant-derived sterols) has also been used to treat BPH. This mixture is often referred to as "beta-sitosterol" (the name of its main component), although other sterols are also present in the mixture. In a 6-month, double-blind study, beta-sitosterol (130 mg per day) was significantly more effective than a placebo, as determined by improvements in urinary symptoms, an increase in the maximum urinary flow rate, and a decrease in post-void residual urine volume.[12] Similar results were reported in another study.[13] Neither of these studies reported any serious side effects.

Another herb known as stinging nettles (*Urtica dioica*) has also been found to be helpful. Several studies show that this herb can increase urinary flow rate, decrease residual urine volume, and sometimes reduce the size of the prostate in men with BPH.[14]

The best-studied (and possibly most effective) herbal remedy is saw palmetto, which was discussed previously. Some of the prostate formulas on the market contain various combinations of the herbs that have been mentioned. Additional research is needed to determine whether such combinations are more effective than any one of the herbs alone. Until that research is done, we advise our patients to make sure that their herbal prostate formula contains a therapeutic dose of at least one of the herbs that are known to be effective (usually saw palmetto).

Conclusion

IN OUR EXPERIENCE, at least two-thirds of men with symptoms of BPH obtain gratifying and long-lasting relief by following a natural-treatment program. Equally important, the natural approach to prostate health is generally safe and is not particularly expensive. Of the approximately 350,000 prostate operations performed each year in the United States, many or even most could be avoided if physicians would routinely offer these simple and safe natural remedies.

Summary of Recommendations for Treating Benign Prostatic Hyperplasia

PRIMARY RECOMMENDATIONS:

- Diet: Avoid margarine, partially hydrogenated vegetable oils, and fried foods; keep high-cholesterol foods to a minimum.

- Zinc (picolinate or citrate), 30 mg, 2 to 3 times per day for 3 months, then 1 to 2 times per day, depending on response.

- Balance zinc with copper: 2 mg of copper per day with 30 mg of zinc per day; 3 to 4 mg of copper per day with 60 to 90 mg of zinc per day.

- Essential fatty acids, 1 tablespoon per day, alternating flaxseed oil and sunflower oil. Flaxseed oil alone may be preferable for the first few months for individuals who have been consuming a typical American diet.

- Balance essential fatty acids with vitamin E, 400 IU per day.

- Saw palmetto, 320 mg per day of an extract standardized to contain 85% fatty acids.

OTHER RECOMMENDATIONS:

- *Pygeum africanum,* 50 to 100 mg, 2 times per day, of an extract standardized to contain 14% triterpenes.

- Beta-sitosterol (phytosterols), 60 to 130 mg per day (in divided doses).

- Stinging nettles (*Urtica dioica*), dosage depending on the preparation used.

- Amino acids (glycine, alanine, and glutamic acid—brand name, Prostex), 2 tablets (approximately 375 mg per tablet) 3 times per day for 2 weeks, then 1 tablet 3 times per day for maintenance.

BIRTH DEFECTS

PREGNANCY IS AN *extremely delicate process. The embryo, which starts out as just a few cells, undergoes rapid growth and complex transformations. Pregnant mothers also experience dramatic changes in their physiology. Pregnancy is accompanied by increased nutritional requirements, since the mother must feed both herself and the rapidly growing fetus.*

If the fetus does not receive adequate amounts of all essential nutrients, structural abnormalities may occur. Birth defects can also result from excessive exposure to various toxic substances, including alcohol, certain prescription drugs, and large doses of vitamin A. The health of the pregnant mother also depends in large part on maintaining proper nutritional status.

DR. WRIGHT'S CASE STUDY

Diana and John Moscone came in together, looking quite serious. Diana spoke first. "My aunt had two children with spina bifida," she said. "They both died of complications of their problems. John and I've been married for 7 years, and we're ready to have our first child. We don't want to have that happen to our child! I read 2 or 3 years ago that the Public Health Service concluded that folic acid prevents birth defects. When I talked to my mother about it, she gave me a copy of your 1984 book. You had a whole chapter in there about preventing birth defects with folic acid!"

"Government 'authorities' are usually the last to know," I replied.

"Diana started taking folic acid right away," John said. "I did, too, I figured it wouldn't hurt me any. But then we decided to make an appointment, just in case there were other things we could do that the Public Health Service or FDA or whomever doesn't know yet."

"Or isn't telling us," Diana said.

"Glad you came in because there certainly are other things. Folic acid is very important, but we really need to start with basic diet first."

Diana and John looked at each other. "We knew this was coming," Diana said. "My mother raised me on Adelle Davis, and your articles from *Prevention* magazine. Ever since I left home, she's mostly kept quiet, but when I tell her I'm not feeling well, she always reminds me about whole foods and no sugar. . . ."

"And lately my mother's joined her," John added. "She just started on the natural-food thing three years ago, but she's a fast learner. When we visit them, my father is always grumbling about how there's no decent junk food in the house any more."

"Then you both know the basics," I said.

"Even if you haven't been applying them to your-selves, I'm glad you're going to give your children the best possible start. And of course, it'll do you some good, too.

"As your mothers say, whole, unprocessed foods are basic. Make sure you have plenty of vegetables and fruits. Sources of essential fatty acids—fish, unroasted nuts and seeds, salad oils . . . are important. Include egg yolks and soy lecithin—these are the only dietary sources of phospholipids, which are crucial to nerve-cell membranes. Animal proteins are OK, just don't make them the majority of your diets.

"If you buy anything in a package, read the label every time! Eliminate any chemical addi-tives—colorings, flavorings, preservatives, aspar-tame, any synthetic chemical. They're probably more dangerous to a developing infant than to anyone else. Use as many organic foods as you can; fortunately even supermarkets are carrying more of them. No sugar; raw, filtered honey or molasses are OK in small quantities. No refined-flour products, and watch out for hydrogenated or partially hydrogenated vegetable oils! They contain unnatural molecules that are likely to ac-cumulate in a baby's brain and nervous system."

Diana was taking notes. "We've started in this direction," she said. "Still a way to go, though."

I waited until she finished. "Once the diet's under control, the supplements will actually do more good," I said. "Folic acid is first. Please use 1 milligram—that's 1,000 micrograms—every day. Next, vitamin B_{12}, 500 micrograms daily. Last in this group, zinc, 30 milligrams daily. Use the picolinate form." I turned to John. "Please make sure you take this group, too."

"I will, but I thought it was more important for mothers."

"Folic acid, vitamin B_{12}, and zinc are all vital to DNA metabolism. DNA is what chromosomes are made of, and these nutrients help ensure nor-mal chromosome division, very important to developing babies. But sperm cells are very rapidly developing cells, too, and these 3 nutri-ents will likely lower the number of abnormal sperm. Less abnormal sperm, less chance of trou-ble from your side of things."

John thought for a moment. "Makes sense."

"It's wisest to 'back up' these nutrients with a good multiple vitamin-mineral. Since you're planning a pregnancy, make sure there are no more than 10,000 IU of vitamin A in any multiple."

"We're already doing that, plus vitamin E, 400 IU per day, and 1 gram of vitamin C twice daily," Diana said. "Mothers."

"Not just your mothers," I said. "Look what you're doing for your own baby before it's even here."

"I'm sure it's worth it," John said.

"Once you're pregnant, Diana will need to add extra calcium and magnesium, and possibly iron."

"That's on Mom's list, too!"

DR. GABY'S COMMENTARY

Nutritional Considerations

STUDIES IN ANIMALS have shown that many different nutrients play a role in normal fetal development. For example, deficiencies of vitamin B_6,[1] magnesium,[2] zinc,[3] pantothenic acid,[4] or folic acid[5] have all been shown to result in birth defects. It is likely that many other nutrients are also important. Pregnant women should therefore emphasize foods that are rich in vitamins, miner-als, and essential fatty acids, such as whole grains, fresh fruits and vegetables, nuts and seeds, and legumes. Protein is also very important; the best sources are meat, chicken, fish, and eggs. Women who are vegetarians must carefully combine their grains and beans in order to achieve adequate protein intake. Even with proper food combining, some vegetarian women may need a protein supplement. To assure adequate intake of vitamins and minerals, a well-formulated prenatal supplement should be used.

Folic acid is of particular importance. This B-vitamin has been shown to prevent the occurrence of neural tube defects (NTDs). The neural tube is the portion of the fetus that develops into the brain and spinal cord. Neural tube defects are among the most common birth defects, and they can result in severe disability or death. In the early 1980s, British doctors performed a double-blind study on women who had previously given birth to an infant with a neural tube defect. In the study, 60 such women were asked to take a folic-acid supplement, and 44 women followed that advice. Another 51 women received a placebo. There were no NTD recurrences among the 44 mothers who took folic acid, 2 recurrences among the 16 women who refused to take the vitamin, and 4 recurrences among the 51 women given a placebo. The reduction in NTD incidence due to folic acid was statistically significant.[6] In a more recent study, supplementing with folic acid also prevented NTDs in women who had no prior history of the problem.[7]

Because of these findings, the United States Public Health Service issued the following policy statement regarding folic acid: "All women of child-bearing age in the United States who are capable of becoming pregnant should consume 0.4 mg of folic acid per day for the purpose of reducing their risk of having a pregnancy affected with spina bifida or other NTD's [neural tube defects]."

In other studies, blood levels of vitamin B12[8] and zinc[9] were significantly lower in mothers who gave birth to a baby with an NTD, compared with the levels in women who gave birth to a healthy baby.

Vitamin A: What Level is Safe?

ONE NUTRIENT THAT might actually cause birth defects is vitamin A. According to a recent study, pregnant women who took supplements containing more than 10,000 IU of vitamin A per day had an increased risk of delivering a baby with defects such as cleft lip, cleft palate, or abnormalities of the heart.[10] Only vitamin A in supplement form (as opposed to vitamin A in the diet) was associated with an increased risk (suggesting, perhaps, that the increased risk may have resulted from some other characteristic of supplement takers, rather than from the vitamin A per se). In 2 other studies, women who took more than 10,000 IU of vitamin A per day had a lower risk of delivering a baby with one of these birth defects, compared with women who took no vitamin A supplement[11] or less than 5,000 IU per day.[12]

How do we resolve these contradictory studies? There is no question that very large doses of vitamin A can cause birth defects; that has been demonstrated repeatedly in animal studies. However, we do not know what is the optimal amount of vitamin A for pregnant women; nor do we know what is the maximum safe level. Nearly everyone agrees that 10,000 IU per day is safe. If there is a medical reason to take larger amounts of vitamin A during pregnancy, the risks should be carefully weighed against the benefits. It may be appropriate, for example, for pregnant women who are infected with the HIV virus to take extra vitamin A (perhaps 25,000 IU per day). That is because low levels of vitamin A, which are common in HIV-infected women,[13] are associated with an increased risk of transmitting HIV to the infant.[14] When in doubt, one can measure the vitamin A level in the blood. In addition, it may be possible to reduce the risk of vitamin A toxicity by taking other nutrients. For example, supplementing pregnant rats with B-vitamins greatly reduced the capacity of large doses of vitamin A to cause birth defects.[15]

Summary of Recommendations for Preventing Birth Defects

- Avoid nutrient-depleted foods, such as refined sugar and other refined carbohydrates, processed foods, and alcohol.

- Emphasize nutrient-dense foods such as whole grains, fruits, vegetables, nuts, and seeds.

- Consume eggs and other animal proteins in moderation.

- Add a high-potency multiple vitamin/mineral that contains at least 0.4 mg of folic acid, 50 mcg of vitamin B_{12}, and 15 mg of zinc.

- Do not consume more than 10,000 IU of supplemental vitamin A per day without medical supervision.

BURSITIS

A BURSA IS *a fluid-filled cavity situated near tendons, joints, and bone in areas where friction would normally develop. The numerous bursae in the body reduce friction and enhance the mobility of joints and tendons. When a bursa becomes inflamed, it is called bursitis. The most common type of bursitis occurs in the shoulder around the deltoid muscle, and is referred to as subdeltoid or subacromial bursitis. Conventional treatment for bursitis includes rest, physical therapy, anti-inflammatory drugs, and in some cases injection of cortisone-like drugs into the bursa.*

DR. WRIGHT'S CASE STUDY

"It's my shoulder," George Orloff said. "It's hurting pretty bad again, especially if I try to move it. I've been getting bursitis on and off for years, and I'm getting very tired of it. I thought I'd give this natural-medicine thing a try."

"How long have you had bursitis?"

"Nearly 10 years. First time, I was 63. Doctor gave me a cortisone shot, it went away, but came back again in a couple of months. Doctor gave me another cortisone shot, and told me I'd better not have any more because too many cortisone shots weren't good for me."

"Especially when you likely weren't getting cortisone . . ."

He looked surprised. "I was told it was—and some of my friends have had cortisone shots for bursitis, too."

"Real or identical-to-natural cortisone has rarely been injected since the early 1950s. Since then it's artificial, patentable, cortisone-like molecules such as triamcinolone or dexamethosone,

considerably more powerful than natural cortisone and which can cause much more damage. Unfortunately, doctors and pharmacists have inaccurately called them cortisone, giving real cortisone an unnecessarily bad reputation . . . but that's not why you came in. Sorry. So after your second injection, then what?"

"Luckily, I didn't have any more attacks for about 2 or 3 years. The next time it wasn't too bad, so I just loaded up on aspirin for a couple weeks. I've taken aspirin or some prescription anti-inflammatory whenever it hit ever since. The last couple years that hasn't been working very well—like this time. So I thought I'd try here."

"Do you get much gas or indigestion?"

He frowned. "Yes, but . . . what's that got to do with bursitis?"

"Perhaps quite a bit. Are you less energetic than you think you should be?"

"That's what my wife says, but I'm 73, lots of people my age slow down, and get indigestion."

I smiled. "True. But let's see what we can do about it all."

"Let's work on the bursitis first, OK?"

"Of course, but it's all part of the same problem."

We covered the rest of his health history, and a physical exam. He was acutely sore when pressed at the point of the shoulder on the right, and couldn't raise his arm to level with the shoulder. It hurt too much.

"Well, what'll I do? Is there a natural pain reliever for bursitis?"

"Not really a pain reliever, but something that almost always works. The nurse will teach you how to give yourself vitamin B_{12} injections."

"Vitamin B_{12} injections? What are those supposed to do?"

"Relieve your bursitis."

"Vitamin B_{12}?"

"Yes. Works nearly every time. Dr. Klemes of New York City reported on it in the late 1950s."

"1950s? If it works that well, why didn't I get it in the 1970s and '80s?"

"Even in 1996, doctors don't read as much about natural treatments as they might. And it isn't patentable. But don't worry, I've asked dozens of people to use it, and so far it's worked every time. Please inject 1 cc (1,000 micrograms) of vitamin B_{12} daily."

"It's injected into my shoulder?" Mr. Orloff asked.

"No—into the side of your upper leg. The nurse will show you how. Then for added insurance, we'll have you rub DMSO on your shoulder. DMSO reduces inflammation and speeds healing."

"DMSO? My vet told me to use DMSO on my dog."

"Works just fine on people, too. Helps reduce inflammation, swelling, and accompanying pain. Rub a 50%-DMSO solution over the sore area several times daily. And make an appointment for a stomach-acid test."

"Doc, I've heard some weird stuff today—vitamin B_{12} for bursitis, DMSO like I use on my dog, but a stomach-acid test?"

"Every one of those dozens of people whose bursitis got better with vitamin B_{12} has had a significant impairment of stomach function. Many have no useful function at all. That's at least partly where your gas and indigestion are coming from—but more importantly, you've likely been absorbing sub-normal quantities of many nutrients including vitamin B_{12} for at least the 10 years you've had bursitis. No wonder your energy is low. Actually, I'm surprised more hasn't gone wrong by now."

With daily vitamin B_{12} injections, Mr. Orloff's bursitis pain was substantially less within 3 days and gone in 10 days. Since his stomach-function test was substantially abnormal, he was advised to continue vitamin B_{12} injections (with folic acid) each week. It's been 7 years, and he hasn't had a bursitis attack since. As a "bonus," the correction of his digestive problem has eliminated his indigestion and gas, and his energy level has increased considerably.

DR. GABY'S COMMENTARY

NATURAL MEDICINE OFFERS two simple and effective treatments for bursitis. Both treatments should only be undertaken in consultation with a doctor who is knowledgeable about natural medicine.

Vitamin B_{12}

IN 1957, DR. I.S. Klemes reported that vitamin B_{12} was an effective treatment for bursitis. He gave intramuscular injections (not into the bursa) of vitamin B_{12} to 40 patients with acute bursitis (36 subdeltoid bursitis, 3 of the hip, and 1 of the elbow). The dosage was as follows: 1,000 mcg per day for 7 to 10 days, then 3 times a week for 2 to 3 weeks, then once or twice a week for 2 to 3 weeks. The frequency of injections was adjusted according to the degree of improvement. Nearly all of the patients improved after receiving these injections. Reduction of pain and other symptoms occurred rapidly, and patients often experienced complete relief within several days. In cases where calcium deposits were present, follow-up X-rays showed a considerable reduction in the amount of calcification, presumably indicating a reversal of the disease process.[1]

Although this study dealt only with acute bursitis (the kind that flares up and then goes away), we have found that chronic bursitis (the kind that persists for a long period of time) often responds as well as, or better than, the acute cases. No one knows how vitamin B_{12} works for bursitis. However, the frequency of the injections appears to be more important than the amount given. For example, 1,000 mcg injected daily is more effective than 3,000 mcg given every third day.

DMSO

DIMETHYLSULFOXIDE (DMSO) is a unique compound extracted from wood pulp. When applied to the skin, it penetrates into the deeper tissues, where it exerts potent anti-inflammatory effects and promotes tissue healing. A twice-daily application of a 50 to 70% solution of DMSO for a few weeks over the area of inflammation often provides long-lasting relief of acute or chronic bursitis.

Individuals must take several precautions when using DMSO. First, because it is a solvent and penetrates the skin, DMSO can carry dirt or microbes through the skin into the bloodstream. It is therefore important to clean the applying hand and the application site thoroughly with soap and water before administering DMSO. Additionally, this compound can cause irritation or mild burning of the skin, similar to a "sunburn" sensation. This effect is concentration-related; most people who experience a problem with a 70% solution can tolerate a 50% solution. DMSO is sold as a 99% solution, which must be diluted to 50 to 70% by adding water. This dilution should be performed carefully, since the addition of water to DMSO causes the solution to become warm or hot for several minutes. Although DMSO can be obtained without a prescription, over-the-counter products may contain impurities (which could conceivably be carried into the bloodstream). We advise our patients to obtain DMSO from a compounding pharmacist. DMSO has an odor similar to that of garlic. Several minutes after applying the compound, individuals may notice a garlic taste in the mouth. If you wish to use DMSO, we recommend that you seek the advice of a physician knowledgeable in its use.

Summary of Recommendations for Treating Bursitis (under medical supervision)

- Vitamin B_{12} injections.
- Dimethylsulfoxide (DMSO), 50 to 70% solution, applied topically to affected area, 2 to 3 times a day for 1 to 3 weeks.

APHTHOUS ULCERS *(commonly known as canker sores) are small lesions that occur on the mucous membranes of the mouth, lips, or tongue. These ulcers typically last several days to two weeks and are extremely painful. Aphthous ulcers may recur frequently; indeed, in some cases, new lesions continue to appear even before the old ones have had a chance to heal.*

The cause of aphthous ulcers is not known, although allergy or autoimmunity is thought to be involved. Herpes viruses have been isolated from certain types of mouth ulcers, but the consensus is that aphthous ulcers are not caused by a virus.

Local anesthetics such as Xylocaine can be applied to the ulcers to relieve the pain. However, the anesthetic has to be applied repeatedly, since its effect wears off rapidly. Drugs that suppress the immune system are also helpful in some cases. However, because of their potential to cause side effects, these drugs are reserved for the most severe cases. In conventional medicine, recurrent aphthous ulceration (RAU) is often a frustrating condition, both for the patient and the doctor.

DR. WRIGHT'S CASE STUDY

"Remember me?" Linda Ebersole asked. "I was here last year with Emily. Her eczema's all gone, so I decided to come in for myself this time. I get these canker sores . . ."

"You mentioned that when you were here with Emily, didn't you?"

"Yes, but I thought with all the allergy work we'd have to do for Emily . . ."

"Like mother, like daughter. Now it's your turn to work on allergies."

"Me?"

"Sure. Food allergies are frequently a cause of recurrent canker sores. I assume yours are recurrent, or you wouldn't be here."

"Recurrent isn't the word for it. They're more like continuous. There's hardly a time I don't have one or several."

"How long have you been getting canker sores?"

"Since my late teens, and I'm 29 now. Before Emily was born, they'd come and go—sometimes a lot, sometimes not for months. But since she was born, they haven't quit! That's over 4 years with a sore mouth."

"Have you quit milk and dairy along with Emily?"

"I got all the milk out of the house, and the cheese, too, but. . . ." She looked a little embarrassed, "I have this weakness for yogurt. I eat that nearly every day. But I didn't realize food allergies could cause canker sores."

"They do. But there are other factors, too.

Once you've been tested for food allergy, please see our nutritionist for an allergy-avoidance diet of your own. We'll work on desensitization, too, but it frequently takes longer for adults to respond than children."

"As long as it works sooner or later. I wouldn't like several years of diet restriction."

Mrs. Ebersole had a total of 7 obvious open canker sores on her gums and inside her cheeks. We finished checking things over and went back to my office.

"Have you put anything on those canker sores?" I asked.

"They've given me several things, but only the pain-killer ointment does anything."

I started making a list for her. "Until you get your allergies under control, use a half-and-half mixture of preservative-free zinc oxide and vitamin E oil from capsules. Rub the mixture into each sore as soon as it occurs. But avoiding and desensitizing allergies will help the most in the long run. In addition to working on your allergies, there are several supplements you should use. First, zinc again . . ."

"For me, too? You gave that to my daughter for her eczema."

"You too. Zinc promotes healing of ulcerations anywhere, including these. Thirty milligrams of zinc twice daily until you're better for several months. Use zinc picolinate; it assimilates well."

"I didn't expect my problems would have the same solutions as my daughter's."

"There are a lot of parallels."

"What else do I need?"

"Remember we'll need to check copper levels. When you take zinc, it's important to make sure it's 'in balance' with copper. Also, *Lactobacillus acidophilus,* a "friendly" bacteria. Years ago, Harvard researchers reported that use of acidophilus would promote rapid resolution of canker sores."

She shook her head. "Another interesting coincidence; you recommended the same treatment for my daughter."

"Now, some items that just apply to you. Let's check your serum ferritin. Many folks with canker sores need more iron, and the 'ferritin' test helps let us know. Also, since they're harmless, start in with folic-acid drops—a total of 10 milligrams daily, and vitamin B_{12} drops, a total of 5,000 micrograms daily. Mix them together in lukewarm or cool water, swish them around your mouth awhile, and swallow. Studies have shown both B_{12} and folic acid are helpful in eliminating canker sores."

"What's with the 'swish and swallow?'"

"Folic acid is absorbed especially well into oral tissues, which is right where it's needed in canker sores. It's also very helpful systemically."

"Is that all?"

"There's one other problem common to both eczema and canker sores that we may need to check into if you don't clear up entirely."

"Wait—I think I remember—is that about poor stomach function?"

"You have a good memory! It's been my observation that any condition which gets better with iron, folic acid, and vitamin B_{12} has a higher association with stomach malfunction, too, since stomach acid is required for the absorption of each of these nutrients."

"Sort of reasoning backward from effective treatment to possible problem leading to the need for the treatment."

"Right."

"And I should remember to supplement my good diet with a broad-spectrum multiple vitamin-mineral."

"Right again."

Her canker sores responded quickly, clearing in 3 months with allergy elimination, desensitization, zinc, iron, folic acid, vitamin B_{12}, and *Lactobacillus acidophilus,* but she still has one very occasionally when "I'm not quite as careful with my diet as I am with Emily's."

DR. GABY'S COMMENTARY

FORTUNATELY, THE SUCCESS rate for treating RAU using natural medicine is considerable. We have found that a combination of dietary modifications and nutritional supplements is helpful for the majority of individuals with RAU, and in many of these patients, the problem disappears completely.

Dietary Considerations

THE IMPORTANCE OF dietary factors in preventing canker sores has been shown in several studies. In one study, 12 patients with RAU went on a diet that eliminated common allergens. After 6 to 8 weeks on the diet, 4 patients were entirely symptom-free and 1 had marked improvement. By retesting foods individually, 4 of the 5 patients who improved were able to identify the foods that were causing their ulcers.[1]

In another study, 20 patients with RAU eliminated all of the gluten (wheat, oats, barley, and rye) from their diet. In 5 (25%) of the patients, the ulcers disappeared completely. In each of these 5 cases, retesting of gluten confirmed its causative role.[2] In view of the fact that these patients had been suffering from RAU for an average of more than 11 years, the results with the gluten-free diet were especially gratifying.

In our experience, the most common foods that trigger canker sores are wheat, citrus fruits, and chocolate. However, many other foods may also be involved, depending on the individual's particular sensitivities. One of the elimination diets I have used in my practice is presented in appendix A. Some doctors use other tests for allergy and sensitivity, as well as desensitization techniques. The reliability and effectiveness of some of these methods is controversial. (See chapter 3 for additional discussion.)

Nutritional Supplements
Zinc

HEALING of many different types of ulcers, including RAU, has been shown to be promoted by zinc. In one study, 17 patients with RAU received 50 mg of zinc per day. If no improvement occurred after 3 weeks, the dose was increased to 50 mg, 3 times a day. Of those 17 patients, 12 (71%) reported a 50 to 100% reduction in the number of ulcers. Individuals with low levels of zinc in their blood were more likely to respond to zinc supplements than were patients with higher zinc levels.[3]

Other Nutrients

DEFICIENCIES of one or more of the following—thiamin, riboflavin, vitamin B_6, folic acid, vitamin B_{12}, and iron—have been found in some individuals with RAU.[4,5] In one report, as many as 17%, 62%, and 44%, of patients with RAU were deficient in iron, folic acid, and vitamin B_{12}, respectively.[6] Like zinc, some of these nutrients play a role in the healing process. In these studies, supplementing with the nutrients that were in short supply frequently enhanced healing and prevented recurrences of RAU.

Using "Friendly" Bacteria

LACTOBACILLI, the bacteria used to make yogurt, are known to have a number of health-promoting effects. In one study, individuals with RAU chewed and swallowed 2 to 4 tablets of a lactobacillus product, 3 times a day for 2 to 3 days. In a large proportion of these cases, the soreness was relieved within 48 hours, and the lesions healed more rapidly than usual.[7]

Herbal Supplements
Licorice Extract

HERBALISTS have long known that licorice can promote the healing of ulcers and other conditions of the oral cavity. However, the use of licorice as a medicinal agent has been limited by concerns about potential side effects. Licorice contains a compound called glycyrrhizin, which has properties similar to those of cortisone. In large doses, glycyrrhizin can cause high blood pressure, potassium deficiency, and heart problems. Fortunately, scientists discovered a way to remove about 97% of the glycyrrhizin from licorice, without destroying its tissue-healing effects. This extract, known as deglycyrrhizinated licorice (DGL), has been found to be a safe and effective treatment for both peptic ulcers (see the chapter on peptic ulcer) and aphthous ulcers. In one study, 20 patients with an acute aphthous ulcer gargled 4 times a day for 7 days with 200 mg of powdered DGL dissolved in about 6 ounces of water. Three-quarters of the patients experienced a 50 to 75% reduction in pain within 24 hours of starting treatment, with complete healing by the third day.[8]

Check Your Toothpaste

SODIUM LAURYL SULFATE, a detergent used in many brands of toothpaste, can strip away the protective coating that lines the mouth, rendering the area more susceptible to ulceration. When individuals with RAU changed to a toothpaste that did not contain sodium lauryl sulfate, the number of aphthous ulcers fell by 64%.[9]

Summary of Recommendations for Treating Canker Sores (Aphthous Ulcers)

PRIMARY RECOMMENDATIONS:

- Work with food allergies.
- Avoid toothpastes that contain sodium lauryl sulfate.
- Take a high-potency multiple vitamin/mineral.

OTHER RECOMMENDATIONS:

- Additional vitamin B-complex, zinc, and/or iron in selected cases.
- For treatment of active lesions: *Lactobacillus acidophilus*, and deglycyrrhizinated licorice (DGL), 200 mg in 6 ounces of water. Use as mouth-rinse/gargle, 4 times a day for up to 7 days.

MANY PEOPLE DO *not appreciate the fact that cholesterol is essential for life. This steroid compound contributes to the structural integrity of cell membranes and serves as a precursor for the synthesis of steroid hormones such as cortisol, DHEA, estrogen, testosterone, and progesterone. If the diet does not contain any cholesterol, then the liver manufactures some and supplies it to the rest of the body. However, as with other essential biochemicals (such as glucose), too much can be a bad thing. It is well known that high serum-cholesterol concentrations are associated with an increased risk of developing cardiovascular disease.*

Not all forms of cholesterol in the bloodstream are "bad." Serum cholesterol can be divided into several subgroups, including low-density lipoprotein (LDL) cholesterol (which correlates with increased risk of heart disease) and high-density lipoprotein (HDL) cholesterol (which correlates with decreased risk). Because of these associations, doctors look for ways to reduce total- and LDL-cholesterol levels, while increasing HDL cholesterol.

Animal studies suggest that cholesterol itself is actually a relatively benign molecule, but oxidized cholesterol is extremely toxic to blood vessels.[1] Since the cholesterol that circulates in the bloodstream is constantly in contact with oxygen, there is a tendency for cholesterol to undergo spontaneous oxidation. Therefore, the main problem with high serum cholesterol may be that more of it is available to be converted to blood-vessel-damaging cholesterol oxides. If that is the case, then supplementing with anti-oxidants (such as vitamin E, vitamin C, selenium, and carotenoids) might at least partially counteract the adverse effects of elevated serum cholesterol by inhibiting the conversion of cholesterol to cholesterol oxides. That possibility was supported by a study of 16 European populations, in which blood levels of vitamin E were more closely related to heart-disease risk than was serum cholesterol.[2] In addition, the protective effect of fruits and vegetables against heart disease may be attributable in part to the wide array of antioxidant "phytochemicals" that are found in these foods.

DR. WRIGHT'S CASE STUDY

"The doctor I saw for my check-up wants me to take a cholesterol-lowering drug . . ." David MacElroy began.

"And his wife won't let him!" Wendy MacElroy finished. "He finally took a step to check on and protect his health, and I won't let him take that—poison—as a result."

"C'mon, Wendy, it's not poison, it's a medicine," David said.

"I've read the complete drug description in the PDR—the Physicians' Desk Reference—and it certainly is," Wendy replied. "It might lower your risk of dying from cholesterol-related illness, but it raises your risk of dying of something else. It's the same for all those 'cholesterol' drugs. And I know that changing what you eat and taking the right vitamins can control your cholesterol and help you be healthier and probably live longer, too!"

"Don't get excited, that's why I'm here." He turned toward me. "I admit that I've been a 'junk fooder' all my life. Wendy's tried to raise our kids right on really good food, and I haven't been much of a help or a very good example. But I turned 40 this year, and I made up my mind it's time to reform. I haven't told you yet that my father died of a heart attack at 56, and his father died the same way at 61. I figure I can only push it so far."

"Likely you're right. How high was your cholesterol?"

"It was 322."

"And your HDL-cholesterol—the 'good' cholesterol?"

"Thirty-four," Wendy said. "Definitely high risk. I have to give Dave some credit—even before he had his cholesterol checked; I guess it was right after his 40th birthday—I noticed he was cutting back on the hamburgers and grease when we're out."

"Even I know that 'low fat' is the way to go to lower cholesterol, isn't it?"

"Most of the time, but not always. Is there any diabetes in your family?"

"I don't think so. Neither of my parents, or any of my grandparents, as far as I know. Wendy?"

"Don't know why it's always us women who're supposed to know these things," she smiled. "But we do. No one in David's family can think of anyone who's had diabetes." She paused. "Why does that make any difference?"

"Individuals with diabetes in their families frequently have their cholesterol levels—and triglycerides as well—raised mostly by sugar, refined carbohydrate, and carbohydrate in general in the diet, and less by dietary fat."

"Really? Maybe that's why my friend Molly

has been so frustrated with her cholesterol. It just won't come to normal, and she's been the strictest low-fat person I know for several years. But her mom has 'maturity' diabetes . . . but back to Dave. He should be on low-fat, right?"

"Sounds like that's right for him."

"OK, so I'll ease back on beef and pork, eliminate the eggs and butter, use margarine and low-fat milk, cut way back on ice cream, eat more chicken and turkey—is that the general idea?"

"We'd better review 'good' fats and 'bad' fats and a few related topics. Generally speaking, the 'bad' fats—the ones we want to reduce—are the saturated fats, and the 'good' fats are the unsaturated fats. You're right about beef and pork—their fat content is all 'saturated', so cutting these foods back is wise. Actually, the fats in chicken and turkey are mostly saturated, too, there's just less of it. But there's one 'animal protein' that contains almost entirely 'good', unsaturated fats . . ."

"That's fish, isn't it?" Wendy asked.
"Yes."

"Well, Dave likes salmon and halibut . . ."

"And marlin and swordfish and mahi and nearly any fish but cod," David said. "It's just hard to find those in a 'fast-food' format—but I like 'em, and I'll do it, as long as I can have some chicken and turkey, too."

"No problem. Now, about margarine, butter, milk, and other dairy, and eggs. First, margarine is worse for us than butter. It does contain unsaturated fats, but some of them are *trans*-fatty acids, which are probably worse than eating saturated fat itself. If you must use one or the other, butter's better, but mostly avoid it. For home use, you could make 'better butter', a mixture of butter, beneficial oils, and lecithin, first suggested by Adelle Davis . . ."

"My mother has all her books, I'll look it up!" Wendy exclaimed.

"There's not much to say about milk, except that it belongs in little cows and not in little people—or big ones for that matter. There's even good reason to suspect that homogenized milk is a cause of atherosclerosis, independent of its fat content. Stop milk—just say no!"

Dave looked bothered. "What about cheese and ice cream?"

"Dave really likes ice cream," Wendy said.

"That part's easy. There are terrific alternative products. We've put Rice Dream, Ice Bean, and similar products to the 'children's party' test, and they always disappear completely."

"That's the best test there is," Wendy agreed. "Where do we get them? And what about cheeses?"

"Natural-food stores. And once Dave's cholesterol is under control, a little cheese occasionally will likely be tolerable. Now, about those eggs—eat 'em!"

David looked puzzled. "Why's that? I thought eggs were full of saturated fat and cholesterol."

"The 'average' egg has approximately 300 milligrams of cholesterol, but more importantly, the 'average' egg contains approximately 1,500 milligrams of phospholipids. It's a bit technical, but those phospholipids more than offset any possible adverse effects of egg cholesterol. Even more importantly, phospholipids have a unique function in keeping brain-cell membranes healthy. Eggs and soy are the only dietary sources of phospholipids. Since most of us still don't eat soy products—although for you it actually would be a good idea, since soy protein has been shown to lower serum cholesterol—if we eliminate eggs, we're eliminating the only dietary source of nutrients crucial to brain cells."

"I need all the brain protection I can get," David said.

"Me too! I never recommend eliminating eggs except as a 'last resort.'"

Wendy reviewed her notes. "Let's see—much more fish, chicken, turkey, less beef and pork, add some soy protein, no milk or dairy except maybe a little cheese later on, eat those eggs . . . and you didn't mention it yet, but on the 'positive' side, lots of vegetables, fruits, and whole grains—and eliminate sugar, white flour, and food chemicals."

"Excellent summary, and you're right, I should have emphasized the vegetables, fruits, and whole grains first. I also should mention other foods which lower cholesterol. In addition to soy protein, garlic, onions, oat bran, carrots, and alfalfa sprouts are all beneficial."

"Now, what about supplements?"

"There are so many vitamins, minerals, and botanicals known to lower serum cholesterol that drugs are virtually never a necessity. Let's see, there's inositol hexanicotinate, lecithin, pantethine, L-carnitine, beta-sitosterol, calcium, and chromium. Then, to raise HDL cholesterol, the 'good' cholesterol, there's magnesium, vitamin C, chromium, lecithin (or phosphatidylcholine), and vitamin E. Then there are botanicals, including gugulipid, garlic oil, ginger, pectin, fenugreek powder, reishi mushroom, silymarin, turmeric, *Garcinia camboga,* artichoke . . ."

"Whoa," David exclaimed. "If you or Wendy think I'm going to take all that stuff . . ."

"No, of course not. Just illustrating why drugs are hardly ever necessary. We'll keep it a lot simpler. Besides, if you're serious about reforming your diet . . ."

"I am, I am. I've passed the big 4-0. I'm not a kid anymore."

"Then supplementation will be less necessary. So: please start with vitamin E—the 'mixed tocopherol' type—400 IU daily. There are several studies show that vitamin E lowers heart-attack risk by a very significant percent."

"Next, inositol hexanicotinate, 600 milligrams, twice daily. It's helpful for lowering serum cholesterol, and a much safer form of niacin when higher quantities are necessary."

"Third, vitamin C. For now, please use 2 grams twice daily. Also, please get a high-potency multiple vitamin/mineral with at least 200 micrograms of chromium and 300 to 400 milligrams of magnesium. You may need to get a separate multiple mineral if you can't find those in a vitamin-mineral combination. Lastly, lecithin. Remember those phospholipids for brain cells?

Besides eggs, soy lecithin is the only other diet source. Might as well protect those brain cells and increase your HDL cholesterol with the same item. Please obtain the 19-grain capsules, and for now, take 2 twice daily."

"That's it?" Wendy asked.

"Along with real diet change, that should do the job. If not . . ."

"I know, there are 50 million more supplements I could take," Dave said.

After 6 months, Dave's total cholesterol was down to 237 mg/dl, and his HDL cholesterol had risen to 41 mg/dl. At the end of a year, his numbers were 188 and 46, respectively, and his risk of following his father and grandfather to an early cardiac death was substantially reduced.

DR. GABY'S COMMENTARY

WHILE LOWERING ELEVATED serum cholesterol seems like a good idea, the outcome (in terms of heart disease and mortality) depends on how you do it. In one study, men with heart disease were assigned to receive either no dietary advice (control group) or a low-fat diet supplemented with unsaturated fat (corn oil). Although treatment with corn oil reduced serum cholesterol, it also nearly doubled the incidence of heart attacks, compared with the control group.[3] This adverse effect of corn oil may have resulted from a depletion of vitamin E (unsaturated fats increase vitamin E requirements). Another possibility is that ingesting large amounts of corn oil (about 4 tablespoons per day in this study) upset the balance between omega-3 and omega-6 fatty acids. These two types of essential fatty acids, which are classified according to their chemical structure, are each important for cardiovascular health. However, the typical Western diet already appears to contain too many omega-6 fatty acids (found in corn oil, sunflower oil, and safflower oil) relative to the amount of omega-3 fatty acids (found in fish oil, flaxseed oil and, to a lesser extent, soybean oil). Creating a further imbalance by taking a corn-oil supplement might cause a relative deficiency of omega-3 fatty acids, which could adversely affect the heart.

Studies using cholesterol-lowering drugs have also produced conflicting results. For example, long-term treatment with clofibrate did not im-prove coronary mortality and actually increased the death rate from other causes. Administering cholestyramine (Questran) did reduce heart-disease deaths, but did not significantly reduce total mortality, because deaths from other causes were increased. The newer "statin" drugs (such as pravastatin and simvastatin) have produced more encouraging results—reducing both coronary and total mortality. However, the long-term safety of these drugs has not been demonstrated, and there is concern that they may cause cancer.[4]

While the evidence indicates that most of us should aim for a serum cholesterol level near the lower end of the normal range (such as 150 to 180 mg/dl), we should seek to attain these levels in ways that do not cause adverse effects. Fortunately, there are a number of safe, natural ways to lower total and LDL cholesterol and/or raise HDL cholesterol, through both diet and natural treatments.

Dietary Considerations
Foods to Eat, Foods to Avoid

A CHOLESTEROL-lowering diet should be low in total fat and refined sugar (refined sugar lowers HDL cholesterol in some individuals).[5] Specific foods that have been shown to reduce serum cholesterol include soy products, carrots, oat bran, yogurt, walnuts, garlic, and onions. High-fiber foods (such as whole grains, legumes, fruits, and vegetables) may also help lower cholesterol levels. In one study, the cholesterol-lowering effect of a diet high in fruits, vegetables, and nuts was 34 to 49% greater than what would have been predicted from the fat content of the diet.[6] Boiled (unfiltered) coffee contains at least two compounds that raise serum cholesterol, whereas filtered coffee has little or no effect on cholesterol levels. Ingesting one or two alcoholic beverages per day may increase HDL cholesterol; however, there is still no firm proof that drinking alcohol prevents heart disease. Although eggs contain a large amount of cholesterol, eating eggs does not seem to raise serum cholesterol levels in most people.[7]

Role of Food Allergies

FOOD allergy may also be a cause of elevated serum cholesterol. In one study, 7 patients with multiple food allergies followed a diet in which most of the calories came from beef fat. The patients were also given various nutritional supplements. Although such a diet would normally have been expected to increase serum cholesterol, the average level actually fell from 263 to 189 mg/dl.[8] Evidently, eliminating the biochemical stresses associated with repeated allergic reactions helped lower serum cholesterol, although the nutritional supplements may have had an effect, as well.

Nutritional Supplements
Pantethine

A NATURALLY occurring derivative of the B-vitamin pantothenic acid, pantethine plays a role in the metabolism of fat and cholesterol. Several studies have shown that pantethine can reduce serum cholesterol levels by about 10 to 20%, while increasing HDL cholesterol by 10% to as much as 38%.[9, 10, 11, 12] These results are similar to those seen with many cholesterol-lowering drugs. Pantethine has not been reported to cause any significant side effects, even with long-term use. Unlike pantethine, pantothenic acid does not affect serum cholesterol levels.

Niacin and Chromium

NIACIN (nicotinic acid) is recognized in conventional medicine as an effective cholesterol-lowering vitamin. Large doses (such as 3 grams per day) can substantially reduce cholesterol levels and may increase HDL cholesterol; however, at those doses, niacin sometimes puts stress on the liver or causes other side effects. Smaller amounts (such as 1,300 mg per day) have been shown to reduce serum cholesterol by an average of 11%.[13] Even lower doses of niacin can reduce serum cholesterol if chromium is taken at the same time. In one report, a daily dose of 100 mg of niacin and 200 mcg of chromium reduced serum cholesterol from 399 to 280 mg/dl in one patient and from 337 to 260 mg/dl in another.[14] This combination treatment probably works by promoting the production of glucose-tolerance factor, a molecule that enhances the action of insulin. Unlike niacin, niacinamide does not decrease serum cholesterol.

Inositol hexanicotinate, a compound that consists of niacin plus the B-vitamin inositol, can be used as an alternative to niacin. Inositol hexanicotinate does not typically cause the "niacin skin flush" (an uncomfortable skin reaction that often occurs after taking niacin and lasts about 20 to 30 minutes) and has not been associated with liver toxicity. However, this compound does not appear to be as effective as niacin at lowering serum-cholesterol levels. In addition, there is not enough published research to know whether inositol hexanicotinate is completely safe for the liver.

Calcium

IN a double-blind study, 56 patients with high serum cholesterol were randomly assigned to receive calcium (as calcium carbonate), 400 mg, 3 times per day, or a placebo for 6 weeks, and the alternate treatment for an additional 6 weeks. Compared with the placebo, calcium reduced LDL cholesterol by 4.4% and increased HDL cholesterol by 4.1%. The ratio of LDL to HDL cholesterol decreased significantly with calcium treatment (suggesting a reduction in cardiac risk).[15] The mechanism by which calcium affects cholesterol levels is not fully understood, although it may bind cholesterol and fats in the intestinal tract, thereby preventing their absorption.

Other Nutrients

VITAMIN E has been shown to increase HDL cholesterol levels, but only in relatively young individuals (around age 30) who have abnormally low HDL cholesterol.[16] Vitamin C at a dose of 1 gram per day increased HDL-cholesterol levels in elderly men and women with heart disease and in elderly men (but not women) without heart disease.[17] In another study, 16 patients with elevated LDL- and low HDL-cholesterol levels received approximately 400 mg of magnesium per day for 4 months. Total cholesterol decreased significantly from an average of 297 to 257 mg/dl, while HDL cholesterol increased significantly from 35.2 to 46.7 mg/dl.[18] Other nutrients that may lower serum cholesterol and/or raise HDL cholesterol include copper, lecithin, and essential fatty acids. L-carnitine has been shown to have a beneficial effect on both total- and HDL-cholesterol levels; however, in some cases L-carnitine causes a paradoxical worsening of cholesterol levels. An herb known as gugulipid (*Commiphora mukul*) has been shown to reduce serum cholesterol by more than 20%, without producing any significant adverse effects.[19] Beta-sitosterol, a steroid found in many plant foods, has also been reported to lower serum cholesterol. In selected cases, thyroid hormone is an extremely effective cholesterol-lowering agent.

Conclusion

THE POTENTIAL BENEFITS of any cholesterol-lowering regimen (particularly drug therapy) should be weighed against its risks. A number of dietary modifications and nutritional supplements can reduce serum-cholesterol and/or increase HDL-cholesterol levels. Many of the nutrients discussed in this chapter also have been shown to prevent heart disease in ways that are unrelated to their effect on serum cholesterol. Antioxidants are especially important, as they may prevent cholesterol from being converted to dangerous cholesterol oxides.

Summary of Recommendations for Improving Cholesterol Levels

- Diet: Avoid refined sugar, refined flour, foods high in saturated fat and cholesterol (with the possible exception of eggs), margarine and partially hydrogenated vegetable oil, and unfiltered coffee. Emphasize fruits, vegetables, whole grains, nuts, seeds, legumes (particularly soy), and fish. Work with food allergies in selected cases.

- Pantethine, 300 mg, 2 to 4 times per day.

- Inositol hexanicotinate, 500 to 600 mg, twice daily, plus chromium, 200 to 500 mcg per day. An alternative to this regimen is 100 mg of niacin per day, plus 200 to 500 mcg of chromium per day. Larger doses of niacin are more effective, but should be monitored by a doctor.

- Calcium, 600 to 1,200 mg per day, plus magnesium, 300 to 500 mg per day.

- Other nutrients or herbs that may reduce total-cholesterol levels include L-carnitine (results are unpredictable), beta-sitosterol, gugulipid (*Commiphora mukul*), and essential fatty acids (results with fish oil are unpredictable).

- Other nutrients that may increase HDL cholesterol levels include vitamin C, vitamin E, L-carnitine (results are unpredictable), chromium, and lecithin.

- Antioxidants such as vitamin C, vitamin E, selenium, and carotenoids might help minimize the adverse effects of elevated serum cholesterol.

CHRONIC FATIGUE SYNDROME

🌿 CHRONIC FATIGUE SYNDROME *(CFS) is a condition that causes severe fatigue and various "flu-like" symptoms, including sore throat, swelling of the lymph nodes, low-grade fever, joint pains, muscle aches, headaches, difficulty concentrating, and poor tolerance to exercise. Chronic fatigue is very common; indeed, it is one of the most frequently reported symptoms in a medical setting. However, most people who experience tiredness—even chronic fatigue—do not have the condition that is currently being called CFS.*

Chronic fatigue syndrome is still poorly understood, and doctors have differences of opinion about how and when it should be diagnosed. Some doctors believe that CFS is not even a distinct entity, but just a new name for the psychosomatic disorder known as neurasthenia, or another manifestation of depression. However, there is evidence that the overwhelming, debilitating fatigue and the associated flu-like symptoms seen in CFS patients are, in fact, distinct from these other conditions.

Many different causes for CFS have been suggested. Research shows that some patients have various abnormalities in their immune system. As a result, some researchers have labeled CFS "chronic fatigue and immune dysfunction syndrome" (CFIDS). Other studies indicate that patients with CFS tend to be deficient in cortisol—the body's natural cortisone-like hormone made by the adrenal glands.[1]

Certain viruses, particularly the Epstein-Barr virus (EBV, the virus that causes mononucleosis), are thought to play a role in CFS. However, 90% of American adults have been exposed to EBV at some time during their lives, and it is not always clear whether antibody tests for EBV indicate an active infection or merely past exposure. Therefore, researchers are still not sure what role, if any, EBV and other viruses play in the average case of CFS.

Conventional treatment for CFS is generally unsatisfactory, although anti-inflammatory drugs and anti-depressants may help to some extent. Sometimes, for no apparent reason, CFS just goes away by itself after several years. In other cases, however, the symptoms persist and remain debilitating.

DR. WRIGHT'S CASE STUDY

"I know what's the matter with me," Dora Kilcoyne declared. "I've been thoroughly examined, tested, and inspected by no less than 37 doctors over the last 4 years, including the best clinics here in Seattle, over at the University, and even the Mayo Clinic. I've got all the papers and reports here . . ." she rummaged in a small suitcase, pulling out several file folders ". . . if you want to see them. Maybe they'll do you more good than they've done me. All I've gotten out of all of this so far . . ." she waved at the stack of folders ". . . have been several recommendations for antidepressants and a series of vitamin B_{12} shots. At least the B_{12} shots have done me a little bit of good, so I thought what the heck, you guys are supposed to be the experts on vitamins and minerals and all that—why not come over here? My husband's been against it until now because our insurance won't cover me here, but after the Mayo doctor couldn't suggest anything but the B_{12}, he finally said OK, go for it." She paused for breath.

"What have you been told?"

She handed me the stack of files. "You can see for yourself, they've all pretty much agreed I've got chronic fatigue syndrome. I could have told them that from the start. I'd been exhausted and worn out for a year or two before I saw the first doctor, but apparently you have to fulfill certain criteria before you're 'official'. I'm official! Official, but not much better."

I rummaged through the files as she spoke. "Thanks for bringing these in, it makes my job a lot easier. Now all we need to do here is help you get better."

"You're kidding. Four years of doctors and tests and you say it's easy, all we need to do is get you better? You can't mean that!"

"Sorry if I wasn't clear. All this paperwork you've brought in tells us a lot of things that aren't wrong, and as you say, reach a fairly clear consensus about chronic fatigue. With that literally in hand, there's a fairly clear path to follow to recovery. I didn't mean to say that following that path is always easy."

"A fairly clear path? So why haven't I heard about this path to recovery before? Not to be disrespectful, don't get me wrong, but if it's clear, why aren't all the doctors following it?"

I smiled. "Mostly because it doesn't involve drugs or surgery. But they're catching on fast. Let's start with those vitamin B_{12} shots. A few years ago, you probably wouldn't have gotten

them, just the recommendation for anti-depressants. Tell me what they do for you."

"The vitamin B_{12} shots?"

I nodded.

"Actually, I had to ask for those. But the Mayo doctor said why not, they wouldn't hurt, and he'd read they might help, too."

"Right. But how do you feel when you take the shots?"

"Oh yes. Well, the first one gave me quite a lift, but it wore off after a day or two. Now I get a little boost out of them, but there's still a lot missing."

"Chances are that's exactly correct. When injectable vitamin B_{12} has a noticeable effect, it's a strong clue pointing to stomach malfunction, a very common problem in individuals with chronic fatigue. When the stomach malfunctions, it affects not only vitamin B_{12} absorption, but protein digestion, and the extraction and assimilation of many minerals from their food-bound form."

"So chronic fatigue is due to the stomach not working, which causes a form of malnutrition?"

"Yes and no. Much of the effective treatment for chronic fatigue involves nutrients—amino acids, minerals, other vitamins. They're given by injection because they haven't been getting in by the usual route—the stomach and the rest of the digestion. But that doesn't mean that stomach malfunction is the entire cause of chronic fatigue. We also need to take a look at allergies and sensitivities—especially to foods—and at thyroid and adrenal malfunction. All of these are common trouble spots in chronic fatigue."

"I've had my thyroid checked 2 or 3 times I think, just look in those papers. And I think I heard something about adrenal testing, too."

I looked through her paperwork again. "You have had some standard blood tests of thyroid function here and one cortisol stimulation test, but they're certainly not comprehensive or definitive. Years ago, a doctor named Broda Barnes wrote a book on hypothyroidism about the incompleteness of then-current thyroid blood tests. The situation's better today, but these blood tests still don't tell us everything. Similarly, this cortisol stimulation test is OK, but it's incomplete. Dr. John Tintera, and more recently, Dr. William Jefferies have written about more comprehensive overall evaluation and treatment of adrenal malfunction."

"So, I'll need to do those tests over again?"

"Not the exact same ones. To more comprehensively test the function of the adrenal glands, we'll check not only cortisol and cortisone, but other major hormones including DHEA and aldosterone, before and after stimulation with ACTH—the adrenal-stimulating hormone from the pituitary gland. For the thyroid, there are also additional evaluations, including stimulation with "TRH"—thyrotropin-releasing hormone, and the simple procedure of taking your body temperature each day as recommended by Dr. Barnes."

"I hope you're writing this down."

"On this lab test request form . . . adrenal test, thyroid, food allergy and sensitivity testing, stomach test, and the nutrients most affected by stomach malfunction including especially the essential amino acids and minerals. We usually need to look at all of these areas in cases of chronic fatigue."

"Should I go have these done now?"

"Not quite yet. We still need to complete your personal health history and physical exam. Everyone's an individual, and your personal 'recovery path' may have other 'stops' along the way."

Almost a month later, Mrs. Kilcoyne was back. She opened a new file folder containing copies of her recent tests and recommendations. "I think I understand all this, but let's go over it anyway," she said. "The path to my recovery may be clear, but it doesn't look easy, so I want to make sure I get it right."

"OK, let's look at the diet plan first. Apparently, we found quite a number of food allergies and sensitivities. Unfortunately, that's not unusual in chronic fatigue. For the next 6 weeks

or so, it's important to avoid those foods and take the desensitization drops. As the sensitivities clear, it'll be possible to add back more and more of these foods without contributing to your fatigue. Please check back with the technicians about this."

"I'm ahead of you there. In fact, after two weeks I decided to 'cheat' and eat several of the 'not-now' foods. I definitely felt worse. What I'm not clear about is why the nutritionist advised me to eliminate all the sugar, refined carbohydrate, hydrogenated vegetable oils, and food additives and preservatives, too. The test didn't show me allergic to them."

"True, but they're all unnecessary burdens to your immune system—to everyone's immune system in fact—and as long as you're re-arranging your diet for the best of health, you may as well get rid of these 'non-foods', too."

She made a note. "OK, but I want to do some more studying on that. Now, this stomach test. The technician who did this said it wasn't good at all, very low stomach-acid production."

I looked at her test. "It's about average for chronic fatigue. You've started on the hydrochloric acid-pepsin capsules with meals?"

"Yes, and my digestion does feel better. She also told me to continue the vitamin B_{12} shots, but to add a little bit of folic acid to each one. No wonder those shots helped—my stomach wasn't working well, at all!"

"Right. And that's also likely why your essential amino-acid test is so poor. Five of the 8 essential amino acids are low. Have you gotten your individualized amino-acid blend yet?"

"Not yet. It's a little expensive—nearly $200—although I'm told it's a 3 to 4 month supply. I've done a little reading, and amino acids are digested from proteins, and my stomach isn't working well. I can understand how my amino acids might get low. But why can't I just wait for the hydrochloric acid-pepsin capsules to do the job?"

"You could, but it'll take a lot longer. Your

amino-acid blend is individualized—targeted to most effectively make up for the deficiencies found on your test. Since the amino acids require no further digestion, they start working quite rapidly. People with chronic fatigue say they can feel the effects from their individualized amino-acid blends within just a few weeks—both physically and mentally. And if they stop them too soon, they can tell a difference."

"What's too soon?"

"It varies from person to person, but most people don't need them anymore after 6 to 8 months."

"Why are amino acids so important?"

"The essential amino acids are necessary for every protein the body makes—both structural protein like muscle, and functional proteins, such as the hundreds of enzymes contained in every body cell that perform all of our bodies' biochemical functions. Also, amino acids are precursors of neurotransmitters—the molecules that carry the messages between our nerve cells. That's why amino acids are also effective at helping depression."

She made a few more notes. "I assume that's generally why you're recommending these minerals intravenously—because my stomach doesn't work so well, and probably hasn't for quite awhile."

"You're right. We use small quantities of nearly all the essential minerals, repeated once weekly for several weeks. We usually put vitamin B_{12} and other B-vitamins in the IV, too, along with a tiny quantity of hydrochloric acid, which stimulates the white blood cells."

"Your nurse says you've recommended 1 grain of thyroid . . ."

"Based on an overall evaluation of your 'regular' thyroid tests, your TRH stimulation test, and the body temperature record you've turned in."

"The thing I'm most nervous about is this recommendation for cortisol, 5 milligrams, 4 times daily. I've heard all kinds of 'cortisone horror stories' since I started talking to my friends about this possibility. Are you sure I need it?"

"Remember, all of our adrenal glands make cortisone every day. If they didn't, we wouldn't survive. Your adrenal-function test shows a failure of reserve capacity. In other words, when unstressed, your adrenal glands do OK, but instead of responding to stress with considerably increased hormone production, they barely make any more hormone at all—cortisone, cortisol, DHEA, or any of the other hormones tested. So for quickest recovery, it's best to support them with small quantities of identical-to-natural cortisol and DHEA. That way, they don't have to 'produce' all the time, and they can recover themselves. Identical-to-natural cortisol in quantities smaller than what the body makes on its own are just as safe as thyroid hormone in similar quantities, or any other identical-to-natural hormone supplement. This whole concept is discussed in the book *Safe Uses of Cortisol* by Dr. William Jefferies."

"Sounds reasonable, and my test doesn't look good, as you say. But I think I'll look at Dr. Jefferies' book, too, just to calm my friends down if I need to."

With the help of her allergy-free and "junk"-free diet, hydrochloric acid and pepsin to aid digestion, the individualized essential-amino-acid blend, the temporary use of injectable minerals and vitamins, and small quantities of identical-to-natural thyroid and adrenal hormones, Mrs. Kilcoyne reported feeling "just like my old self" within six months. She was able to resume almost all of the foods she'd tested sensitive to without adverse effects within 1 year, and over the course of the next 2 years, she was able to reduce her supplemental amino acids, vitamins, minerals, and identical-to-natural hormones considerably. She continues to do well several years later.

DR. GABY'S COMMENTARY

Nutritional medicine has a great deal to offer individuals suffering from CFS. Even though we do not fully understand this condition, many CFS patients recover their health fully after undertaking a comprehensive program of diet, nutritional supplements, and natural-hormone therapies. Although no single treatment is universally effective, individuals with CFS have a good chance of healing if their body chemistry is balanced properly.

Nutritional Supplements

Nutrient Injections

Injections of vitamins and minerals are helpful for many individuals with CFS. We do not know why injections (as opposed to oral supplements) are necessary for some patients. While impaired digestion and absorption may be a contributing factor, it is also possible that in certain chronic illnesses the cells lose their ability to retain nutrients or to extract what they need from the bloodstream. This sets up a vicious cycle in which nutritional deficiencies lead to worsening illness which, in turn, results in even greater deficiencies. In the face of severe illness, taking nutritional supplements by mouth may not raise blood levels high enough to force the nutrients back into the cells. However, giving the same nutrients by injection will often accomplish what pills cannot.

In one study, patients with CFS were found to have low levels of magnesium in their red blood cells. Magnesium is known to play an important role in energy production, and a deficiency may result in fatigue. Thirty-two patients with CFS were therefore given (in double-blind fashion) either intramuscular injections of magnesium sulfate (1 gram weekly for 6 weeks) or a placebo. Of the 15 patients receiving magnesium injections, 12 (80%) reported more energy, better mood, and

less pain. Fatigue disappeared completely in 47% of these patients. In contrast, only 18% of those given the placebo improved, and none had complete relief.[2]

In our clinics, we have been impressed with the effects of magnesium injections. However, we have also found that a combination of nutrients works better than magnesium alone. In my clinic, I give an intravenous "cocktail" containing magnesium, calcium, B-vitamins, and vitamin C (see appendix B). About half of my CFS patients have noticed a definite and sometimes dramatic improvement after receiving a series (usually 4) of these injections. In some patients, the results appear to be permanent. In other patients, "booster" injections are necessary. Dr. Wright has been using a similar combination of nutrients, but his "cocktail" also includes a number of trace minerals (zinc, copper, chromium, selenium, manganese, and others). Obviously, more research is needed before we will know the best combination of nutrients to give to patients with CFS.

In some patients, we have used intramuscular injections of vitamin B_{12}—either alone or in combination with other B-vitamins. Although these injections may not work as well as the intravenous treatments, they are less expensive, and they can be given outside the office by a nurse or a family member who has been trained in proper injection procedure.

Amino-Acid Therapy

Dr. Wright has been a pioneer in the use of amino acids to treat CFS. Amino acids are the building blocks for every protein made in the body, including the antibodies that fight viral infections. Amino acids are also the precursors (raw materials) for many so-called "neurotransmitters," the chemicals that influence various processes in the brain and central nervous system. A deficiency of amino acids could therefore have a profound influence on immune function, brain chemistry, and general health.

Dr. Wright has found that many patients with CFS have low blood levels of one or more of the 8 essential amino acids. These patients are prescribed a powdered amino-acid mixture, individualized for each patient according to their blood amino-acid pattern. He has found that this treatment increases his success rate and helps patients recover more rapidly. Other doctors have found similar results using amino-acid therapy.[3]

Hormone Therapy
Adrenal Hormones

LABORATORY tests performed on CFS patients often demonstrate a deficiency of one or both of the two major adrenal hormones: cortisol (also called hydrocortisone) and dehydroepiandrosterone (DHEA). A deficiency of either of these hormones can result in fatigue and poor immune function. Cortisol levels tend to be low more often than DHEA levels. When these deficiencies are corrected by appropriate supplementation, the fatigue and related symptoms often improve considerably.

Adrenal hormones, particularly cortisol, can cause serious side effects if used inappropriately. These hormones should not be used to treat fatigue unless a deficiency is demonstrated. In addition, doctors prescribing cortisol should be familiar with the work of Dr. William Jefferies, who has been prescribing low doses of cortisol for more than 30 years without encountering any significant side effects.[4] (See chapter 4 for additional discussion of Jefferies' work.) Of two recent studies that showed cortisol was helpful in CFS,[5, 6] one also found evidence of an adverse effect: the suppression of normal adrenal function. However, some of the patients in that study should not have been given cortisol, because they did not have evidence of a deficiency. In addition, most of the

medication was given in the morning, rather than in 4 divided doses, as recommended by Dr. Jefferies. In our experience, low-dose cortisol therapy is safe, as long as Jefferies' guidelines are followed.

Other Natural Treatments

SOME PATIENTS WITH CFS have food allergies, which can make their fatigue worse and put stress on their immune system. Methods of identifying and working with food allergies are discussed in chapter 3. Dr. Wright has found that many individuals with CFS have hypochlorhydria (low stomach acid). Without adequate stomach acid, absorption of various amino acids, vitamins, and minerals will be impaired. Medically supervised treatment with hydrochloric acid and pepsin may improve overall nutritional status, and thereby improve energy levels and immune function.

Hypothyroidism (a deficiency of thyroid hormone) also may be a contributing factor in some cases of CFS. In addition to fatigue and poor immune function, patients with hypothyroidism often have one or more of the following symptoms: cold hands and feet, constipation, dry skin, difficulty concentrating, hair loss, fluid retention, and menstrual irregularities. Many doctors of natural medicine have observed (although most conventional doctors disagree) that a patient can be clinically hypothyroid and still have normal blood tests for thyroid function[7] (see chapter 4 for more information). Nutrition-oriented physicians may diagnose hypothyroidism on the basis of symptoms, physical examination, and a sub-normal body temperature. Although prescribing thyroid hormone for people with normal lab tests remains controversial, we are convinced that unrecognized hypothyroidism is an important and overlooked factor in some patients with CFS.

Kutapressin is an extract of liver that is being used in some CFS clinics. Kutapressin must be given frequently by injection and is rather expensive. However, some patients who have tried this treatment feel that it has helped them. Another natural treatment for CFS is adenosine. Adenosine is a compound that occurs naturally in the body that enhances immune function and helps fight viral infections. One doctor has reported that adenosine injections are helpful for individuals with CFS.[8] Adenosine is commercially available for intramuscular injection, and is used by some doctors of natural medicine. See the chapter on herpes simplex for additional discussion about adenosine.

Conclusion

CFS IS A complex disorder that probably has many different causes. A comprehensive search by a nutrition-oriented physician may identify deficiencies of adrenal or thyroid hormones, food allergies, impaired secretion of stomach acid, and amino-acid imbalances. When these problems are corrected, patients with CFS often improve. Injections of various vitamins and minerals are also helpful, sometimes resulting in dramatic recoveries.

Although we still have a lot to learn about CFS, the "balancing body chemistry" approach frequently helps restore CFS patients back to good health, without risking serious side effects.

Summary of Recommendations for Treating Chronic Fatigue Syndrome(treatment should be supervised by a doctor)

- Diet: Avoid refined sugar, caffeine, and alcohol. Emphasize whole foods. Work with food allergies.

- Injections of vitamin B_{12}, magnesium, and other nutrients.

- Treatment with cortisol, DHEA, and/or thyroid hormone in selected cases.

- Amino-acid therapy in selected cases.

- Assess digestion and absorption, and use appropriate digestive aids when indicated.

CONGESTIVE HEART FAILURE

CONGESTIVE HEART FAILURE *(CHF) is a common condition in which the heart becomes too weak to pump enough blood to the tissues of the body. Because of this failure of pumping action, blood returning to the heart "backs up," leading to a buildup of fluid (congestion) in the lungs. This "waterlogging" of the lungs causes shortness of breath. Other symptoms of CHF, such as fatigue, weakness, generalized fluid retention, and alterations in mental status, are caused by a lack of blood flow to the kidneys, brain, and other tissues.*

The most common causes of CHF are high blood pressure (which continually overworks and eventually damages the heart), cardiomyopathy (a primary disease of the heart muscle), impaired blood flow to the heart muscle resulting from atherosclerosis (hardening of the arteries), and heart-valve dysfunction. In many cases, CHF is a serious medical condition. In one study, only 20% of a group of men with CHF lived 10 years after being diagnosed, compared with 50% of those who had suffered a heart attack. In people with moderate to severe CHF, 5-year survival was only 10%.

Conventional treatment of CHF includes restriction of dietary salt (sodium chloride) intake. An amount of salt that would be well tolerated by the average healthy person can cause fluid to accumulate in the lungs and elsewhere in someone with CHF.

Studies have shown that a class of drugs known as angiotensin-converting enzyme (ACE) inhibitors (Vasotec, Capoten, and others) can prolong life in individuals with CHF. ACE inhibitors work by dilating arteries, thereby allowing the heart to pump blood with less effort. Another class of drugs, known as beta-blockers, also has been shown to be helpful. Beta-blockers work by reducing the demand on the heart. Diuretics are often prescribed to remove excess fluid from the body, and digoxin is used to stimulate the heart. However, none of these drugs actually improves the health of the heart muscle; they merely allow the body to cope better with a progressively worsening situation.

DR. WRIGHT'S CASE STUDY

Mrs. Helen Livingston walked slowly into my office and sat down carefully. "I'd like to sleep lying down for the years I have left," she said. "Got accustomed to it the first 75 years or so,

and I just can't get to liking sleeping half-way propped up on pillows."

"What happens when you try to sleep lying flat?"

She gave me a sharp look. "Can't breathe right, of course." She paused and relaxed a little. "Forgot I hadn't told you what the problem is yet." She started rummaging around in her large black purse.

"You have a heart problem?"

"Glad you guessed right the first time. Some of these young doctors . . ." She handed me 3 prescription bottles. "Here's what they give me to take. Helps some. I only need 2 pillows to prop me up instead of 3 or 4, but it's still not right."

I read the labels on her prescription bottles, all generic from a large local health care co-operative. "Digoxin, furosemide, and potassium—the usual group for heart failure. Glad they have you on the potassium, too."

She snorted. "I had to fight 'em for that one. They kept telling me my potassium was normal. I asked why did I keep having leg cramps then? It's that diuretic one—furosemide. Every time I take more than one of those water pills, I feel all washed out, no strength, can't get anything done, and my legs cramp something fierce. At least the potassium keeps the cramping under control."

"But you still can't sleep at night lying flat."

"No. The doctor keeps pestering me to take 2 or 3 water pills a day, he says there's still some water in my lungs that needs clearing out, but whenever I do I'm weak as a kitten and can hardly think straight. Seems like those pills just wash the strength and pep right out of me."

"Actually, they do in a way. Potassium's only one of many minerals and other nutrients lost to excess when we take diuretics. We lose magnesium, zinc, thiamine—a whole list of nutrients."

"That's what that Bill Harrison keeps badgering me about, and his pestering is making more sense than that young doctor's. All that doctor ever says is, 'What can you expect at your age, Mrs. Livingston. Take more water pills' and just wait around to die, I suppose! Costs Medicare less that way, too!" She glared at me, readjusted her expression, and continued.

"I saw what your clinic did for Bill a few years back. Near at death's door, now he's out working the yard, fixing the roof, and he's 3 years older than I am. When I first got this congestive heart failure 5 or 6 years ago, he told me to come see you, but Medicare won't cover your type of treatment and the co-op won't either. Bill says he's tired of me complaining about not sleeping flat and if I'm too cheap he'll pay for it himself. I told him these are the 1990s and even an 81-year-old woman like me can take care of herself, thank you. So here I am."

I took the rest of Mrs. Livingston's health history. She'd been basically healthy until age 75 when she first started noticing a little shortness of breath, especially on exertion. She had no chest pain or other symptoms, so she decided "it was just age" until she found she had to sleep sitting up in order to breathe. She also noticed "a little swelling 'round the ankles" and decided she'd visit the doctor. She was promptly hospitalized with a diagnosis of congestive heart failure and given the digoxin and diuretics which "made me lose 15 pounds in 3 days!" Since then, she'd needed no further hospitalization.

On physical examination, the stethoscope disclosed faint sounds of fluid in the lower regions of both lungs. When she took a very deep breath, there was a faint wheeze. "I hear that too, from time to time," she said. "Reminds me there's still a problem." Fortunately, her heart size seemed normal, and there was very little fluid in her legs or elsewhere.

"So, what can you do for me?" she asked. "Any hope of sleeping flat without more water pills? Bill said you'd have a long list of vitamins besides the ones he's talked me into already, so let's get started."

"There's definitely hope of improving your heart function further, and clearing out your lungs, but before we get to supplements, let me go over basic diet first. You probably know it's best to cut back on salt?"

"I may be ancient, but I'm not senile," Mrs. Livingston interrupted. "I'll give you the benefit of the doubt for trying to be complete, but even my 6-year-old great-grandson knows that! So you won't waste anymore of our time, let me bring you up to date on what I'm doing already. Maybe it wasn't obvious in that diet I wrote down. I'm not using a speck of salt, and I'm avoiding salty foods. Bill kept after me 'til I quit using any sugar or refined food, and keeps coming over to read all the labels on everything in my kitchen to make sure. I only tolerate that because he means well, and besides he clears the plumbing for me when it gets clogged. He's got me off margarine and avoiding all that partially hydrogenated vegetable oil in everything. He says it's even worse than saturated fat." She paused, with a questioning look.

"He's right."

"I suppose I'll have to give him the satisfaction of telling him you said so. So all I've got is good healthy food. If you looked at my list, you probably saw I'm taking a strong multiple vitamin and mineral—one of those that comes in 4 capsules. And 400 units of vitamin E, and 1 gram of vitamin C every day. But I told that man I wasn't going any further—even if he comes over and bothers me every day—until I talked to you about it. I'm sure the vitamins I'm taking won't hurt anything, and probably will help, but I don't want to take anything else just on his say-so without making sure it won't interfere with the medicines I'm already taking. They're not doing all I want, but they're better than nothing."

I reviewed my notes. "You've definitely covered all the basics. There are a few lab tests I'd recommend you get done—minerals, amino acids, digestion . . . but I can make quite a number of recommendations now. Most things you can do at home, but one important one should be done here at the clinic." I wrote the recommendation for her. "Please have a series of magnesium injections, intravenously, along with vitamin B_6."

"Intravenous injections? Sounds expensive, and a lot of bother! Why don't I just swallow magnesium pills, instead?"

"For congestive heart failure, magnesium frequently works better when given by relatively rapid IV injection. In heart failure, the heart-muscle cells are sometimes too weak to extract all the magnesium they should from the bloodstream. A fairly rapid IV injection forces magnesium into the heart-muscle cells, helping them to work better and stronger. The shots are a bit of bother, but magnesium, even intravenously, is cheap."

"But if I start won't I need shots forever to maintain the effect?"

"Usually not. Once magnesium's forced into the cells, they continue to take up more magnesium on their own. Also, the other things we'll go over will strengthen your heart muscle, too. It'll just take them a little longer than magnesium injections.

"The rest of these items you can swallow. Start with coenzyme Q_{10}, and use at least 60 milligrams, 3 times daily for now. If you can afford a bit more—maybe 90 milligrams each time, please do. It's quite safe."

"Bill's been saying something about how important an 'enzyme 10' is, but I've ignored him. What's it do?"

"Takes care of congestive heart failure all by itself sometimes. Helps the heart muscle work stronger and more effectively. There are literally dozens of research papers about coenzyme Q_{10} and heart function."

"If there's so much research, why hasn't the co-op doctor told me about it?"

"It's a natural substance, not publicized by the pharmaceutical companies because it's not patentable."

She held up her hand. "I know the rest of that story. What's next?"

"L-carnitine. Please use 250 milligrams, 3 times daily." I wrote a list of the items as we talked.

"That does what?"

"Enables the heart-muscle cells to use more sources of energy, and to burn them all more efficiently."

"Sounds worthwhile."

"Next is taurine, another naturally occurring amino acid like L-carnitine. It's particularly concentrated in the heart—in fact, it's the most abundant amino acid found there. It's known to keep the electrical activity of the heart flowing smoothly and to increase the strength of the heart muscle. Please use 1,500 milligrams twice daily, in between meals."

"In between meals?"

"Yes, but all the rest can be with meals, or not, as you'd like."

"Is that all?"

"One more for now. Please get either the solid extract of hawthorn, and use ½ teaspoon twice daily, or take 250 milligrams of the standardized 10% procyanidin extract of hawthorn, 3 times daily."

"Hawthorn? That's one I haven't heard a word about from Bill Harrison yet—that's just an herb! What's it supposed to be doing?"

"Some of the most powerful and useful human medicines are 'just herbs.' The digoxin you're taking started several centuries ago as 'just an herb' called foxglove. Actually, considerable research has found that hawthorn does safely what several much more toxic drugs do, and several things they can't. It improves energy production in heart-muscle cells, and improves heart-muscle contraction. It dilates coronary arteries, providing more blood flow. It acts as a mild diuretic, can lower cholesterol, and can slow and possibly even reverse atherosclerosis a bit."

"Where's this wonder herb been for all this time?" Mrs. Livingston asked. "Just peaceably growing in hedgerows? I know—not patentable, right?"

"Actually, hawthorn's been used extensively in folk medicine for heart and artery problems for centuries."

"Well, I'm glad you doctor-folk are finally catching on again! Is that everything?"

"For now." I handed her the list, along with another list of recommended laboratory tests. Looking at these, she got up slowly to go, and then sat back down again. She gave me a peculiar look—a combination of an inquiry and her best glare.

"Young man, what's this about a testosterone test? When I said I wanted to sleep lying down flat at night, I meant by myself. Did Bill Harrison have a word with you? Just because I'm a widow, and he's a widower and lives next door . . ."

I laughed. "Nothing like that at all. I haven't seen Mr. Harrison in over a year. No, it's a test I request routinely in congestive heart failure. Remember, our hearts are muscles—specialized muscles all right, but muscles all the same. And testosterone is the body's major muscle builder. Didn't you say you felt a little weaker than you should, even when you don't take extra water pills? When we test people with congestive heart failure, we often find their testosterone levels are much lower than usual for their respective sex. Supplementing identical-to-natural testosterone, done carefully, is often a major help in relieving heart failure."

"When you put it that way, it makes sense. But I don't want to grow a mustache!"

I laughed again. "You won't. First, there's a small amount of testosterone in women's bodies naturally, just as there's a small amount of estrogen in men's. Second, we'll be working with a balanced group of identical-to-natural hormones, not just testosterone. It's simply the most important hormone for strengthening the heart muscle."

"Sounds reasonable, but I'll ask you the details once my test comes back." She put the papers in her purse, and left for the lab.

One week after Helen Livingston's visit, the test results came back, indicating that her serum testosterone level was low. I telephoned in a prescription for a low dose of testosterone. After 3 months, she returned for her follow-up visit and reported she was "feeling much stronger, not taking those water pills at all, and sleeping flat with only one pillow like when I was younger." I recommended she stop the magnesium injections, and substitute magnesium capsules, as well as other minerals indicated by her tests.

At her next visit 3 months later, she reported

she had all her strength back, was working hard around the house and yard, and that "Bill Harrison is a lot better looking than I thought!" Since then, we've only heard from Mrs. Livingston for her testosterone and other hormone prescription refills.

DR. GABY'S COMMENTARY

NUTRITIONAL THERAPY HAS an impact upon the process of congestive heart failure, and helps to restore a failing heart to better health. As with every other organ in the body, the heart has a wide range of nutritional needs. Failure to meet any one of those needs could weaken or damage the heart muscle. On the other hand, supplying the heart with optimal amounts of nutrients will promote better cardiac function and may even prolong life in people with CHF.

Nutritional therapy does not interfere with conventional medications. On the contrary, nutritional therapy may increase the effectiveness and reduce the side effects of some of the medications used to treat CHF. Although there are not as many research studies on nutrients as there are on drugs, the material that has been published about nutrients is straightforward and convincing. Unfortunately, as is often the situation with natural substances, most doctors are unaware of just how much more they could be doing for their patients. Millions of individuals with CHF are therefore being deprived of potentially lifesaving treatments.

Although many different nutrients are essential for heart health, the 3 that stand out the most are magnesium, taurine, and coenzyme Q10.

Nutritional Supplements
Magnesium

MAGNESIUM is required for the production of adenosine triphosphate (ATP), the biochemical "power cell" that stores the energy used by the heart and other tissues. Without adequate magnesium, the heart muscle could not pump properly. Evidence shows that magnesium deficiency is one of the important contributors to CHF. In one study, patients with CHF (due to cardiomyopathy) had 65% less magnesium in their heart muscle than healthy individuals.[1] In another study, the hearts of individuals dying from CHF showed changes similar to those seen in animals fed a magnesium-deficient diet.[2] Magnesium deficiency also increases the risk of heart-rhythm disturbances (arrhythmias), the most common cause of sudden death in heart patients.[3]

Heart patients develop magnesium deficiency for several different reasons. Low dietary intake (too much sugar and fat, not enough whole grains and vegetables) is certainly one factor. Drugs given to patients with CHF, particularly diuretics (water pills) and digoxin, also deplete the body of magnesium. In addition, the failing heart becomes less efficient at hanging onto the magnesium it already has. Thus, a vicious cycle is set up, in which magnesium deficiency promotes heart failure which, in turn, further aggravates magnesium deficiency.

Although there are few published studies on magnesium treatment of CHF, some nutrition-oriented doctors have observed dramatic results using this mineral. In more severe cases of CHF, intramuscular or intravenous injections of magnesium may be necessary to break the vicious cycle of deficiency and disease. I have given magnesium injections to 2 patients who were undeniably in the terminal stages of heart failure. In both cases, they got up from their death beds and went on to live for years. Oral supplementation may be effective in patients with milder cases, or to prevent magnesium deficiency in those at risk. However, when CHF is advanced, magnesium injections are usually necessary, at least in the beginning.

Intravenous injections of magnesium should be given only by physicians who have been trained in their proper administration. Of particular concern is the possibility that giving magnesium intravenously may reduce serum potassium levels,[4] especially in someone whose body supplies of potassium have been depleted by diuretics or other factors. Low serum potassium can result in potentially dangerous arrhythmias in someone who is taking digoxin.

Coenzyme Q10

COENZYME Q10 (CoQ10) is a vitamin-like compound that is produced in the body. It is also present in very small amounts in some foods. Like magnesium, CoQ10 is required for the production of ATP. Deficiencies of CoQ10 have been found in individuals with CHF. In a 1976 study from Japan, 17 patients with mild CHF were given 30 mg of CoQ10 per day. Every patient improved within 4 weeks, and 53% became completely symptom-free.[5] CoQ10 has also been found to help people with severe CHF. In one double-blind study, 641 such patients were randomly assigned to receive either CoQ10 or a placebo for 1 year. The daily dose of CoQ10 was 2 mg per kg of body weight, or about 150 mg per day for a 165 pound individual. The CoQ10 group had a progressive and statistically significant improvement in heart function (as measured by the New York Heart Association functional classification), whereas no change was seen in the placebo group. In addition, the proportion of patients requiring one or more hospitalizations for heart failure was 38% less in the CoQ10 group than in the placebo group (23% vs. 37%). Episodes of pulmonary edema (a life-threatening build-up of fluid in the lungs) were reduced by about 60% in the CoQ10 group, compared with the placebo group.[6] In another study, survival time increased nearly 3-fold when patients with severe heart failure were given CoQ10.[7]

The benefits obtained with CoQ10 are as good as or better than any that have been reported for prescription cardiac medications. The evidence strongly suggests that giving CoQ10 to individuals with CHF will not only improve their health, it will also save money. The results of the study mentioned previously suggest that at least 138 fewer hospitalizations would be required per year for every one-thousand CHF patients who receive CoQ10. Considering an estimated cost of $6,000 per hospitalization and $450 per year for CoQ10 therapy, every dollar spent on CoQ10 would save nearly 2 dollars in hospital costs.

Taurine

TAURINE is an amino acid found in high concentrations in the heart. Although the exact function of taurine is not known, animal studies show that it increases the strength of the heart. Taurine was tested in 7 patients with CHF who were deteriorating despite conventional medical treatment. After supplementing with taurine (2 grams, twice a day), 5 of the 7 patients experienced considerable improvement in the signs and symptoms of CHF. Results were seen within 3 to 21 days.[8]

This promising report was followed by a double-blind study, in which 62 patients with CHF were randomly assigned to receive taurine (2 grams, 3 times a day) or a placebo for 4 weeks. After a 2-week rest period, each patient was given the alternate treatment for an additional 4 weeks. During taurine treatment, patients experienced significant improvements in shortness of breath, palpitations, fluid retention, and chest X-ray findings, whereas they had no such improvements during the placebo period.[9] These studies indicate that taurine is a valuable weapon in the treatment of CHF. No serious side effects were seen in either study.

The main dietary sources of taurine are meat and fish. Taurine is also manufactured in the body from another amino acid, methionine. However, it appears that patients with CHF need more taurine than they can obtain from these sources.

Other Natural Treatments

ALTHOUGH THIAMINE (vitamin B₁) deficiency is a well-known cause of heart failure, deficiency of this vitamin is thought to occur only rarely. However, treatment with the diuretic furosemide (Lasix), a drug often prescribed for CHF, can cause excessive amounts of thiamine to be lost in the urine. In a study of 23 patients receiving long-term furosemide therapy for CHF, 21 were found to be deficient in thiamine. Five of these patients were given thiamine supplements; in 4 of the 5 cases heart function improved.[10]

The amino acid L-arginine has also been investigated as a possible treatment for CHF, because of its ability to dilate blood vessels. In a double-blind study, 15 patients with moderate to severe heart failure received L-arginine for 6 weeks and a placebo for an additional 6 weeks, in random order. The initial dosage of L-arginine was 5.6 grams per day (an amount similar to that in a typical diet), but it was later increased arbitrarily to 12.6 grams per day. Compared with the placebo, L-arginine significantly improved aerobic capacity (as determined by a walking test) and significantly reduced the number of heart disease-related limitations (as assessed by the Living-With-Heart-Failure questionnaire). No side effects were seen.[11] Foods high in L-arginine include nuts, seeds, cereal grains, and peas.

Individuals with CHF are also likely to be deficient in other nutrients. Just as heart failure results in congestion in the lungs, so too can CHF lead to swelling of the intestinal lining and pancreas. Consequently, individuals with CHF may have poor absorption of many different nutrients. In one study, malabsorption was documented in 56% of a group of patients with CHF.[12] Thus, individuals with CHF might benefit from a comprehensive program of nutritional supplementation.

The male hormone testosterone has also been studied in Europe as a potential treatment for heart disease. Testosterone deficiency appears to be relatively common in heart patients, and treatment with this hormone is said to improve various heart and blood-vessel disorders.[13] Measuring free testosterone in the blood is more reliable than measuring total testosterone, because the former is the more biologically active form of the hormone. Testosterone therapy is discussed in chapter 4, and it has been reviewed in a recent book by Dr. Wright.[14]

Hawthorn (*Crataegus oxyacantha*) is one of the most widely prescribed herbs in Europe. It has a long history of use as a "tonic" for various cardiac conditions, including CHF. Hawthorn has been shown to improve blood flow to the heart by dilating the coronary arteries and to increase the contractile strength of the heart muscle.[15] In a double-blind study, 30 patients with CHF were randomly assigned to receive an extract of hawthorn or a placebo for 8 weeks. Compared with the placebo, hawthorn significantly improved subjective symptoms, as well as objective measures of heart function.[16] No significant side effects have been seen with hawthorn. Although the berries, leaves, and flowers all have activity, the most potent cardiac effects appear to reside in the leaves and flowers.

Conclusion

DESPITE RECENT ADVANCES in drug therapy for individuals with CHF, some of the most dramatic effects are still obtained with magnesium, CoQ10, taurine, and other natural substances. These natural treatments are safe, and they can be used in conjunction with conventional therapy. If the medical profession would take a closer look at these treatments, millions of heart patients would benefit. It should be noted that, in most of the studies described above, patients continued their conventional treatments. While some individuals who respond well to natural medicines are able to reduce the doses of—or even discontinue—their prescription heart medications, such changes should be considered only with the supervision and close monitoring of a physician.

Summary of Recommendations for Treating Congestive Heart Failure

PRIMARY RECOMMENDATIONS:

- DIET:

  ➤ Restrict salt intake

  ➤ Consume nutrient-rich foods (i.e., whole grains, fruits, vegetables, nuts, legumes, fish).

- SUPPLEMENTS:
  (to be taken under medical supervision)

  ➤ Magnesium, 400 to 600 mg per day, in divided doses. Reduce dose if diarrhea occurs.

Intramuscular or intravenous injections of magnesium may be advisable in individuals with more advanced cases.

➤ Coenzyme Q10, 30 to 200 mg per day.

➤ Taurine, 500 to 1,500 mg twice a day.

➤ High-potency multiple vitamin/mineral (adjust doses of other nutrients as needed).

➤ Hawthorn (leaf with flower); dosage varies according to the preparation used.

OTHER RECOMMENDATIONS:

- L-arginine, 1 to 2 grams twice a day.
- Testosterone (if blood levels are low).

CROHN'S DISEASE

CROHN'S DISEASE *(also called regional enteritis) is a chronic inflammatory disease of the intestinal tract. The inflammation is usually localized to the small intestine, but it may also affect the colon, esophagus, or stomach. The condition typically begins during early adulthood with symptoms of fatigue, abdominal pain, and diarrhea. Patient's may also experience weight loss, low-grade fever, nausea, vomiting, loss of appetite, and rectal bleeding. The cause of Crohn's disease is unknown, but it has features that suggest either an autoimmune disorder or an infectious disease.*

While some individuals with Crohn's disease experience nothing worse than a periodic flare-up of bothersome symptoms, others develop serious complications including intestinal obstruction, fistulas (abnormal passageways from the intestines to other organs), and severe malnutrition. Other potential complications of Crohn's disease include arthritis, liver disease, and eye damage.

Conventional therapy consists of anti-inflammatory medications and antibiotics. Patients with severe cases may be given drugs that suppress the immune system. Unfortunately, with time, the disease becomes less responsive to medical therapy. More than two-thirds of people with Crohn's disease eventually develop complications that require surgical removal of a portion of the intestine. However, even surgical intervention doesn't prevent recurrences, and as many as 5 to 10% of patients with Crohn's disease ultimately die from complications of the disease.

DR. WRIGHT'S CASE STUDY

"Well, here I am again," Arthur Crandell said. He sat down with his arms crossed. "Ready to go through the whole thing again. Should work just as well the second time, shouldn't it?"

Mr. Crandell hadn't been in for several years, and at that time his Crohn's disease had been under excellent control. So I was a bit puzzled. "Second time?"

He uncrossed his arms. "Yeah, second time. Maybe I'll get it through my head this time, and

if I don't, my wife will do it for me. I just got out of the hospital 3 weeks back. Lost a foot-and-a-half of my intestine, all inflamed with Crohn's."

"Sorry to hear that. Thought you'd been doing well."

"I was, but you know us hard-headed engineers, we need proof. Data. At least that's what I tell myself. Of course, my wife doesn't agree. She says it's 'plain old stubbornness', She says I just don't want to recognize that I can't stay healthy if I eat junk food, or any wheat or grains or milk or ice cream . . . after all, my favorite lunch was a hamburger and a milkshake! That Specific

Carbohydrate Diet is a real bear to stick with."

"It's not easy, but it works, and you were doing well. What happened?"

"Well, as you know, I stuck with it for 3 years, and I was really doing well. Off all the drugs, no pain or spasms, taking my vitamins, minerals, shots, IVs . . . and really resenting the hell out of the routine, to tell you the truth. So first I stopped the shots, then I started getting a little lax on the supplements, and only got a few minor symptoms. But next I started into the junk food and it seemed like I couldn't stop . . . milkshakes, bread, potatoes, lunch meat, ketchup, my old routine. My insides got worse and worse, but I couldn't . . . or maybe wouldn't . . . stop, and then I had the worst pain I've ever had. It was a total intestinal blockage. . . . I hear that's not unusual with Crohn's . . . and they hustled me into surgery, and took that foot-and-a-half out."

"I assume you're back on the Specific Carbohydrate Diet."

"For life, unless somebody comes up with an outright cure for Crohn's. Of course, I've gotten a little help. When I got back from the hospital there wasn't a thing in the house that wasn't allowed on the diet. And Cynthia had called all my friends I ever have lunch with and told them exactly what I should and shouldn't eat. But actually I have enough data, enough proof, for me. Of course Cynthia's version is 'if you hit a mule over the head with a 2-by-4 it'll pay attention'. Well, I'll admit I've been 2-by-4'ed. And once is enough, even for this stubborn ol' mule."

"Have you restarted your vitamins?"

"Yeah." He pulled a list out of his shirt pocket, and put on his glasses. "Let's see, *Breaking the Vicious Cycle*, the book with my diet plan by Elaine Gottschall." He looked at me. "That's first on the list because Cynthia told me to buy another copy, she's about worn out the first one."

"Good! That's THE book to follow for Crohn's disease. Elaine has kept the Specific Carbohydrate

Diet idea alive almost single-handedly since the doctors who created it died."

"I'm glad she did—it worked for me. Now, what's next on the list . . . oh yeah, all that fish oil to settle down inflammation. I can't stand so much cod-liver oil, so I'm using that MaxEPA instead—about 5 grams daily for now. Then there's vitamin A—you said vitamin A helps improve the health of the cells that line the intestines. How much am I supposed to take?"

"Considering your problem, 50,000 IU daily."

"And you said glutamine sort of does the same thing. It's the main fuel for the intestinal-lining cells, so it helps them get healthier too, right?"

"Right. For the next 6 weeks, please use 1 gram twice daily. Then cut back to 1 gram a day."

"OK." He made a note. "Next, zinc picolinate. I remember that was 30 milligrams daily, that helps promote healing."

"Since you've had surgery not long ago, use that one twice a day for the next 6 weeks."

"OK . . . then there's 400 IU of vitamin E to help the vitamin A, and a little bit of vitamin C to help the zinc heal my insides." He looked up from his list again. "You know, this does go on, no wonder I got tired of it . . . folic acid, that liquid type, —5 drops (25 milligrams) daily. And there's the lactobacillus to help keep my intestinal bugs more normal, and a general vitamin and mineral in capsule form for better absorption." He put the list away, and smiled at me. "Did I get that all right, Doc?"

"So far. But speaking of absorption, what happened to the hydrochloric acid-pepsin with meals, and the pancreatic enzymes after meals? Don't you remember the stomach test and that stool test for digestion you had after your first visit here?"

"Don't I! You told me I had hardly any acid at all in my stomach, and there was a lot of undigested food in the stool test."

"Shouldn't those be on your list?"

"This is a shopping list, and Cynthia already stocked up on enough hydrochloric acid-pepsin capsules and digestive enzymes to last for the next several months. I've been taking those since the first meal after I got home."

"And your B_{12} shots with B-complex and folic acid?"

"I'm supposed to get new prescriptions from you so we can start them up. Tell me again why I need shots and can't just swallow them."

"Research has shown that a whole variety of nutrients aren't absorbed properly by folks with Crohn's disease. Folic acid, vitamin B_1, vitamin B_2, vitamin B_6, B_{12}, vitamins C, A, D, K, calcium, magnesium, zinc, selenium. Read Elaine Gottschall's book again. It explains how so many nutrients could be so poorly absorbed. When you were last here, when you were doing so well, do you recall we discussed cutting back again on nearly all your supplements? As the diet takes hold the intestines can heal, they can work better, absorption of nutrients is better from the food itself, and less supplements are needed."

"I remember. I cut back as you said, continued to feel well, and I think I just kept on cutting back on what I was supposed to do until I went way too far. I won't do that again!"

"Remember, after you've been feeling well for six months or so this time, the only things NOT to cut back on, at all, are the Specific Carbohydrate Diet, and the digestive aids—hydrochloric acid-pepsin and pancreatic digestive enzymes. Even sticking to the diet doesn't appear to reduce the need for those."

"Does everyone with Crohn's disease need digestive aids?"

"Not everyone, but most do, and you're in that majority. A minority are OK in that department. Remember we also tested you for food allergies? Most people with Crohn's disease have significant food allergies as well, and notice the difference in their intestinal symptoms when they avoid them or desensitize them. You were in the minority there—not really any food allergy problems."

"For once I got lucky." He looked over his list and notes, and started to go.

"Wait a moment. Don't forget the request for your IVs." I started to write it for him.

"I was hoping you'd forget that, or I wouldn't need it. Can't I get by without the IVs this time?"

"Remember all those minerals and vitamins that people with Crohn's have been found deficient in? Well, we could run tests for every one of them, but it would cost a lot more to do all the tests than just putting all the nutrients into a few IVs and running them in. They're safe, and by putting them in an IV we make sure you're getting 100% of all of them absorbed. That's part of what got you improving so rapidly the first time, and it'll likely do it again."

"OK, OK, it makes sense, and I promised Cynthia I'd do whatever it takes."

As Mr. Crandell had promised, he stuck strictly with the Specific Carbohydrate Diet described in Elaine Gottschall's book. He took his digestive aids, all his supplements, his B-vitamin injections, and his nutrient IVs. After only 4 months, he remarked that he felt "just as well as when I did this the first time." After another 2 months, we cut back each of his supplements somewhat, and he continued to do well. It's been 4 years now, and he remains almost entirely free of the symptoms of Crohn's disease.

DR. GABY'S COMMENTARY

Dietary Considerations

DIET IS EXTREMELY important for people with Crohn's disease, and a specially designed diet can help in alleviating symptoms. Additionally, since individuals with Crohn's disease may be deficient in many nutrients, a number of nutritional supplements are frequently helpful.

The Role of Allergy

FOOD allergy is one of the most important factors for patients with Crohn's disease. The relationship between allergy and Crohn's disease was described more than 40 years ago by the pioneering allergist Dr. Albert Rowe.[1]

In a more recent study, 136 patients with active Crohn's disease were treated with a type of diet known as an elemental diet. Consisting only of amino acids, simple sugars and fats, salt, vitamins and minerals, elemental diets are essentially free of allergens. Of the 93 patients who were able to continue the diet for 14 days, 84% experienced a resolution of symptoms. Half of the patients who responded to the diet were then given steroid treatment and returned to their usual diet. The other half were instructed to introduce one new food daily, and to exclude any foods that precipitated symptoms. This process of food testing revealed a number of common symptom provokers, including: corn, wheat, milk, yeast, egg, potato, rye, tea, and coffee. The patients who were assigned to the diet group remained free of recurrences nearly twice as long as did patients treated with steroids (7.5 months vs. 3.8 months). Of those who continued to follow the diet, 45% remained symptom-free for at least 2 years.[2] Similar results have been reported by other investigators. In one of these studies, brassicas (cabbage, cauliflower, broccoli, brussels sprouts, and turnips) were found to be among the common symptom-provoking foods.[3]

Of the several dozen patients I have seen with Crohn's disease, at least half improved significantly or became completely symptom-free after removing allergenic foods from their diet. One of the elimination diets I have used in my practice is presented in appendix A. Some doctors use other tests for allergy and sensitivity, as well as desensitization techniques. The reliability and effectiveness of some of these methods is controversial (see chapter 3 for additional discussion).

The "Specific Carbohydrate Diet"

ASIDE from allergy, foods can cause adverse reactions in susceptible people in other ways. Nutritionist Elaine Gottschall has pointed out that some individuals with intestinal diseases are unable to digest certain carbohydrates known as disaccharides. Disaccharides contain two individual sugars per molecule (for example, lactose consists of glucose and galactose; sucrose contains glucose and fructose; and maltose and isomaltose each contain two molecules of glucose). Normally, disaccharides are broken down into their component sugars by enzymes present in cells that line the small intestine. However, some individuals may have impaired disaccharide digestion. This may be either a primary problem (as in lactose intolerance) or the result of the intestinal disease itself. Gottschall argues that certain harmful bacteria and yeasts thrive on disaccharides, and that these organisms can colonize and damage the intestinal tract, if provided with enough disaccharides. Thus, a vicious cycle occurs, in which maldigestion leads to overgrowth of harmful organisms, which leads to even more-severe intestinal disease.

Following up on the work of Drs. Sidney V. and Merrill P. Haas, Gottschall developed a low-disaccharide diet (called the Specific Carbohydrate

Diet), which she has found to be extremely helpful for some individuals with Crohn's disease. The only carbohydrates allowed on this diet are those found in fruits, honey, properly-prepared yogurt, and specific vegetables and nuts (even these foods are restricted when severe diarrhea is present). All cereal grains are forbidden. According to Gottschall, many patients with Crohn's disease can be cured by following this diet for two years. By a "cure" Gottschall meant that patients could gradually reintroduce previously forbidden foods without experiencing a recurrence of symptoms. The low-disaccharide diet is described in detail in Gottschall's book, *Breaking the Vicious Cycle*.[4] Because this diet is rather restrictive, it should be supervised by a trained dietitian.

A Yeast Connection?

SOME individuals with Crohn's disease may have an overgrowth of *Candida albicans* (the common yeast germ) in their intestinal tract. Yeast overgrowth may result from antibiotic therapy, from maldigestion of disaccharides, from the use of cortisone-like drugs or birth controls pills, or from a general weakening of the immune system. I have seen one patient with Crohn's disease who had an obvious beneficial response to the anti-yeast medication nystatin, and several others who improved after following an "anti-yeast" program consisting of medication plus a diet free of all refined sugars.

Effect of Refined Sugar

SOME patients with Crohn's disease fare better when they avoid refined sugar. The adverse effect of sugar may be due to its ability to promote the growth of yeast. Additionally, the most commonly used form of refined sugar is sucrose, which is one of the disaccharides that Gottschall found to be harmful. Whatever the explanation, we usually advise patients with Crohn's disease to stay away from sugar.

Nutritional Supplements

INDIVIDUALS WITH CROHN'S disease often have multiple nutritional deficiencies, which can result from diarrhea, malabsorption, and the nutrient-depleting effect of chronic inflammation. Deficiencies of virtually every nutrient have been reported in patients with Crohn's disease. Such deficiencies are likely to be most severe in people who have long-standing diarrhea and inflammation, and in those who have had significant portions of their small intestine surgically removed.

Most patients with Crohn's disease could benefit from a broad-spectrum, high-potency, hypoallergenic multivitamin/mineral formula. Nutrient supplementation may help prevent the decline in immune function that often accompanies Crohn's disease. The minerals zinc and copper, as well as vitamins C, E, and A, and the B-vitamins, all have anti-inflammatory and tissue-healing effects. Supplementing with these nutrients might therefore promote healing of inflamed intestinal tissue and help prevent the formation of fistulas.

Patients with active Crohn's disease and those with a history of intestinal surgery may require relatively large doses of vitamins and minerals—more than one would find in a high-potency multiple. In more severe cases, repeated intravenous injections of vitamins and minerals may be necessary to prevent malnutrition.

Supplementing with vitamin A was reported to induce a remission in one woman with Crohn's disease.[5] Although this report was consistent with the known tissue-healing effects of vitamin A, other investigators have found this vitamin to be ineffective.[6] Fish oil, which has anti-inflammatory activity, has also been tried as a treatment for Crohn's disease. In a double-blind study, 78 patients with inactive disease were randomly assigned to receive 4.5 grams of a fish-oil concentrate per day or a placebo for 1 year. Of the patients receiving fish oil, only 28% had a relapse, compared with 69% of those in the placebo group (a statistically significant difference).[7]

Conclusion

CROHN'S DISEASE CAN be a serious medical condition, which often fails to respond to conventional therapy. Fortunately, we have seen a relatively high success rate by treating patients with dietary modification and nutritional supplementation. In my experience, at least half of patients with Crohn's disease improve and many become completely symptom-free. I had not been aware of the Gottschall diet until recently. However, in Dr. Wright's experience, the success rate with Crohn's disease is even higher when disaccharide intolerance is taken into consideration.

Summary of Recommendations for Crohn's Disease

- Diet: Avoid refined sugar. Work with food allergies. Follow a low- or no-disaccharide diet in selected cases.

- Fish-oil concentrate, 3 to 6 grams per day. Balance with vitamin E, 400 IU per day.

- High-potency multiple vitamin/mineral. Additional amounts of vitamins A, C, E, and B-complex, zinc, copper, and other nutrients may be helpful. In some cases, nutrient injections may be necessary.

- Anti-yeast medication in selected cases.

- Assess digestion and absorption; use appropriate digestive aids when indicated.

DIABETES

DIABETES MELLITUS IS *a disease that affects more than 10 million Americans. It is characterized by ele-vated blood levels of glucose (sugar), one of the main sources of energy in the body. The term "diabetes," which means "to run through," refers to the large volume of urine that is excreted in severe cases. The word "mellitus," which means "sweet," refers to the taste of the urine when sugar is present.*

Long-term consequences of diabetes include atherosclerosis (hardening of the arteries), heart disease, neuropa-thy (nerve damage), nephropathy (kidney disease), retinopathy (damage to the retina of the eye), and cataracts. These problems are more likely to develop if blood-sugar levels remain chronically elevated than if they are kept closer to the normal range. Therefore, one of the main treatment goals for diabetics is to maintain blood glucose in a tight range—as close to normal as possible. Patients with adult-onset (type 2) diabetes can often accomplish that goal by means of dietary and lifestyle changes alone. Patients with juvenile-onset (type 1) diabetes are depen-dent on insulin, although it is often possible to reduce their insulin requirement with a program of diet and sup-plements. Reducing the insulin requirement is a desirable objective, since excessive insulin levels may be one of the factors contributing to the development of heart and blood-vessel disease.

DR. WRIGHT'S CASE STUDY

"I guess I should have expected it," Orphelia Hampton said. "My mother and grandmother both got sugar problems past age 55 or so. But I've been working 2 jobs, last 2 children at the university—so I thought I was just feeling poorly from overwork. Then they had one of those sugar and cholesterol screening programs at the mall a few weeks back, and Daniel, he's my youngest, he said 'why not get it checked, momma', so I did, and my sugar was over 200. 'Course I wasn't fasting, so I went to the doctor and had it done first thing in the morning, and it was still way too high—184. My cholesterol was high, too.

The doctor said these days as long as the fasting sugar isn't over 200, they usually don't prescribe pills or insulin shots, just go to some diabetes classes if I want, and try to lose some weight, that would probably help. I've always had a problem with that, same as Momma and Grandmomma, too."

"Have you started a diet program?"

"No, that's partly why I'm here. My oldest daughter, LaDonna, she's changed into a regular health nut since she started having her children, she's got 3 now. She nursed them all for nearly 2 years, won't let any cow-milk stuff in the house, 'cause she read that black folks have a particular problem with it. She don't allow any sugar or junk food with chemicals. She's been all over my telephone since I found out, advising me on what to do. She lives in Philadelphia, sees one of those good health doctors there. She asked and he said I should come here."

"So you've already eliminated the sugar and white flour?"

"I've made a start, but you know it's hard. Sometimes I get cravings, and every once in a while if I don't eat for a few hours I get real light-headed and a little weak and the sugar cravings get real hard then."

"Sounds like you have a little low blood sugar, too."

"Can I have high sugar and low sugar all at the same time?"

"Definitely, though low-blood-sugar episodes often start years before diabetes—high blood sugar—comes on, and lessen as diabetes worsens."

She thought for a moment. "Now that you mention it, I've haven't had as many spells like that the last year or two." She paused again. "But you know, I'm confused. LaDonna's been sending me books and articles and things about diabetes diets and vitamins and minerals and all that. . . . There's so much, I just don't know what to do. One book says lots of whole grains and beans and fruits and vegetables, and another one says don't do that, eat a lot of protein and cut down on the carbohydrates. I can't do both of those at once."

"Those are the two basic approaches: high complex carbohydrate and high protein, low carbohydrate. Before choosing one or the other, it's best to have a little more information. We need to know about your insulin response to sugar and carbohydrates."

"My insulin response?"

"Insulin is one of the hormones that regulates blood sugar."

"I know that much, anyway. But if my sugar's high, it means I don't have enough insulin, right? I recall Grandma took insulin shots in her later years. So I must have low insulin, too."

"Not necessarily. Since your blood sugar problem—and your mother's and grandmother's, too—came on after age 55, it's likely that you

have 'type 2' diabetes. In type 2, insulin levels are often too high, and go up much more rapidly in response to sugar and carbohydrate intake."

"So if there's too much insulin, how come the sugar's high, too?"

"The insulin's not being used properly by the cell membranes, so the insulin can't take the sugar from the blood into the cells as it's supposed to."

"So the sugar sort of 'backs up' in the blood?"

"Exactly. What's worse, our bodies keep making more and more insulin to try to 'force' the sugar from the blood into the cells. The excess insulin causes other problems, including high blood pressure and cholesterol abnormalities—specifically, lower levels of 'good' HDL cholesterol and higher levels of the 'bad' type."

"My blood pressure has been creeping up over the past few years. The doctor says it's my weight, mostly. And my cholesterol is a little worse."

"It's even possible that some of your weight problem is due to the excess insulin response to sugar and carbohydrate. There's some evidence that people with the genetic—family—tendency towards type 2 diabetes store body fat at a greater rate than others do."

"No wonder I seem to get fatter from breathing food fumes. But what does it have to do with which type of diet is better for me?"

"Please have a glucose-insulin tolerance test done. Once we see how much insulin your body makes in response to a standard amount of sugar, we can make a more informed choice."

Ten days later, Mrs. Hampton was back. "I've been working hard on cutting out the sugar, 'cause that's one thing all the health books and articles agree on."

"For sure. I hope you're also getting rid of processed foods, and anything with artificial flavor, color, or preservatives."

"LaDonna's been on me about that. That girl . . . in college it was coffee and cigarettes, pizzas and sodas . . . now she's lecturing me on health food!"

"I'm glad she's changed . . . it's better for her family, too."

"That's why she did it, she says. Babies sure do change a woman. Now how was that glucose-insulin tolerance test of mine? Do I go high complex carbohydrate or low carbohydrate, high protein? And what vitamins and minerals do I take? LaDonna already sent me a bottle of chromium pills." She showed them to me. "But I been holding off 'til I talked to you."

"Your test shows considerably more insulin response to the sugar challenge than usual."

"So I got plenty of insulin, but my cells just pay it no mind, and the sugar's 'backing up' in my blood?"

"You've got it."

"So what do I do to get those cells to pay attention?"

"In your case, with your blood pressure and cholesterol rising, and a weight problem, as well as the type 2 diabetes—it's probably best to follow the restricted-carbohydrate approach."

"If I remember from what you said last time, more sugar and carbohydrates bring out more insulin, and now you're saying this test shows more insulin's the last thing I need."

"Right."

"So less carbohydrate's the way to go for me for now."

"Please check with our dietitian about the details. She's a much better cook than I am."

"Now what about vitamins, minerals, and all that? Should I take this chromium LaDonna sent?"

"There are so many nutrients shown to be helpful in type 2 diabetes that taking them all individually would be a real chore. You can find in natural-food stores several high-potency 'multiple' formulas designed specifically to aid in blood-sugar control. Look for one with extra chromium and biotin."

"LaDonna was right about that chromium, wasn't she?"

"Yes. Chromium is one of the more important nutrients for type 2 diabetes. Chromium helps to restore the cell-membrane response to insulin."

"So, no sugar, emphasize whole foods, no chemicals in my food, restricted carbohydrates, and a multiple specially made for people with blood-sugar troubles. Is that everything?"

"There are 2 nutrients to use individually, as there usually isn't enough of them in any 'blood-sugar multiple'. The first is niacin. With chromium, niacin forms part of a molecule called 'glucose-tolerance factor', the molecule that helps insulin do its job in the cell membrane."

"So, both chromium and niacin will get my cells to pay attention to the insulin again, and maybe the insulin levels will go down?"

"And your blood sugar, too, as the insulin takes it out of the bloodstream and into the cells more efficiently."

"One of the articles LaDonna sent me says niacin lowers cholesterol. Will that work for me?"

"Since it's likely that excess insulin is behind both situations, it's likely that niacin and chromium will help both the sugar and cholesterol situations. But of course we'll need to do follow-up testing to make sure. For now, please use niacin in the form of inositol hexanicotinate, providing 600 milligrams of niacin daily."

"Inositol hexanicotinate? I'm lucky I can pronounce that."

"It appears to be a safer form of time-release niacin. But since it's possible to take too much niacin, we'll check liver function tests when we check your cholesterol and blood sugar. Lastly, take 1 tablespoon of flaxseed oil daily. Or if you prefer capsules, take 4 of the 1,000 milligram size twice daily."

"That helps the cells use insulin, too?"

"Yes."

"Aren't they in the 'multiple' formula?"

"It's very difficult to get essential fatty acids into a multiple vitamin and mineral formula, since they're oils."

It's been 6 years since Mrs. Hampton started her program to control her type 2 diabetes. Her fasting blood sugar ranges from 120 to 150—not 'perfect'—but considerably better. Her blood pressure fell slowly, and normalized in 18 months. Her cholesterol also normalized. Although as she says, "I could still stand to lose more weight," she's lost 40 pounds.

DR. GABY'S COMMENTARY

DIETARY FACTORS ARE important in diabetes. Depending on an individual's insulin response, either a high-fiber, high-complex-carbohydrate diet or a low-carbohydrate, high-protein diet may be needed. Additionally, research has shown that a number of different nutrients play a role in regulating blood-sugar levels. Many of these nutrients are in short supply in the typical American diet. Supplementing with appropriate vitamins and minerals may therefore be of value in the treatment of diabetes.

Dietary Considerations

BASIC MEASURES THAT individuals can take to control diabetes include maintaining ideal body weight, exercising regularly, and avoiding refined sugars and caffeine. For many diabetics, blood sugar can be controlled to a large extent by consuming more foods that contain complex carbohydrates and fiber, such as whole grains, fruits, vegetables, legumes, nuts, and seeds. Legumes (beans) are especially important for diabetics. Studies have shown that ingesting a bean dish helps prevent blood-sugar elevations not only at that meal, but at the following meal, as well.[1] One of the ways I have helped diabetics lower their blood sugar is to have them eat a helping of beans at breakfast and another helping at supper. There are many different beans from which to choose, including soybeans, navy beans, kidney beans, mung beans, black beans, and lentils.

Not everyone responds well to a high-fiber, high-complex-carbohydrate diet. Some individuals, like the patient described by Dr. Wright, do better on a low-carbohydrate, high-protein diet.[2] As Dr. Wright mentioned, a glucose-insulin tolerance test may help determine which diet is preferable for a particular patient. However, as is often the case in medicine, sometimes the best test is trial and error.

Nutritional Supplements
Chromium

IN animal studies, diets deficient in chromium resulted in hyperglycemia (high blood sugar).[3] Chromium is a component of a molecule in the body called glucose-tolerance factor, which is known to enhance the blood-sugar-lowering action of insulin.[4] Chromium deficiency appears to be common in the United States. One dietary survey revealed that 90% of American diets contained less than the minimum suggested daily intake for chromium.[5] Good sources of chromium include brewer's yeast, eggs, and whole grains. White bread contains 71% less chromium than whole wheat bread.

In a double-blind study, daily administration of 200 mcg of chromium resulted in a significant reduction in blood-sugar levels in elderly women with borderline diabetes.[6] In a study of 180 patients with type 2 diabetes, a chromium dose of 1,000 mcg per day was more effective than 200 mcg per day at reducing blood sugar.[7] Several other studies on chromium and blood sugar have produced conflicting results. In some of the negative studies, a poorly absorbed form of chromium (chromium chloride) was used, and the dosage may have been too low. We prefer the better-absorbed forms of chromium, such as chromium picolinate, chromium aspartate, or chromium polynicotinate. The optimal intake of chromium varies from person to person. For most individuals, 200 to 500 mcg per day is adequate; however, in our experience, some patients appear to need 1,000 mcg per day or more.

Recently, a few scientists have expressed concern that long-term use of large doses of chromium, particularly chromium picolinate, may cause chromosomal abnormalities. That concern is based on test-tube studies that used extremely large concentrations of chromium picolinate. This problem has not actually been shown to occur in humans or experimental animals. Toxicity studies in animals have shown that chromium is remarkably safe; it has one of the lowest toxicity profiles of all the essential trace minerals. Picolinate is a normal breakdown product of the amino acid tryptophan that appears to function in the body as a mineral carrier. It therefore seems unlikely that supplementing with a small amount of picolinate would cause adverse effects. Nevertheless, to be on the safe side, individuals wishing to supplement with more than 200 mcg of chromium per day should consult a practitioner who is trained in nutritional medicine.

Niacin

As a component of glucose-tolerance factor, niacin plays an important role in carbohydrate metabolism. Many of the refined foods consumed by Americans are depleted of niacin. Grains and other foods that are "enriched" usually contain added niacinamide, but that form of vitamin B₃ cannot be converted by the human body into niacin. Most vitamin supplements also contain niacinamide, rather than niacin. Although niacinamide is capable of performing most of the functions of vitamin B3, a small amount of niacin seems to be necessary for blood-sugar regulation.

In one study, 16 elderly individuals received either 200 mcg of chromium, 100 mg of niacin, or both, daily for 28 days. Fasting plasma-glucose levels and glucose tolerance were unaffected by either chromium or niacin alone. However, when these nutrients were taken together, the individuals experienced significant improvements in both fasting blood sugar and glucose tolerance.[8] Based on the results of this study, it appears that a small amount of niacin (such as 20 to 100 mg per day) should be included in any supplement program designed to regulate blood sugar.

Biotin

THIS B-vitamin plays a role in the metabolism of glucose within the cell. Administering biotin to genetically diabetic mice improved glucose tolerance and lowered insulin resistance.[9] In one human study, 7 insulin-dependent diabetics were removed from insulin therapy and treated with biotin (16 mg per day) or a placebo for 1 week. Fasting blood-glucose levels rose significantly in patients given the placebo, but decreased significantly in those treated with biotin.[10] In another study, serum biotin levels were significantly lower in 43 patients with non-insulin-dependent (type 2) diabetes than in healthy individuals. Eighteen diabetics were given 9 mg of biotin per day for 1 month, along with an antibiotic that prevents biotin from being degraded by intestinal bacteria. Ten other patients received a placebo. After one month, the average blood-glucose level fell 45% in the group receiving biotin, but did not change in those given the placebo.[11]

In our experience, it is not necessary to take an antibiotic along with biotin. We have seen a few patients who had a clear reduction in blood sugar after taking 10 to 20 mg of biotin per day.

Vitamin E

PLASMA levels of vitamin E were found to be significantly lower in a group of diabetics than in healthy individuals. In a double-blind study, administering 900 mg of vitamin E per day for 4 months to type 2 diabetics significantly improved both glucose tolerance and insulin action.[12] Therefore, supplementing with vitamin E appears to be worthwhile for diabetics.

Other Important Nutrients

RESEARCH has shown that many other nutrients play a role in regulating blood-glucose levels. These include vitamin B₆, zinc, copper, magnesium, manganese, and vitamin C.[13]

A small proportion of diabetics have a genetic disorder that causes them to accumulate iron in their tissues. Since iron overload can actually cause or aggravate diabetes, all individuals with diabetes should have their iron status determined by a standard laboratory test. Iron should not be included as part of a multiple vitamin-mineral formula unless this genetic disorder has been ruled out.

Herbal Supplements

GYMNEMA SYLVESTRE is a woody climber that grows wild in certain areas of India. The leaves of this plant have been used for several centuries by traditional medical practitioners to control diabetes. In experimental animals made diabetic by administering a pancreas-damaging chemical, treatment with *Gymnema sylvestre* promoted repair and/or regeneration of the insulin-producing cells of the pancreas.[14] Type 1 diabetics given an extract of this herb for 6 to 8 months experienced, on average, a 23% reduction in fasting blood glucose and a 25% decrease in insulin requirement.[15] Type 2 diabetics given the same extract for 18 to 20 months also showed a significant reduction in blood-sugar levels; 5 of 22 patients were able to discontinue their blood-sugar-lowering medication and all of the others (except one) were able to reduce the dosage.[16]

A Cautionary Note

INDIVIDUALS WHO ARE taking medication for diabetes should never make dietary changes or take nutritional supplements without medical supervision. If the diet and supplements work the way they are supposed to, then the dosage requirement for anti-diabetes medications could change, and a dangerous fall in blood sugar could result. In addition, the kidneys of individuals with advanced diabetes may be too weak to process the large amount potassium that is contained in a high-complex-carbohydrate, high-fiber diet. Potassium has, on rare occasions, been known to build up to dangerous levels when individuals with late-stage diabetes changed their diet. To be on the safe side, diabetics should consult their doctor before changing their diet or taking supplements.

Conclusion

A CAREFULLY PLANNED dietary program, combined with appropriate nutritional supplements, will often produce significant improvements in the blood-sugar level of diabetics. Since the optimal treatment may vary from person to person, it is advisable for diabetics to seek the help of a knowledgeable nutrition-oriented practitioner.

In the next chapter, we will learn that treating diabetes involves more than just controlling blood sugar. There is growing evidence that specific nutritional supplements may help prevent some of the complications of diabetes, including eye and kidney damage, nerve problems, and cardiovascular disease.

For Summary of Recommendations for Treating Diabetes, see the following chapter.

DIABETES *(preventing complications)*

IN THE PREVIOUS *chapter, we discussed ways in which diabetics can lower their blood sugar (glucose). It is well known that keeping blood-glucose levels close to the normal range will reduce the incidence of diabetic complications, such as heart disease, neuropathy (nerve damage), cataracts, retinopathy (disease of the retina), and nephropathy (kidney damage). Therefore, one of the main treatment strategies for diabetics is to keep blood sugar tightly controlled.*

However, even tight control does not completely eliminate the risk of organ damage that can result from diabetes. Other biochemical changes occur in diabetes that are only partly related to blood-glucose levels. Addressing these abnormalities may greatly increase the likelihood that a diabetic will live a normal life.

DR. WRIGHT'S CASE STUDY

"My blood sugar's a lot better now," Mr. Takajima reported. "I've finally gotten rid of all the sugar, processed foods, and food chemicals— my wife made sure of that. I'm taking that niacin, inositol hexanicotinate . . . whatever. Also, the flaxseed oil, and the multiple vitamin and mineral for blood-sugar troubles, with extra chromium. And I'm feeling a lot better, too. More energy, my vision's a little less blurry, I lost some weight . . . just generally better all 'round. Now, you told me when I got all of this under control, we should talk about preventing complications of this diabetes. I've been putting it off, the business is picking up, but my wife told me I'd better come in or else. She didn't say what else, but I got the idea."

"You told me you have . . . or had . . . older relatives with diabetes? Let's see . . ." I looked through his record. "Your mother's had lens-

replacement surgery, both eyes, for cataract and now she's losing her vision to retinopathy. . . . Her older brother had diabetic neuropathy, severe nerve pain, and then a leg amputated, and died of a clot after surgery. Her younger brother's had bypass surgery. And your grandmother, your mother's mother, died of a heart attack. Enough complications to prevent, all right."

"I probably forgot to tell you about my grandmother on the other side. She got what she called 'a little sugar' when she was past 70, and finally died of kidney failure. My wife reminded me that kidney failure is another possible complication of diabetes, and to make sure to tell you."

"She's right." I made a note, and checked his lab reports. "No sign of kidney problems on your tests so far, but unfortunately most routine tests for kidney function aren't very sensitive."

"So what do I do? Somehow I suspect it involves swallowing a lot more vitamin and mineral supplements."

"And botanicals—herbals—too! But it's

certainly easier to swallow a lot of supplements every day than suffer one or more of the diabetic complications your relatives have had. Before we get to supplementation, though—aren't you also taking digestive aids?"

"Oh, yeah, but those are almost automatic now and besides they're not really nutrients, so I forget to mention them. You said the first time I was here that most diabetics have problems with digesting and assimilating nutrients, and that could lead to as many problems in the long run as eating wrong or not taking any vitamins. So I took that test for stomach acid, and the other tests for pancreas function and digestion in general. And I'm taking the betaine hydrochloride and pepsin to make up for my weak stomach, and the pancreatin because my pancreas wasn't doing too well making digestive enzymes."

"Good. Since your stomach function was weak, we asked you to start on vitamin B_{12} injections with folate, didn't we?"

Mr. Takajima looked embarrassed. "I've only taken 1 or 2 of those. I developed an aversion to needles the first time I ever saw a doctor."

"Let's start with more reasons for vitamin B_{12} injections. Remember your mother's retinopathy, and her brother's neuropathy? There's evidence that vitamin B_{12} can help prevent both of these problems."

"Really? Guess I better just do it . . . maybe my wife can do it for me?"

"No reason why not, if it's easier for you."

"I've been thinking—what about the rest of the B-complex?"

"Vitamin B_6 may help prevent diabetic neuropathy, too—along with biotin. For now, the amounts in the 'blood-sugar multiple' should do the job. As we grow older, the absorption of other B-vitamins gets more problematic, so we often add them to the injection along with the B_{12} and folate."

"How about the retinopathy and cataracts? I really don't want anything to happen to my vision."

"Besides vitamin B_{12}, magnesium is advisable.

There's evidence of low magnesium in diabetic retinopathy and microangiopathy—that's disease of the small blood vessels in the back of the eye and likely elsewhere."

"Should I take extra magnesium?"

"There's likely enough in your 'multiple'. It has 400 milligrams."

"Anything else for my eyes?"

"Several nutrients in the multiple—vitamin B_2, selenium, vitamin C, vitamin E, and zinc—all help in cataract prevention. However, please get some bilberry—that's a botanical concentrate also called European blueberry. Make sure it's standardized—a usual standardization is 25% anthocyanosides. For now, take 80 milligrams, twice daily. One study shows that bilberry, when used in combination with vitamin E, slows the progression of existing cataract. There's every reason to expect bilberry to be preventive, also." I wrote it down. "There's another, broader, and very important reason to use bilberry routinely in diabetes."

"What's that?"

"In diabetes, there's a gradual thickening of the substance surrounding the smallest blood cells, called the 'basement membrane'. As it thickens, it's harder and harder for nutrients to move from the bloodstream into the cells, and for waste products and metabolites to move from cells back into the bloodstream. This is particularly a problem in diabetic nephropathy—diabetic kidney disease."

"But it could affect blood vessels over the entire body, and more or less 'gum up' the entire small-blood-vessel system, couldn't it?"

"Very likely."

"Would it hurt if I took a little more of the bilberry?"

"No."

"It's just a concentrate from blueberries—isn't it remarkable what it can do?"

"And it's very unlikely any synthetic drug will ever be able to do the same, especially without side effects."

"Is that all?"

"Not yet. Even though vitamin C is in the multiple, it's wisest to use extra. Please use another gram—1,000 milligrams, twice daily. Vitamin C can help prevent cardiovascular problems."

"I've read and heard about vitamins C and E to prevent heart and blood-vessel disease everywhere . . . radio, TV, newspapers. . . . Should I take extra vitamin E, too?"

"Your 'blood-sugar multiple' has 400 IU of vitamin E. For now, that's likely enough, but we'll do a platelet-aggregation test to be sure."

"Platelet what?"

"Aggregation. That's a measurement of 'stickiness'. Many diabetics have excessively 'sticky' platelets, leading to microvascular (small blood vessel) disease. Vitamin E can significantly reduce platelet aggregation, 'stickiness'. Other nutrients do this job also: the flaxseed oil you're already using, magnesium . . . also gamma-linolenic acid, or GLA."

"You haven't mentioned GLA yet. Is that in the multiple?"

"Haven't I?" I checked Mr. Takajima's list. "No. And it's not in the multiple. . . . Well, I'll add it now. Please use gamma-linolenic acid, 120 milligrams daily. Evening primrose, borage, and black-currant-seed oils are all good sources."

"Why won't just flaxseed oil do the job?"

"GLA can also help prevent diabetic neuropathy. Flaxseed oil does not contain any GLA and hasn't been shown to prevent neuropathy."

"Let's see . . . in addition to my digestive aids, there's all that stuff in the 'blood-sugar multiple', inositol hexanicotinate, flaxseed oil, vitamin B_{12}, bilberry, vitamin C, and GLA . . . anything more?"

"At least one more, and possibly two. The first is the amino acid taurine. It'll help prevent retinal and heart problems, and very likely help improve gallbladder function. Taurine is frequently low in diabetics."

"And the other?"

"This one we'll need a test for, as it's a hormone—testosterone."

"What does testosterone do for diabetes?"

"A Danish physician, Dr. Jens Moller, discovered that testosterone had powerful effects in diabetes, helping to improve overall carbohydrate metabolism, and specifically reversing diabetic vascular disease. He published two books with pictures showing complete reversal of gangrene in diabetic feet."*

"Gangrene? Reversal of gangrene? Why wasn't that done for my uncle?"

"The very large majority of American doctors have just started to look at natural treatments, including natural testosterone. And testosterone isn't the only so-called 'alternative' treatment that can save a gangrenous diabetic foot or leg: Chelation therapy has been doing that for more than 30 years."

Mr. Takajima shook his head. "My uncle died just 20 years ago. But since I have no gangrene, why should I need to worry about testosterone now?"

"In natural medicine, it's been observed over and over again that if a large amount of a vitamin, mineral, botanical, or other natural supplement will successfully treat a problem, a small, steady amount will likely prevent it. But in the case of testosterone or other hormones, it's rarely wise to use them unless levels are low in the first place."

"But not with vitamins and minerals?"

"No. Natural-medicine doctors have known for years—and universities are just learning—that extra amounts of vitamins and minerals far beyond the so-called 'RDA' can have powerful preventive and therapeutic effects with minimal 'side effects', especially when compared with synthetic pharmaceuticals."

"So I'll have my testosterone checked?"

"Right." I marked a lab request form, and Mr. Takajima got up to go.

---

*Dr. Moller's two books are available in reprint form from the Barnes Foundation, Box 98, Trumbull, Connecticut, 06611; (203) 261-2101, fax: (203) 261-3017.

There's no way to tell in advance whether Mr. Takajima will develop complications from his diabetes. Only long-term research studies can show how well this type of preventive nutritional program really works. But Dr. Gaby and I believe that if such studies were done properly, the outcome would be extremely favorable!

DR. GABY'S COMMENTARY

DIABETICS ARE AT risk for a number of complications and conventional medicine offers little in the way of prevention. Fortunately, a growing body of research suggests that nutritional supplements may be of value in preventing such complications.

Preventing Two Kinds of Organ Damage
Sorbitol Damages Cells

SCIENTISTS have identified two main processes that lead to diabetes-related organ damage. One is the accumulation of sorbitol in certain tissues and organs. Sorbitol (the same compound used in "sugarless" gum) is manufactured in the body from glucose. When glucose levels are elevated inside the cells, sorbitol is produced faster than it can be broken down. Since sorbitol cannot cross cell membranes, it builds up inside the cells. The accumulated sorbitol draws water in by the process known as osmosis. Sorbitol-induced osmotic swelling is believed to be one of the main causes of tissue damage in diabetics. (Ingested sorbitol does not cause this problem, because it does not enter the cells.)

One way to minimize sorbitol accumulation is to reduce its production by keeping blood-glucose levels low. Another strategy is to inhibit the conversion of glucose to sorbitol or to enhance the breakdown of sorbitol. Vitamin C apparently performs one or both of these latter functions, since it has been shown to lower intracellular sorbitol levels without affecting blood sugar. In one study, supplementing with vitamin C prevented the accumulation of sorbitol in the lens of the eye in diabetic guinea pigs.[1] Presumably, this effect of vitamin C would reduce the risk of cataracts developing. In another study, treatment of diabetics with 2,000 mg of vitamin C per day for 3 weeks reduced the average sorbitol concentration in red blood cells by 44.5%.[2] If vitamin C affects other tissues the same way, then taking 2,000 mg of this vitamin per day should help prevent some of the complications of diabetes. It should be noted that diabetics have a higher-than-normal requirement for vitamin C,[3] probably because glucose (which is structurally similar to vitamin C) competes with the vitamin for entry into cells.

Glycosylation: The "Browning" Reaction

GLYCOSYLATION is the other reaction that is thought to cause organ damage in diabetics. Glycosylation refers to a sugar molecule binding irreversibly to a protein molecule. Glycosylation of protein is known to bakers as the "browning reaction," since the binding of sugar to protein in the baking process causes browning to occur. In the body, this metaphorical "tanning of one's inner hide" leads to tissue damage and premature aging.

Glycosylation occurs in all human beings, but it takes place at a faster rate in people who have elevated blood-sugar levels. While reducing the blood sugar will decrease the rate of glycosylation, other measures can also be taken to slow the reaction. Studies have shown that vitamins B_6, E, and C are all capable of inhibiting glycosylation (measured as glycoslyated hemoglobin or albumin) in diabetics. The effective dose of vitamin B_6 was 50 mg, 3 times a day.[4] Vitamin E inhibited glycosylation at doses of 600 and 1,200 IU per day, but the higher dose was slightly more effective than the lower dose.[5] Vitamin C reduced protein glycosylation when given at a dose of 1 gram per day.[6] Although it is possible that lower doses of these nutrients, when taken in combination, would also prevent glycosylation, the research done so far has focused only on one vitamin at a time.

It is noteworthy that each of these vitamins has also been shown to prevent heart disease (a common side effect of diabetes). Vitamins E and C function as heart-protecting antioxidants and as mild blood thinners. Vitamin B_6 helps break down homocysteine, a byproduct of amino-acid metabolism that leads to heart disease.

Nutritional Supplements
Flavonoids Promote Tissue Integrity

DIABETICS frequently have reduced integrity of capillaries and connective tissue. These abnormalities can lead to retinal hemorrhages, blood-vessel damage, or other problems. In addition to vitamin C, flavonoids play an important role in enhancing tissue strength. Flavonoids are present in a wide variety of fruits and vegetables. One particularly potent flavonoid is present in bilberry (the European blueberry). In one study, the tissue abnormalities seen in diabetics were largely reversed by treatment with an extract of bilberry.[7] Administering bilberry extract to diabetics with eye disease also reduced the tendency of their retinal tissue to bleed.[8] Other food-derived flavonoids have also been shown to improve capillary integrity.[9]

Some B Vitamins and Gamma-Linolenic Acid Help Neuropathy

DIABETIC neuropathy can cause severe pain, tingling, numbness, and weakness. Conventional therapy, which consists primarily of medications to relieve pain, is often ineffective. A number of different nutrients have been found to relieve diabetic neuropathy. Although it is not always clear how these nutrients work, they are safe and are therefore worth a try.

In one study, 3 patients with diabetic neuropathy were treated with the B vitamin biotin, beginning with intramuscular injections and followed by 5 mg per day by mouth. Within 4 to 8 weeks, the patients experienced marked improvements in painful muscle cramps, numbness, tingling, and other nerve-related symptoms.[10]

As early as 1951, vitamin B_{12} injections were reported to be helpful for diabetic neuropathy. Of 12 patients who received a series of vitamin B_{12} injections, 7 had complete or almost complete relief of symptoms.[11] The treatment seemed to work best when the injections were given frequently.

Research has also demonstrated a beneficial effect of evening primrose oil (EPO), a source of a fatty acid called gamma-linolenic acid (GLA). In a double-blind study, 111 patients with mild diabetic neuropathy were randomly assigned to receive 12 capsules of EPO per day (providing 480 mg of GLA per day) or a placebo for 1 year. Of 16 measures of nerve function that were assessed, all 16 improved in the group treated with EPO, whereas 15 of these parameters became worse in the placebo group.[12] Similar benefits were reported with EPO in another study.[13] Borage oil is a less-expensive source of GLA than EPO. However, it is not certain whether GLA is the only active ingredient in EPO, and borage oil has not been tested as a treatment for diabetic neuropathy.

Vitamin B_6 has also shown to be effective against diabetic neuropathy. Of 10 diabetics treated with 50 mg of vitamin B_6, 3 times a day, everyone had a complete resolution of their symptoms of neuropathy.[14] However, other investigators found that vitamin B_6 had little or no effect on neuropathy.[15]

Nutrients for Retinopathy

DIABETICS are often deficient in magnesium, and the deficiency is most severe in those with retinopathy.[16] Although there is no proof that supplementing with magnesium will prevent retinal damage, magnesium deficiency should not go untreated.

According to some reports, vitamin B_{12} injections may also be beneficial. In one study, 15 type 1 (juvenile-onset) diabetics with retinopathy received 100 mcg of vitamin B_{12} per day, mixed with their daily insulin injection. After 1 year, all signs of retinopathy had disappeared in 7 of 15 patients.[17] Similar results were reported in another study.[18]

The amino acid taurine may also help prevent the decline in visual function that is associated with diabetes. Research has shown that low blood levels of taurine are common in diabetics.[19] Since this nutrient is required for normal vision, as well as for a healthy heart, supplementation may be worthwhile. A dosage of 500 mg, 3 times a day, was found to normalize low taurine levels in diabetics. The main dietary sources of taurine are meat and fish.

Preventing Heart Disease

DIABETICS are at increased risk of developing heart disease. Many of the nutrients discussed in this chapter may help prevent heart disease. Other important nutrients for the heart include folic acid, zinc, copper, chromium, and coenzyme Q10.

Conclusion

THE RESEARCH I have reviewed in this chapter and the previous one demonstrates that diet and nutritional supplementation can do a great deal of good for diabetics. However, diabetics wishing to go on a nutrition program should seek professional help, because the treatment can be quite complicated and may require adjustment of medications. In addition, as I pointed out in the previous chapter, some diabetics have weak kidneys and must proceed with extreme caution. When these considerations are taken into account, nutritional therapy can help most diabetics lead healthier, and possibly longer, lives.

Summary of Recommendations for Diabetes

(NOTE: All recommendations should be medically supervised)

PRIMARY RECOMMENDATIONS:

- DIET

  ➤ Avoid refined sugar and other refined carbohydrates, caffeine, and alcohol.

  ➤ For most individuals, a diet high in fiber and complex carbohydrates is preferred. Some people, particularly those with insulin resistance, experience better blood-sugar control with a low-carbohydrate diet.

- SUPPLEMENTS

  ➤ Chromium (picolinate, aspartate, or polynicotinate), 200 to 1,000 mcg per day. Chromium may help control blood-sugar levels more effectively when niacin (30 to 100 mg/day) is also supplemented.

  ➤ Vitamin C, 1,000 to 3,000 mg per day.

  ➤ Magnesium, 300 to 600 mg per day.

  ➤ Vitamin E, 400 to 800 IU per day.

  ➤ Vitamin B_6, 50 to 150 mg per day.

  ➤ Biotin, 10 to 20 mg per day in selected cases.

  ➤ High-potency multiple vitamin-mineral formula that includes trace minerals. Iron should not be included unless iron-storage disease has been ruled out. Adjust doses of other nutrients according the amounts in the multiple.

  ➤ *Gymnema sylvestre* in selected cases. (See previous chapter.)

OTHER RECOMMENDATIONS:

- Taurine, 500 to 1,500 mg per day.
- Vitamin B_{12} injections in selected patients with neuropathy or retinopathy.
- Evening primrose oil in selected patients with neuropathy.

EAR INFECTIONS

"OTITIS MEDIA" IS *the medical term for inflammation of the middle ear. "Otitis" means inflammation of the ear, and "media" refers to the middle ear. Otitis media is one of the most common medical problems in children, exceeded only by colds and sore throats. By 2 years of age, nearly one-third of all children will have had 3 or more episodes. The annual cost of diagnosing and treating this condition is more than $2 billion.*

There are 2 main types of otitis media. The first type, acute otitis media (the classic acute ear infection), is diagnosed when there is fluid in the middle ear accompanied by pain, bulging of the eardrum, or drainage of pus. The second type, otitis media with effusion (OME, or serous otitis media), refers to fluid in the middle ear without signs or symptoms of an ear infection. OME tends to be a more chronic problem, often persisting for months, during which time the fluid in the ears makes it difficult to hear.

Acute ear infections are typically treated with antibiotics, although such infections usually run their course without treatment. Doctors disagree about whether long-term antibiotic therapy is advisable for children who suffer recurrent ear infections. Although such treatment does prevent recurrences, the benefits are limited, since only 1 of every 9 children treated shows evidence of improvement.[1]

An even more controversial treatment involves placing tubes in the ears of children with chronic OME. The purpose of inserting tubes is to allow the pressure to equilibrate on both sides of the eardrum, thereby improving hearing and preventing problems with speech development and learning. However, putting a hole in the eardrum also provides an avenue through which bacteria can enter the middle ear. In addition, recent evidence shows that the improvement in hearing lasts only 6 months and that, in the long run, putting tubes in the ears might actually make hearing worse.[2] Furthermore, there is no good evidence that chronic OME causes any kind of permanent problem.[3] Therefore, putting tubes in a child's ears may not be appropriate in many cases. Nevertheless, most "experts" still recommend using tubes, even though they admit that their opinion is not supported by scientific research.[4]

DR. WRIGHT'S CASE STUDY

"We just don't want tubes put in Joshua's ears," Donna James said. "But he just keeps getting earaches. He had the first one when he was only 6 months old, and he's had over a dozen of them since. We've given him gallons of antihistamines and antibiotics, but the infections just keep coming back. Now the pediatrician says the only thing to do is to put tubes in his ears, to 'keep them drained'. She says there's fluid behind his eardrums all the time now, and that makes them get infected easier."

"Did you ask why the fluid's there all the time?"

"She said something about the eustachian tubes being too small to drain to the inside."

"There's likely another cause for that—a cause that tubes in the ears does nothing to change. Also, several research studies have shown that tubes in the eardrums don't do any good, and may actually do some harm. That research has been out there for several years. I'm surprised that anyone's still recommending them."

"The pediatrician said there's nothing else to do. That's why we're here. My husband and I weren't happy with that."

I made a note, and turned to Joshua. "How old are you, Joshua?"

He held up 3 fingers. "Three."

"He'll be 4 in 4 months."

"And what do you eat for breakfast?"

Joshua giggled, put his thumb in his mouth, and looked at his mother.

"He usually has one of those dry cereals—not the sugar-frosted ones—with milk. Sometimes eggs and toast and orange juice."

"Lunch?"

"A sandwich and milk."

"Peanut butter?"

"And jelly," Joshua said.

"Is there anything else?" his mother asked. "Also an apple or some other piece of fruit."

"And at dinner?"

"Well, we're cutting back on beef and pork, so we have more chicken, turkey, and some fish. I make sure we have vegetables or a salad, and usually rice or potatoes."

"Do you use whole grain bread and rice, or white flour and white rice?"

"Usually white rice, and the bread is some of each. Joshua's father doesn't like whole wheat."

"Does Joshua drink soft drinks?"

"Sometimes. Usually the cola kind."

"What about snacks?"

"He gets his share of cookies and ice cream,

but I make sure he gets carrots, celery, and fruit, especially during the daytime."

I scribbled a few more notes. "You said Joshua got his first ear infection at 6 months. How long did you nurse him?"

"Actually, his first ear infection was at 6 months and 2 weeks, just 2 weeks after I went back to work. I stayed home for the first 6 months, and nursed him, but it was really going to be difficult after that, so I started him on a formula just before he was 6 months old."

"Cow milk formula?"

"To start. After 2 or 3 earaches, we switched to a soy formula but it didn't seem to make any difference."

"When did he start on solid food?"

"About 8 or 9 months."

"Do you have any problems with your health?"

"I'm a little more tired than I'd like, but otherwise I'm fine."

"Joshua's father?"

"He's fine."

"How about Joshua's grandparents?"

"My mother has mild diabetes—just diet and some pills—no insulin. My father's OK as far as I know, but he won't go to a doctor unless he's practically dying. Joshua's other grandfather died of a heart attack before Joshua was born, and his other grandmother had breast cancer, but she's fine now. Oh—she has some kind of sinus problems, too."

"Does anyone in the family have allergies?"

"My husband has a little sneezing and hay fever in the spring, but not much. He says it was much worse when he was growing up."

I asked a few other health-background questions about Joshua, then asked him and his mother to go to an examination room.

His eardrums both had fluid behind them—the right more than the left. He had dark circles (often called "allergic shiners") under both eyes, as well as "Dennié's lines" (tiny horizontal creases) in both lower eyelids. There were a dozen or so small bumps scattered over the backs of both upper arms; overall, Joshua's skin was a bit on the dry side. Otherwise, his examination was normal.

"Joshua appears to have allergies," I observed.

His mother looked puzzled. "How can you tell just by looking at him?"

"Those dark circles under his eyes, they're usually called 'allergic shiners', especially in small children. The other common causes of dark circles under the eyes besides allergy include chronic lack of sleep, pregnancy, and hormone treatment."

She laughed. "He's certainly not pregnant or taking hormones, and he gets plenty of sleep."

"Also, each of his lower eyelids has several small horizontal creases called 'Dennié's lines', for a Dr. Dennié who originally discovered that they were usually associated with allergy. Actually, though, I knew that Joshua has allergies when you told me he's had recurrent ear infections—allergy is almost always part of the cause of this problem."

"Really?"

"Really. Just think for a moment—what happens to his father's nose and sinuses when he's exposed to his springtime allergies?"

"He gets all stuffed up . . . "

"And Joshua's eustachian tubes and ears?"

"Oh—they get all stuffed up!"

"Which makes a perfect breeding ground for germs."

"Makes sense. So, we'll check him for allergies?"

"Yes."

"Isn't that awfully tough on a 3-year-old?"

"We don't use skin testing for allergies. No needles."

She relaxed. "Good. What else?"

"It'll be tough, but please eliminate all the refined sugar and refined carbohydrates from his diet."

"All the sugar? Why's that?"

"Sugar interferes with the immune system. Careful experiments performed 20 years ago showed clearly that ingesting sugar interferes with the normal germ-destroying ability of white blood cells for 3 to 5 hours. Remember, the average soft drink has several teaspoons of sugar, as does the average dessert. So, please read all the labels on any packaged food and eliminate anything with sugar. Of course, no 'soft drinks', and remember, most commercial fruit drinks contain a lot of added sugar. If Joshua drinks fruit juice, please make sure it's the whole fruit."

"What if we make our own in a blender, and add some water?"

"Sounds OK."

"So, no sugar, eliminate allergies once we find out what they are . . . what about vitamins and minerals?"

"They're next. First, zinc." I checked Joshua's weight in his record. "Please give him 30 milligrams of zinc (as zinc picolinate) daily. The capsules are small, but you can empty one out into juice if he can't swallow it."

"What does zinc do?"

"Helps improve the function of the immune system in a number of different ways—helps increase resistance against infection. Next, vitamin A—at Joshua's weight—20,000 IU daily for the next few months."

"How many months?"

"We'll keep an eye on those little bumps on the skin on the back of his upper arms. Those are usually signs of insufficient vitamin A. But even if he didn't have those, I'd recommend extra vitamin A, anyway. Research has shown that animals and children deficient in Vitamin A get more ear infections.

"Vitamin C is next. At his size, please give him 500 milligrams, twice daily. If he shows any signs of catching a cold or other infection, increase the vitamin C to 500 milligrams every hour or two while awake until he's better."

"Isn't that quite a lot?"

"If it's too much, he'll get gas or loose bowels, and it's time to back off. But it isn't harmful."

"Zinc, vitamin A, vitamin C, no sugar, no allergies. I hope he doesn't have too many allergies. It's going to be very difficult to eliminate very many foods from his diet."

"Even if there are quite a number, almost all of them can be desensitized within 4 to 8 months."

"Without needles?"

"Drops under the tongue."

"Sounds easy enough. But still, that's a lot to do; I hope there's not too much more."

"Just one more thing for now—a good general multiple vitamin-mineral—both to make up for what's not in the food, and to 'back up' the individual nutrients."

"That's it?"

"Most of the time, that'll do the job."

Joshua's mother got up to go. "It's worth it if Joshua stops having ear infections."

Joshua turned out to be allergic to cow's milk, corn, chicken, oranges, peanuts, and 9 more foods. I asked his mother to eliminate them until they were desensitized, except for the cow's milk, which I usually don't recommend drinking at all. After doing some reading, she decided to eliminate all the sugar and refined food from her whole family's diet. We continued all the supplements for 9 months before cutting back, except for the extra vitamin A, which was cut back to 10,000 IU daily at 5 months, as the bumps on the skin of the back of his upper arms had disappeared by then.

The fluid behind Joshua's eardrums was no longer visible at 6 months, and his "allergic shiners" faded, but they didn't totally disappear. Most importantly, he stopped having earaches entirely, and still hasn't had another in 4 years since his first visit.

DR. GABY'S COMMENTARY

WITH ALL THE research pointing to allergies and other dietary considerations as the cause of ear infections, it is surprising how many doctors still insist that tubes are the only effective treatment. Like Joshua, with careful attention to diet and the use of supplements, children need not suffer from this painful condition.

Dietary Considerations
Effect of Sugar

FORTUNATELY, good results in treating ear infections can usually be obtained, if individuals pay careful attention to diet and nutrition. We have observed that restricting or eliminating refined sugar from the diet often reduces the incidence of ear infections and effusions. That clinical finding may be explained by the fact that eating sweets has an adverse effect on the immune system. In one study, healthy young adults drank 24 ounces of a cola beverage (containing about 66 grams of sucrose). Within 45 minutes, the ability of their white blood cells to engulf bacteria dropped by about 50%.[5]

Other scientists found that ingesting 100 g of some other sugars, including glucose, fructose, honey, and even orange juice, had a similar effect.[6] This decline in immune function was greatest about 2 hours after ingestion of the sugar, and it persisted for at least 5 hours. In another study, the ability of rats to manufacture antibodies was reduced by 50% when their diet contained as little as 10% sucrose. Larger amounts of sugar impeded antibody production even more.[7]

Some children appear to be more sensitive than others to the effects of sugar. In these children, even small amounts of sugar will cause problems. I suspect that eating sweets has several different effects on the body, depending on both the amount consumed and the individual's susceptibility to sugar. First, as mentioned above, large amounts of sugar have a direct suppressive effect on the immune system. Additionally, moderate amounts consumed for long periods of time may also suppress immune function directly, probably more in some people than in others. Finally, eating sugar can have an indirect effect, by depleting the nutrients that the body needs to support a healthy immune system. Sugar provides virtually no vitamins or minerals at all; therefore, if your diet contains 19% sugar (the average amount found in the American diet), you will be getting about 19% less vitamin C, zinc, vitamin A, vitamin B$_6$, folic acid, and other key nutrients. Since each of these nutrients plays a role in immune function, deficiencies might render you more susceptible to infection or allergies.

Small amounts of sugar probably have little direct effect on the immune system or nutritional status of healthy children. However, some children develop symptoms after ingesting even small quantities of sugar. Apparently, these children are allergic to (or have some other type of sensitivity to) sugar.

The Role of Food Allergy

FOOD allergy is probably the most important—and definitely the most overlooked—factor in children who suffer from recurrent ear infections or chronic OME. In our experience, at least 75% of children with these problems see a marked improvement after the offending foods are identified and removed from their diet. As with other food-allergic conditions, the most common symptom-evoking foods are sugar, dairy products, wheat, corn, egg, citrus fruits, and chocolate. I typically recommend an elimination diet, in which all the common allergens are avoided simultaneously. In most cases, the symptoms improve or disappear within 3 weeks. At that point, foods are tested individually, watching for a recurrence of symptoms with each food challenge.

One of the elimination diets I have used in my practice is presented in appendix A. Some doctors use other tests for allergy and sensitivity, as well as desensitization techniques. The reliability and effectiveness of some of these methods is controversial (see chapter 3 for additional discussion).

I once saw a 3-year-old girl who had suffered for 2 years from frequent recurrences of ear infections. Her pediatrician had prescribed continuous antibiotic therapy (amoxicillin), because whenever the child had tried to stop taking the antibiotic, another infection developed within a few days. She began an elimination diet, and amoxicillin was discontinued 1 week later. During the following week, while the child was still on the elimination diet, no symptoms occurred. However, within 20 minutes of testing corn, she was crying from ear pain, and within 60 minutes, pus was coming out of her left ear. The removal of corn products from her diet eliminated her ear problems, and she has remained free of infections (without the use of antibiotics) for 5 years.

Doctors who maintain that food allergy is not a scientifically documented cause of otitis media have not been keeping up with the medical literature. A relationship between food allergy and OME was reported as early as 1942.[8] More recently, Italian researchers provided evidence that allergy causes the eustachian tubes to swell, thereby blocking the outflow of fluid from the middle ear.[9]

A study published in 1994 validated what innovative practitioners have been saying for a long time. Of 104 children with OME, 81 (78%) tested positive for food allergies. Among those 81 children, exclusion of the offending foods from the diet for 11 weeks led to significant improvement in 70 cases (86%). Subsequent challenges with suspected foods led to a flare-up of otitis in 66 (94%) of 70 cases.[10] This report confirms our own impression that the vast majority of children with chronic OME improve significantly when food allergy is considered and the offending foods are eliminated.

Nutritional Supplements

NUTRITION-ORIENTED DOCTORS frequently recommend supplements to help fight infections and allergic conditions. Vitamin C is particularly useful; not only does this vitamin stimulate the immune system, it also has an antihistamine effect.

Zinc and vitamin A have been shown to enhance immune function and to help fight infections.

Although no studies have specifically addressed the effect of these nutrients on acute otitis media or OME, it has been shown that elderly people who take nutritional supplements have about a 50% reduction in the incidence of infections.[11] Older people tend to have lower levels of various vitamins and minerals, compared with younger adults. Children with recurrent ear problems are also likely to have nutritional deficiencies. Continually having to fight infections and allergic reactions probably puts added stress on a child's nutritional status. Furthermore, ingesting allergenic foods may cause damage to the stomach and small intestine, resulting in reduced absorption of vitamins and minerals. Therefore, supplementing with a broad-spectrum hypoallergenic multiple vitamin/mineral is a good idea for most children with chronic ear problems. It may also be helpful to use additional zinc, vitamin A, and vitamin C. However, because too much vitamin A or zinc can be toxic, the appropriate doses of these nutrients should be discussed with a knowledgeable practitioner.

Conclusion

SCIENTIFIC RESEARCH AND clinical experience have shown that dietary modification, combined in some cases with nutritional supplements, is an effective treatment for most children suffering from recurrent otitis media. Doctors who ignore these simple, nontoxic treatments and emphasize antibiotics and surgical implantation of tubes are certainly achieving less-than-optimal results and are exposing their patients to needless risk and expense. We are hopeful that the day will come soon when conventional medicine will take a closer look at the nutritional approach to recurrent otitis media.

Summary of Recommendations for Preventing Ear Infections

- Diet: Eliminate refined sugar and refined flour. Work with food allergies.

- Multiple vitamin/mineral (adjust doses of other nutrients as needed).

- Vitamin C, 100 to 500 mg twice a day, depending on age and body weight.

- Vitamin A and zinc (consult a nutrition-oriented doctor for appropriate doses).

ECZEMA

ECZEMA (ALSO KNOWN as atopic dermatitis) is one of the most common skin disorders in children. In some children, the itchy, red, crusty lesions of eczema are only a minor problem. However, in more extreme cases, the itching and pain can be so severe that it interferes with the child's life.

Eczema usually responds well to steroids (cortisone and related drugs), either applied to the skin or taken by mouth. However, the condition often returns as soon as the medication is discontinued. In addition, prolonged use of steroids can cause a number of serious side effects, ranging from diabetes to cataracts. Safe and effective alternatives to steroid treatment are therefore needed.

DR. WRIGHT'S CASE STUDY

"We actually have two appointments," Linda Ebersole said. "Emily's first, though. I'll come in later. Emily has eczema, I have canker sores. I thought we might as well try to get her better with natural treatment. We're certainly not doing so well with the regular approach."

"Please tell me about Emily's skin problems."

"OK. As I said, she's 4. She started having eczema at just 6 months. At first it was just in front of her elbows, but then it spread to the spaces between her fingers, behind her knees, and at the worst—when she was 2 and a half—she had spots of it all over her body. She was scratching so much she got it infected and had to be on antibiotics for 3 or 4 months. She's been given a lot of treatments, mostly synthetic cortisones. Those keep the eczema down, but they never cure it."

"Not a surprise; eczema certainly isn't due to a lack of synthetic cortisones. How long did you nurse Emily?"

Linda looked uncomfortable. "Three months. Since I've been reading about natural health care I wish I could go back and do it over again. I understand now that our intestinal tracts just aren't ready to handle food until one year of age or so. But I had to go back to work . . ."

"Make sure to apply what you've learned for your next child. But please don't punish yourself over the past, especially when you didn't know better. It won't help Emily now. So, have you had her tested for allergies?"

"Actually, that's one of the reasons we're here. My reading on natural health care tells me that eczema's due to allergy, particularly food allergy. But nearly all the doctors I've taken Emily to say food allergy has very little to do with eczema—and besides testing for food allergy isn't all that accurate anyway."

"Depends on how it's done. But you're right, eczema is usually triggered and perpetuated by food allergy. Since you've been reading in this area, have you tried eliminating various foods?"

"Yes, and the only one we can tell makes a difference is milk and dairy. After her worst eczema at two and a half, I started my reading, and we took Emily off milk. She's been significantly better, never all over her body again, but we can't tell a difference with other foods. That's another part of why we're here—we heard from our neighbors that food-allergy testing and treatment really made a difference for their son."

"We check everyone with eczema for allergy and sensitivity, and always find it. Once Emily's been tested, please see our nutritionist for an allergy-avoidance diet. We'll get to work on desensitization, too. If desensitization goes as usual, after a few months, many or most of the allergic reactions will be gone, and she can resume eating many of those foods without getting eczema."

"Good. I wasn't looking forward to years of diet restriction."

We went to an exam room. Emily had red cracked skin between the fingers of both hands, and red, rough areas on her wrists and on the skin in front of both elbows. There were faint rednesses behind her knees, and the skin behind her right ear was cracked. We finished checking things over and went back to my office.

"In addition to working on Emily's allergies, there are several supplements for her to take. First, zinc, 15 milligrams 3 times daily, at least until she's been better for several months. Use zinc picolinate, it assimilates well. Remember, zinc stimulates healing of skin and body-lining surfaces. Next, to help heal Emily's eczema, she'll need a supplemental source of essential fatty acids, such as flaxseed oil. Some children with eczema need particular forms of oils, such as evening primrose, black currant, or borage oil—all of which contain gamma-linolenic acid, also called GLA. There's a blood test that will tell us which one Emily needs."

"Anything else?"

"We'll need to check copper levels. When you take zinc, it's important to make sure it's 'in balance' with copper."

"That's all for her eczema?"

"Yes, and one more thing—give her *Lactobacillus acidophilus*—a special type called *Lactobacillus GG.* French researchers reported that this type appears to help improve eczema. Also, Emily's been on antibiotics . . ."

"Early on in my reading I came across the information about antibiotics and replacement with *Lactobacillus acidophilus.* Since it's safe, I put Emily on it right away. It improved her bowel movements, which had gotten irregular after the antibiotics. I still give it to her when I see a problem in that area. I'll switch to the 'GG' type now."

"Now let's make a list of more minor, but still important supplements for Emily. In addition to zinc, essential fatty acids, and the *Lactobacillus GG,* please give her vitamin A, 15,000 IU daily. It'll help the zinc in healing her skin. Also give her vitamin E, 200 IU daily—vitamin E should be taken any time we take extra essential fatty acids. It helps to prevent free-radical formation. Vitamin E also protects vitamin A against rapid oxidation. Lastly, vitamin C, perhaps 500 milligrams daily.

"There's one other problem that we may need to check into if Emily's eczema doesn't clear up entirely."

"What's that?"

"The possibility of stomach malfunction, with an underproduction of hydrochloric acid and pepsin. In 1931, this was shown to occur frequently in more severe childhood eczema.

Emily's eczema cleared entirely in 7 months with allergy avoidance, desensitization, zinc, evening primrose oil, *Lactobacillus GG,* and vitamins A, E, and C. With her mother's supervision of her diet and nutrition, it hasn't returned.

DR. GABY'S COMMENTARY

Food allergies are frequently a contributing cause of eczema, particularly in children. As with Emily, a combination of dietary changes and nutritional supplements can be effective in treating eczema.

Dietary Considerations
Role of Food Allergy

A number of studies have demonstrated that food allergy is an important triggering factor in causing eczema in many children.[1, 2] Food allergy also appears to play a role in adult eczema, but not as often as in children. However, in some studies, food allergy was not found to be a common cause of eczema.

These conflicting reports may be explained, at least in part, by differences in how food allergy was diagnosed. Skin tests, as performed by conventional allergists, frequently give incorrect results. Surprisingly, the observations of a child's parents are also unreliable in many cases. Chronic food allergies are often hidden and may therefore not be apparent, even to someone who is looking for them very carefully. These hidden allergies can be "unmasked" by a medically supervised elimination diet, followed by individual food challenges. When the search for food allergies is done correctly, and the offending foods are eliminated, many children with eczema improve.

One of the elimination diets I have used in my practice is presented in appendix A. Some doctors of natural medicine use other tests for allergy, as well as desensitization techniques. The reliability and effectiveness of some of these methods is controversial (see chapter 3 for additional discussion).

Nutritional Supplements
Essential Fatty Acids

Essential fatty acids (EFAs) play an important role in promoting healthy skin. Some children with eczema appear to have a defect in their ability to utilize EFAs. As early as 1933, EFA supplements were found to aid in the healing of skin lesions in children with eczema.[3] More recent studies have produced similar results,[4, 5, 6] although some other studies failed to show any benefit.

In our experience, EFA supplements do help many (but not all) children with eczema. Good sources of EFAs include sunflower, safflower, soybean, cod-liver, and flaxseed oils. These oils contain different proportions of omega-6 and omega-3 fatty acids, and the optimal supplement may vary from person to person. In some cases, evening primrose oil or borage oil, which contain a fatty acid called gamma-linoleic acid (GLA), may be preferable to the other oils. Normally, the body converts linoleic acid (found in all of the oils listed above except cod-liver oil) into GLA, which is believed to play an important role in healing eczema. However, some individuals appear to have difficulty converting linoleic acid to GLA. In those cases a supplement that contains preformed GLA would be desirable. It is not always easy to predict whether someone will require evening primrose or borage oil, or whether the other, less expensive, oils will be sufficient. Lab tests that measure blood levels of EFAs may provide useful information, although one may also identify the most effective supplements by a process of trial and error. A practitioner trained in nutritional medicine can help you choose the most appropriate EFA supplement. Please remember that taking EFA supplements increases the body's requirement for vitamin E.

Zinc

Zinc is known to be beneficial for a number of different skin conditions. Although there are no published studies on the treatment of eczema with zinc, in our experience it appears to be helpful.

The combination of zinc and EFAs is usually more effective than either one alone. The dosage of zinc varies with a child's age and body weight, and should be supervised by a health-care professional.

Other Nutrients

VITAMIN A and vitamin C are often used by nutrition-oriented doctors to help skin lesions heal. Some studies suggest that vitamin A is of value in the treatment of eczema.[7, 8]

Summary of Recommendations for Treating Eczema

PRIMARY RECOMMENDATIONS:

- Work with food allergies.

- Zinc (balanced with copper) and essential fatty acids (balanced with vitamin E); forms and dosages as recommended by a nutrition-oriented practitioner.

OTHER RECOMMENDATIONS:

- Vitamin A, vitamin C; dosages as recommended by a nutrition-oriented practitioner.

EMPHYSEMA AND CHRONIC BRONCHITIS *(chronic obstructive lung disease)*

CHRONIC BRONCHITIS AND *emphysema are two different lung disorders, which often occur in combination and result in obstruction of the airways. When bronchitis and emphysema occur together, the condition is called chronic obstructive lung disease (COLD—formerly called chronic obstructive pulmonary disease, or COPD). Chronic bronchitis is characterized by excessive production of mucus in the bronchial passages, and it is sometimes associated with chronic infection and/or asthma. Emphysema is a distention of the air spaces, with destruction of portions of the alveoli (the small sacs in the lungs through which air exchange takes place). Cigarette smoking is the most important contributing factor to the development of COLD, but other environmental exposures also appear to play a role. In its advanced stages, COLD can lead to severe disability and death from respiratory failure.*

Conventional treatment of COLD includes bronchodilators (drugs that open up the bronchial passages) and cortisone-like drugs, which reduce inflammation. While these medications may provide varying degrees of symptom relief, they also can cause a number of different side effects, including heart-rhythm disturbances (bronchodilators), diabetes, osteoporosis, and cataracts (cortisone-like drugs).

DR. WRIGHT'S CASE STUDY

Erwin Jangaard looked blue; not bright blue, but more a dull, mottled blue with red tones, darker around his lips and cheeks, a little lighter on the rest of his face. The skin of his hands was more red with blue mottling, lighter on his fingers, where yellow-brown-orange cigarette stains also appeared. He was obviously working hard for each breath. His wife Ingrid was with him, and spoke first.

"Erwin just won't quit smoking," she said. "His breathing just gets worse and worse, and now the doctor is telling him he might need an oxygen tank soon with that tubing and the horrible little prongs in his nose! I insisted he come here so maybe he could improve his health a little, maybe postpone the oxygen tank a few years—and maybe buy a little more time for him to quit smoking."

"Actually, I've quit dozens of times," Edwin said. "The trouble is staying stopped." He paused for breath. "I don't know why I just can't stay away for more than a week or two, but I just haven't been able to."

"How long have you been smoking?"

"Since I was 13, and I'm 67. Both my parents smoked, and 3 grandparents; must be a family tendency, too."

"Sounds that way. How many cigarettes a day, average, the last few years?"

"At least I've cut down. The last 10 years or so it's been a pack a day. Before that it was over 2 packs a day for years."

"Do you have both bronchial obstructive disease and emphysema?"

"That's right. The doctor calls it 'COPD with emphysema.'"

"I assume you're taking medications?"

"I brought them," Ingrid said, and handed me two prescription bottles. One was for a bronchodilator, the other a patentable, unnatural form of cortisone, fortunately at a relatively low dose.

"About average treatment," I said.

I asked about Mr. Jangaard's health history. The only useful information was a history of numerous childhood ear infections.

"How could that relate to my problem now?" he asked.

"Nearly all children with recurrent earaches have allergies, including food allergies. Allergies hardly ever go away completely. Sometimes they 'go underground', sometimes the symptoms change, but they're usually 'lurking in the background' of health problems later in life. If that unnatural cortisone is actually doing you any good, at least part of what it's doing is suppressing allergy symptoms. So, please have allergy and sensitivity testing done."

"I've been telling Erwin that for years," Ingrid said.

"What would allergies do?" he asked.

"Increase bronchial secretions and congestion, possibly constrict the bronchial tubes a little."

"OK. What else?"

"Besides eliminating allergies and sensitivities, which will directly help your lungs, cleaning up your diet will help your health. And strengthening your health in general will help you fight this problem better."

Erwin looked at Ingrid. "No more junk food, right?"

"Right!" Ingrid exclaimed. "And you agreed, remember. If you can't quit smoking and you're looking at oxygen, and I'd be looking at those prongs in your nose, we're going to do everything else." She turned to me. "I've told Erwin no sugar, no white flour, low saturated fat, no food chemicals, only whole fresh foods, no frying . . . we've been doing that as much as I could anyway—now it'll be 100%."

Erwin sighed. "And now for a list of vitamins—a mile long," he observed.

"Only half a mile," I said. "But they'll likely do you some good, particularly as your records say you're not taking any except vitamins E and C right now."

"That's Ingrid's doing. She said she doesn't want me to have a heart attack, too."

"Those vitamins will lower your chances. I'll write down other things for you. First, to help the function of your breathing muscles a little, magnesium (citrate), 200 milligrams, twice daily, and L-carnitine, 250 milligrams, 3 times daily. Secondly, to thin and loosen bronchial secretions so you can 'get them up and out' better, N-acetylcysteine, 500 milligrams twice daily, in between meals, and SSKI—that's saturated solution of potassium iodide, a prescription item—6 drops daily in liquid, to start. Later, you'll probably taper that one down a bit. Incidentally, the iodide in the bronchial secretions inhibits the growth of bacteria, and other microorganisms.

"Third, to improve the health of the cells lining the bronchial tubes and the rest of the lungs, vitamin A, 50,000 units daily, and lecithin, 2 of the 19-grain capsules twice daily. Vitamin E helps here, too. Please make sure that's 400 IU daily, in addition to whatever's in the multiple vitamin. Fourth, extra copper and zinc. Copper is especially important to maintaining elastic tissue, and with emphysema, much of the lung elasticity is lost. We want to protect as much of the rest as possible. Also, over time, N-acetylcysteine depletes copper and zinc from our bodies, so you'll need zinc, too. Please use 4 milligrams of copper (sebacate) and 30 milligrams of zinc (picolinate) daily."

"How much vitamin C?" Ingrid asked.

"At least 2,000 milligrams, 3 times daily."

"Why so much?" asked Erwin.

"For a smoker, that's a minimum. Among other things, it's needed to help clear all the toxins, it protects the arteries . . ."

"OK, OK. I can hear you thinking, 'Why doesn't he stop smoking?' I'm surprised you didn't lecture me first thing."

"Well, I planned to mention it, but I thought you likely knew, so why start with that?"

"Thanks for giving me credit for having some brains. To save time, I will consider myself lectured."

"OK. Last item, a high potency, combination vitamin and mineral." I handed him the list of recommendations. He started counting.

"That's 9 different things."

"Not so bad, Erwin. I take 14," Ingrid said. "Remember, these are nutrients, not drugs."

"One precaution," I said. "Since there's quite a bit of iodide in the SSKI, please have a thyroid test done, and then we'll check it at intervals as necessary."

———

Ten weeks later, Mr. Jangaard was back. Although there was still a slight blue-red tinge to his skin, it was definitely less, and it was much less mottled. His hands had better color, too, although the cigarette stains were the same. His breathing was much less labored.

"And I walked around the building 5 times before we came in just to make it comparable with last time," he said.

"Everyone says Erwin's looking so much better!" Ingrid exclaimed.

"And I feel a lot better, too," Erwin said. "Maybe there's something to this healthy food thing after all."

"Likely so," I said. "And it's certainly better than drugs and an oxygen bottle."

"So do I just continue?" Erwin asked.

"Let's see . . . your thyroid test is here, it's fine. Yes, please continue everything. However, there is another treatment that my colleague Dr. Davis Lamson has been working with recently. It's been doing very well; I think you should try it."

"Another pill?"

"No, a metabolite, a molecule our bodies can make—glutathione. You actually inhale it 2 or 3 times daily. There's been quite a bit written about this treatment recently in medical journals."

"In medical journals?" Ingrid asked. "I've seen glutathione in natural-food stores for years—in capsules of course. Supposed to be a powerful antioxidant, isn't it? And it's in medical journals?"

"More and more natural-treatment research is appearing in major medical journals. Universities seem to be trying to make up for all the time they've lost since the 1940s—time spent ignoring or criticizing natural medicine."

"No apologies for that, are there?" Ingrid noted.

"No, and no credit given either—but back to Mr. Jangaard. Please check with Dr. Lamson's assistant for instructions about the inhaled glutathione.

———

Two months later, Mr. Jangaard was back. Nearly all the blue-red tinge was gone from his face and hands, and only a faint trace remained around his lips. His breathing was obviously better than at his last visit.

"The lung doctor can hardly believe how well I'm doing. I had a change he could notice after my diet change and all the pills, and another really noticeable change when I started inhaling the glutathione," he said. "When I told him this glutathione thing was in regular medical journals, he didn't believe me, but then he looked it up and called me back. He says he's going to use it for all his other patients.

"I can tell I've still got emphysema—it's still harder breathing in and out than it should be. And I understand that part of my lung damage is permanent. But the obstruction part is so much improved. And I'm sure you've noticed I'm not having to pause to breathe every few words."

"Sure did."

"Before, I felt hopeless. I figured I was done for anyway, so why work so hard to quit smoking? You know—the condemned man and his final smokes. But now, I'm starting to make plans for the next few years, and I'm quitting! Finally, once and for all."

"He's down to 8 a day," Ingrid said. "I'm so proud of him! And he's not cheated on anything once. He's even able to walk to the park with our grandchildren again."

"And I never, ever smoke in front of them anymore!"

DR. GABY'S COMMENTARY

ALTHOUGH COLD (particularly the emphysema component) is generally considered irreversible, evidence shows that nutritional therapy can be used to relieve symptoms and possibly to slow or halt the progression of the disease.

Dietary Considerations

INDIVIDUALS WITH EMPHYSEMA are frequently underweight and suffer from generalized malnutrition, even when they are consuming a diet that would be adequate for healthy people. Malnutrition increases the risk of respiratory infections, and it may contribute to lung dysfunction. Patients with COLD should therefore make sure to consume adequate amounts of protein and calories, as well as whole foods (which contain more vitamins and minerals than processed foods).

Role of Allergy

FOR many patients with COLD, symptoms such as shortness of breath, wheezing, and other respiratory symptoms can be reduced by avoiding allergenic foods, combined in some cases with treatment of environmental allergies. Dr. Albert H. Rowe, a pioneer in the field of food allergy, treated 60 patients with COLD by means of an elimination diet (pollen desensitization was also given to 20% of the patients). Symptom relief ranged from "good" to "marked," and it persisted for as long as 4 years.[1] The benefits of allergy control appear to be due to a reduction in bronchial spasm, decreased swelling of the mucous membranes, and less mucus production.

Nutritional Supplements
N-acetylcysteine (NAC)

N-ACETYLCYSTEINE (NAC) is a derivative of the amino acid cysteine, and it performs two different functions that may be beneficial for the lungs. First, NAC acts as a mucolytic agent—a compound that breaks up mucus in the respiratory tract, thereby allowing the mucus to be cleared more easily from the bronchial passages. Second, NAC participates in the synthesis of glutathione, a powerful, naturally occurring antioxidant that protects the lungs against toxins and free radicals.

In one study, 1,392 patients with chronic bronchitis received 200 mg of NAC, 3 times per day for 2 months. Of those patients, 87% showed an improvement in symptoms, including less severe coughing, greater ease of expectoration, and less shortness of breath. Side effects, reported by 19% of the patients, included nausea, vomiting, abdominal pain, dizziness, headache, and dry mouth. Most of the patients who experienced side effects did not consider them severe enough to warrant discontinuing treatment.[2] In a double-blind study using the same dosage regimen, patients receiving NAC had 19% fewer flare-ups of bronchitis and 25% fewer days taking antibiotics, compared with patients given a placebo. However, the differences were not statistically significant.[3] While these studies suggest that NAC may be of value in treating chronic bronchitis, additional research is needed before this treatment can be considered "proven."

Because NAC binds to zinc and copper, long-term use of NAC might lead to depletion of these minerals. Individuals taking NAC should therefore include a multiple-mineral formula or zinc and copper in their supplement program.

Magnesium

A DEFICIENCY of magnesium (documented by low magnesium concentrations in muscle-biopsy samples) was found in 15 (47%) of 32 patients hospitalized with severe COLD. Patients with low concentrations of magnesium required longer hospital stays, compared with patients who had normal magnesium levels.[4] This study suggests that magnesium deficiency may increase the severity of COLD.

Magnesium promotes healthy lung function in at least 2 ways. First, this mineral acts as a bronchodilator, preventing the bronchial passages from going into spasm.[5] Second, magnesium plays a key role in the production of energy, which is needed by the chest-wall muscles and the diaphragm to perform the work of breathing. For individuals with chronic lung obstruction who must labor especially hard to pull in each breath of air, any reduction in the severity of obstruction or any improvement in respiratory-muscle strength would be worthwhile. In a double-blind study, individuals with low magnesium levels had an increase in the power of their respiratory muscles after receiving an intravenous infusion of magnesium. This effect was not seen in healthy individuals with normal magnesium levels.[6]

I have given intramuscular injections of magnesium and B-vitamins to one patient and intravenous injections of magnesium, B-vitamins, and vitamin C to a second patient with severe COLD. Both patients reported that their breathing was less labored and their strength and stamina improved; this effect typically lasted 1 to 2 weeks.

Other Nutrients

COENZYME Q10 and L-carnitine are vitamin-like compounds that occur in small amounts in food and are synthesized in the body. Both of these compounds play a role in energy production and may therefore be helpful for individuals with COLD. In one study, administering L-carnitine (2 grams, 3 times per day for 7 days) increased the exercise tolerance of patients with chronic lung disease.[7]

In another study, serum concentrations of coenzyme Q10 were lower in patients with COLD than in healthy individuals. Administering coenzyme Q10 (90 mg per day for 8 weeks) to these patients significantly increased the amount of time the patients could exercise on a treadmill.[8] While small amounts of coenzyme Q10 and L-carnitine can be obtained from the diet, the amounts needed to treat COLD are much greater; therefore, supplementation is required.

Copper plays a role in promoting the integrity of lung tissue. Guinea pigs fed a copper-deficient diet developed emphysema.[9] In addition, the lung function of healthy humans was shown to increase with increasing copper concentration in the drinking water.[10] The typical American diet contains only about 1 mg of copper per day, whereas the RDA is 2 mg per day. Thus, it seems worthwhile for COLD patients to take a multiple vitamin/mineral formula that contains at least 1 mg of copper. Food sources of copper include nuts, legumes, vegetables, eggs, and meat.

Other nutrients that may improve the integrity of respiratory tissue or increase the body's resistance against infection include vitamin C, vitamin A, zinc, vitamin E, and lecithin.

Prescription-strength iodine (in the form of saturated solution of potassium iodide—SSKI) is used by some doctors to enhance the flow of bronchial secretions. Although this treatment is often quite helpful, large doses of SSKI can affect thyroid function or cause other side effects, and should therefore be monitored closely.

Glutathione

As mentioned above, glutathione plays a crucial role in the natural antioxidant-defense system, which helps prevent oxidation damage to lung tissue. Studies have shown that glutathione can be delivered by aerosol directly to the lungs, and that it remains fully functional as an antioxidant when administered this way.[11]

One of our colleagues, Dr. Davis Lamson, has been administering glutathione by aerosol to patients with COLD, some of whom have shown rather dramatic clinical improvements.[12] However, additional research is needed to confirm the long-term effectiveness and safety of this treatment.

Glutathione aerosol can be obtained by prescription from a compounding pharmacist. The dosage used by Lamson is 2 ml twice daily of a solution containing 60 mg of glutathione per ml. As improvement occurs, the frequency of administration is reduced, and the treatment is then continued as needed.

Conclusion

ALTHOUGH CHRONIC OBSTRUCTIVE lung disease is generally considered irreversible, there is evidence that dietary modification and nutritional

supplements can relieve symptoms and make breathing easier. While long-term studies have not been done, it is conceivable that nutritional therapy may also slow or halt the progression of the diesease.

Summary of Recommendations for Treating Emphysema and Chronic Obstructive Lung Disease

- Diet: Consume adequate amounts of protein and calories. Work with food and environmental allergies.

- N-acetylcysteine (NAC), 600 to 1,000 mg per day in divided doses. With long-term use of NAC, supplement with zinc and copper.

- Magnesium, 300 to 600 mg per day.

- L-carnitine, 500 to 1,500 mg per day.

- Vitamin C, 1,000 to 3,000 mg per day.

- Coenzyme Q10, 60 to 100 mg per day.

- Other supportive nutrients include vitamin A, vitamin E, lecithin, zinc, and copper. Doses of vitamin A greater than 15,000 IU per day in elderly individuals should be monitored by a doctor.

- High-potency multiple vitamin/mineral (adjust doses of other nutrients as needed).

- Intramuscular or intravenous injections of nutrients in selected cases.

- Saturated solution of potassium iodide (by prescription), in selected cases.

- Glutathione aerosol (by prescription), in selected cases.

EPILEPSY

THE TERM "EPILEPSY" *is derived from a Greek word that means "seizures." Epileptic seizures result from a disturbance in the electrical activity of the brain. They can manifest as loss of consciousness, convulsions, abnormal movements, sensory changes, hallucinations, confusion, or a host of other symptoms. There are many different causes of epilepsy, including birth injury, head trauma, brain tumors, disorders of metabolism, alcoholism, and drug addiction. However, for a large proportion of epileptics, the cause cannot be determined.*

In most cases, epileptic seizures are not in themselves dangerous. However, loss of consciousness and uncontrolled movements can result in injury either to the person suffering the seizure or to others. Consequently, epileptics must remain free of seizures for a number of years before they are allowed to drive an automobile or engage in other potentially injurious activities. Patients can take a number of medications, which can effectively control seizures. However, not everyone responds to drug treatment and some patients suffer side effects from the medications.

DR. WRIGHT'S CASE STUDY

"I just don't feel as well as I think I should," John Toricelli said. "There's not really anything specific the matter. I'm starting to suspect some of it might be the medicine I'm taking, but I've taken it for years—ever since I was a kid, and if I don't I have seizures. So if that's it I don't know if there's anything to do about it, but I thought I'd come in and find out."

"What are you taking?"

"Dilantin, 100 milligrams 4 times a day and phenobarbital, 60 milligrams twice daily. My neurologist says that's 'old-fashioned', but it does the best for me."

"How long have you been taking them?"

"Twenty-two years or so, since I was 2 or 3 years old—but not as much of course, back then." When I was 13 or so my seizures got worse so a neurologist had me try several other medicines—Tegretol, Depakote, and other things—but none of them worked as well for me. So we ended up just increasing the Dilantin, and that does the best for me."

"Do you have any seizures now?"

"Not very often—unless I forget to take the medicine."

"Grand mal seizures?"

"Yeah, but they're not so bad anymore, and don't last as long. My parents say when I first started having them it was really scary, and they lasted a long time."

"You said nothing specific is bothering you—but can you give me any more details at all?"

"Well . . . maybe it's a matter of not as much

energy as I think I should have at my age . . . or maybe as much as my friends have. And I just don't seem to have the drive, you know what I mean? I'm single, and all my single guy friends are working really hard trying to get ahead. When they're off work and doing sports or something, they're doing that really hard, too. I try, but after awhile I can't push myself to keep up, even though I really want to. I don't know how else to explain it. Oh . . . and I can't seem to think as clearly as I did a few years back. I catch myself in mistakes I shouldn't be making. Actually, that worries me the most."

"Are your parents well? And what about grandparents?"

"Mom said you'd ask, so she wrote it out." He handed me a sheet of paper.

"Let's see—your mother's well, your father has a mild case of high blood pressure, your mother's mother developed diabetes after age 60 and had a heart attack, her father died of cancer. Your father's mother had a stroke, and your father's father is well at 87. No brothers or sisters?"

"They tried, but it didn't happen."

"Do you eat much sugar and sweet things?"

John looked embarrassed. "I knew you'd ask. When my seizures got worse when I was around 13, Mom really got on my case about all the candy I was eating. She said it was probably making my seizures worse. I was stubborn and didn't want to quit, and the doctor said it had nothing to do with it so of course I believed the doctor. I guess I was doing some of the 'teen rebellion' thing, too. But since I left home, I've found out my mother is really smart about health things, and I've been cutting back on some of the sugar lately. It's hard, though."

"Certainly is. But in families with diabetes, low blood sugar is more likely, and low blood sugar certainly can aggravate seizures." I made a note. "Do you eat very many vegetables?"

"Not really. Actually, I made a list for you. Mom said I should."

His list showed hamburgers, french fries, milkshakes, doughnuts, candy, pizza, chicken, cheese, bread, apples, bananas, and occasional salads.

"I know I'm not eating the best," he said. "That's partly why I'm here. Even if I can't get off these medicines, I'm hoping I'll feel better if I change my diet. Mom hasn't bugged me for a few years, but I know she's ready to help anytime."

"You're not living at home?"

"No, an apartment with a roommate, but I'm not there a lot, and I don't cook well."

"Our nutritionist can help you with a 'healthy single person's quick diet', too, but check with Mom first."

"I will."

"Do you have any allergies?"

"Not as far as I know."

"None in your family? Asthma, hay fever, eczema, skin rashes?"

"Not unless Mom wrote it down. Do allergies have something to do with seizures?"

"Sometimes. Infrequently, allergies can be a major trigger for seizures. But, of course, it's more likely if you or a family member have allergies."

We finished the rest of his health history, then I did a physical exam. Everything appeared normal. Since he'd been on Dilantin for so long, I made sure to check his gums carefully.

"My neurologist does that, too. He says he's glad I haven't had any gum enlargement from the Dilantin like some people do."

We finished his check-up and went back to my office.

"Well, what do I do?"

"First, let's deal with the nutritional side effects of Dilantin and phenobarbital. Both of these medications interfere with the absorption and/or metabolism of vitamin B_{12}, folate, calcium, and vitamin D. Just to make sure they're absorbed, we'll ask you to take a few injections of vitamin B_{12} and folate, and then continue with 2,000 micrograms of vitamin B_{12} and 5 milligrams of folate daily." I wrote these down for him.

"Why do you want me to take shots first?"

"To make sure they're absorbed. Besides anti-seizure medications, many other things can impair their absorption, and like many other

B-vitamins, folate and B_{12} are particularly important to mental alertness and clarity. Many individuals who've been taking anti-seizure medicine tell me that B_{12} and folate injections really help them mentally."

"What about the calcium and vitamin D?"

"Let's wait until we see a magnesium test first. Magnesium deficiency can aggravate or even cause seizures. Your diet hasn't been very good for magnesium—it's found a lot in deep-green vegetables. In a way, additional calcium could aggravate a problem of low body-magnesium supplies. Vitamin D increases calcium absorption, so it could do the same."

"Makes sense." He thought for a minute. "If my seizure medicine can interfere with these nutrients, could the nutrients interfere with the seizure medicine?"

"A really good question! For awhile, it was thought that more than a small amount of folate might interfere with Dilantin's activity, but follow-up studies showed this to be very unusual."

"Any other tests besides magnesium?"

"Several other mineral deficiencies can cause or contribute to seizures. Magnesium and manganese seem particularly important, but low copper, zinc, and selenium can play a role, also. For highest accuracy, we'll use a test called 'Accu-min', which checks magnesium in mononuclear white cells, manganese and zinc in white cells, copper in red blood cells, and selenium in hair."

"I won't even try to remember that—just give me the lab form. Do I need a blood-sugar test?"

"If we did one, it should be a glucose-insulin tolerance test for greatest accuracy. The alternative is just to eliminate sugar and refined carbohydrate."

"Mom's been telling me that for years. Maybe I'll skip the test and just do it. Is there anything else?"

"Yes. For some people, the amino acid taurine can lessen seizures. Although a relatively large but safe quantity—3 grams daily. . . . Extra vitamin B_6 is often helpful, and dimethylglycine, DMG, a natural metabolite, helps a few patients."

"How can I tell what helps me?"

"Some are guided by tests, some by just trying it."

"Well, I guess I'll get these mineral tests done, get the shots, and check back when the tests are done."

His white-cell magnesium and manganese tests were both low; the rest of his minerals were well within normal. In addition to manganese (50 milligrams daily, as manganese citrate) and magnesium (300 milligrams daily, as magnesium citrate), he was asked to take a multiple vitamin-mineral containing 400 IU of both vitamins D and E, and a larger than usual amount of all the B-complex vitamins. Mr. Toricelli found that the vitamin B_{12} and folate injections helped him keep "mentally clearer" than the same oral supplement, so he learned to give himself the injections. Dimethylglycine was not helpful for him, but taurine (1,500 milligrams twice daily in between meals) did help. He also took 600 extra milligrams of calcium, and 100 extra milligrams of vitamin B_6 twice daily.

With all the supplements, he was able to carefully (over 18 months time) eliminate phenobarbital and cut his Dilantin to 100 milligrams, 3 times daily while maintaining the same seizure control. He also reported a noticeable improvement in energy and "drive," as well as a distinct lessening in "unnecessary mental errors" at work.

DR. GABY'S COMMENTARY

Various diets and nutritional supplements have been used to treat people with epilepsy. Although the nutritional approach is not a cure-all, for some people, this approach can help control seizures or reduce the severity of drug side effects.

Dietary Considerations
The Hypoglycemia Connection

Severe hypoglycemia (low blood sugar) is a well-recognized cause of seizures. It is therefore possible that a milder reduction in blood sugar (as one might see in so-called "reactive hypoglycemia") might make an epileptic more susceptible to having a seizure. In some patients, a decline in blood sugar was associated with brain abnormalities that showed on an electroencephalogram (EEG).[1] Although there is not a lot of research in this area, we advise epileptic patients to follow a "hypoglycemia diet" (i.e., avoid refined sugar, caffeine, and alcohol, and eat small, frequent meals). Such a diet will not cause any harm, and it might help the patient control seizures.

The Role of Food Allergy

Food allergy has also been shown to be an important factor in some patients with epilepsy. In one study, 63 children with epilepsy followed an elimination diet for 4 weeks, then added back one food at a time. Of the 18 children who had epilepsy alone, none improved. However, of the 45 children with epilepsy who also had symptoms that suggested food allergy (i.e., recurrent migraines, abdominal symptoms, or hyperactivity), 80% had fewer seizures while on the diet and 56% became seizure-free. Most of these children reacted to several foods and, in the group as a whole, 31 different foods provoked seizures. In double-blind food challenges, seizures recurred in 8 of 16 children after the ingestion of the offending foods. In contrast, no seizures resulted from ingestion of a "placebo" food.[2] This study demonstrates that food allergy is a major cause of seizures in more than half of epileptic children. Individuals who have symptoms that suggest allergy (such as migraines, abdominal pain, hyperactivity, nasal congestion, recurrent ear infection, or asthma) are likely to improve on an allergy-avoidance diet, whereas children who do not have such symptoms will probably not respond.

The Ketogenic Diet

The ketogenic diet[3, 4] is a diet that is very high in fat (87% of total calories) and low in protein and carbohydrate. This diet is called "ketogenic" because it promotes the formation of ketones (partial-breakdown products of fatty acids) in the body. For reasons that are not well understood, the presence of ketones prevents seizures from occurring. The ketogenic diet has been used since the 1920s. For many patients who fail to respond to drugs, the diet has produced complete seizure control. Generalized seizures and myoclonic seizures respond best to this diet, whereas absence seizures (petit mal) do not typically improve.

The ketogenic diet is unpalatable and difficult to prepare; however, absolute adherence is necessary for it to work. Recently, a type of fat known as medium-chain triglycerides (manufactured from coconut oil) has been incorporated into the ketogenic diet, and this change has allowed the diet to be less restrictive and easier to tolerate. The ketogenic diet is deficient in several vitamins and minerals, and it is quite complicated to administer. For these reasons, this diet must be supervised by a well-trained dietitian.

Nutritional Supplements

Vitamin B6

BETWEEN 1951 AND 1953, an infant formula that was inadvertently deficient in vitamin B6 was being sold in the United States. Many children who consumed this formula developed epileptic seizures, which disappeared when they took a vitamin-B6 supplement.[5]

A vitamin B6 deficiency severe enough to cause seizures is uncommon among healthy people who consume a normal diet. However, some individuals have a genetic abnormality that causes them to need unusually large amounts of vitamin B6. These individuals suffer from recurrent seizures (usually beginning during infancy) which can be controlled completely by administering this vitamin. Although vitamin B6-dependent epilepsy is uncommon, it should be considered in any child who has seizures that are difficult to control.[6]

Vitamin B6 may also be helpful for some epileptics who do not have classic vitamin B6-dependent seizures. In one study, a tryptophan-load test was performed on 43 epileptic patients. In that test, the patient ingests a dose of the amino acid L-tryptophan and the urine is then collected to measure the various metabolites (breakdown products) of tryptophan. The excretion of elevated amounts of certain metabolites is considered evidence of vitamin B6 deficiency. Of the 43 patients tested, 26 (61%) showed evidence of vitamin B6 deficiency. Of patients with an abnormal test who received vitamin B6 (160 mg per day), about half showed a reduction in seizure frequency. Some of these patients were able to discontinue their anti-epileptic medication. In contrast, none of 7 patients with a normal tryptophan-load test responded to vitamin B6.[7]

Vitamin E

IN a double-blind study, 24 children (ages 6 to 17 years) with epilepsy who had failed to respond to anti-epileptic drugs received 400 IU of vitamin E per day or a placebo for 3 months. In 10 of the 12 patients who were given vitamin E, compared with none of 12 patients in the placebo group, a greater-than-60% reduction in seizure frequency was seen. The difference in response rate between the two groups was statistically significant.[8] Vitamin E treatment had no effect on blood levels of anticonvulsant medications. We do not know how this vitamin improves seizure control.

Manganese

ANIMALS fed a manganese-deficient diet had increased susceptibility to convulsions. In human studies, blood levels of manganese were lower in epileptic children than in healthy children.[9, 10] The reduction in manganese levels was not related to treatment with any particular anticonvulsant medication. In a case report, a 12-year-old boy with poorly controlled epilepsy experienced a reduction in seizure frequency after receiving 20 mg of manganese per day.[11]

Other Nutrients

RESEARCH has shown that magnesium[12] may be helpful in selected patients with seizures. The amino acid taurine has also been reported to reduce seizure frequency,[13] although other studies have found taurine to be ineffective. If taurine does work as a treatment for epilepsy, it probably acts by stabilizing the electrical activity of the brain.

Supplementing with dimethylglycine, an amino-acid derivative that occurs naturally in the body, was reported to produce a dramatic reduction in seizure frequency in one patient.[14] However, follow-up studies with dimethylglycine were unable to confirm this initial report.

Nutritional Supplements and Epilepsy Medications
Preventing Drug Side Effects

THE anticonvulsant drug Dilantin reduces blood levels of folic acid in about 75% of patients. A deficiency of folic acid can cause various psychological disturbances, some of which are common in epileptics. In one study, folic-acid levels were lower in epileptic patients with severe psychological problems than in those with normal mental function.[15] This finding suggests that folic-acid therapy may improve mental function in patients taking Dilantin. Folic acid may also help reverse the abnormal proliferation of gum tissue (known as gingival hyperplasia) that is seen in many individuals who take Dilantin.[16]

Malabsorption of vitamin B_{12} has also been observed in individuals taking anticonvulsants.[17] Although this defect in absorption can usually be corrected by supplementing with folic acid, taking extra vitamin B_{12} would also be a good idea.

Anticonvulsant medications may also promote vitamin D deficiency, which can lead to a softening of the bones (osteomalacia). In patients receiving anticonvulsants, treatment with vitamin D has been reported to increase bone mass.[18]

Drug-Nutrient Interactions

JUST as Dilantin therapy can cause folic-acid deficiency, taking large amounts of folic acid may interfere with the effect of Dilantin (and possibly other anticonvulsants). In several studies, supplementing with 15 mg of folic acid per day increased seizure frequency in drug-treated epileptics. In other studies, however, the same dose of folic acid had no effect on the number of seizures. Lower amounts of folic acid, such as 1 mg per day, have not been reported to increase seizure frequency.

Treatment with the anticonvulsant drug valproic acid has been shown to reduce blood levels of carnitine. Children who develop fatigue while taking this medication may have a carnitine defi-ciency.[19] Treatment with L-carnitine at a dose of 15 mg per kg of body weight per day will effec-tively reverse the symptoms of carnitine deficiency within one week. It is not known what amount of L-carnitine is needed to prevent a deficiency in individuals taking valproic acid.

There is also evidence that taking large amounts of vitamin B_6 may reduce blood levels of Dilantin and phenobarbitone (another anticonvulsant medication). Therefore, even though vitamin B_6 has an anticonvulsant effect, it could conceivably aggravate seizures in some drug-treated epileptics.

Because of these complex interactions, the nutritional treatment of epilepsy should always be supervised by a nutritionally oriented doctor.

Conclusion

DIETARY MODIFICATIONS AND nutritional supplements can help some epileptics control seizures or reduce the side effects of anticonvulsant medications. However, epileptics should never discontinue or reduce the dose of medications without the approval of their doctor. In addition, because of potential drug-nutrient interactions, nutritional treatment of epilepsy should be closely monitored by a qualified medical practitioner.

Summary of Recommendations for Treating Epilepsy

(NOTE: Treatment should be supervised by a nutritionally oriented doctor)

DIET:

- A "hypoglycemia diet" (i.e., avoiding refined sugar, caffeine, and alcohol, and eating small, frequent meals) may be helpful for individuals with evidence of poor blood-sugar regulation.

- Avoiding allergenic foods may be beneficial in selected cases.

- A "ketogenic diet" (supervised by a trained dietitian) may be considered for difficult-to-treat patients, particularly children aged 2 to 5 years.

SUPPLEMENTS:

- Supplements that may be helpful include vitamin B_6, vitamin E, manganese, magnesium, taurine, and dimethylglycine. The appropiate dosages of these nutrients should be determined by a physician.

DRUG-NUTRIENT INTERACTIONS:

- Some anticonvulsant drugs may cause deficiencies of folic acid, vitamin B_{12}, or vitamin D.

- Treatment with valproic acid may deplete carnitine.

- Large doses of folic acid or vitamin B_6 may interfere with the effects of some anticonvulsant drugs.

FIBROCYSTIC BREAST DISEASE

ALTHOUGH 1 IN 9 *American women will develop breast cancer at some time in their lives, cancer is not the most common disorder of the breast. Fibrocystic breast disease (also called cystic mastitis or mammary dysplasia) is a benign condition that affects a large proportion of women during their ovulatory years.*

Symptoms of fibrocystic breast disease consist primarily of tenderness (ranging from minor to severe) and lumpiness of the breasts. These symptoms tend to be most pronounced just before and during the first few days of the menstrual period and often become less severe or disappear about a week after the onset of menstruation. Fibrocystic breast disease is thought to be caused by excessive estrogenic stimulation of the breasts, or by an exaggerated response by breast tissue to estrogen.

Although some studies suggest that fibrocystic breast disease is associated with an increased risk of developing breast cancer, other studies have failed to find such an association, and the issue remains unresolved. However, doctors cannot always distinguish benign breast cysts from cancer. Consequently, many women with cystic breasts must undergo repeated breast biopsies and cyst aspirations to rule out cancer.

DR. WRIGHT'S CASE STUDY

"I want to hug my husband and children on more than 1 or 2 days each month without hurting," Jenny Bauer said. "It's getting worse all the time. For awhile, I thought the vitamin E my gynecologist told me to take was helping, but now it's worse than ever. She tells me it'll get better after menopause, but that's 15 or 20 years away! My friend said you helped her, so I thought I'd at least try, even though her problem wasn't near as bad as mine is."

"You have fibrocystic breast disease?"

"Oh, excuse me, I didn't say, did I? Yes."

"How long has it been a problem?"

"Let's see, I'm 36 . . . almost 20 years. I went to a doctor when I was 17 and my breasts started to hurt a little before periods. That doctor said a lot of women have lumpy breasts, mine weren't too bad, and besides there wasn't anything to do about it, so I might as well learn to live with it. For about 10 years I only had a little soreness before my menstrual periods, but since then it's steadily been getting worse."

"Still worst before periods?"

"I can't even sleep on my chest before my periods, it hurts so bad then. And if my husband even touches my breasts—well, it makes sex awfully tricky most of the time. Most of the rest of the month, it's a little less, and 2 or 3 days when I only hurt a little."

"Any other problems with your health?"

"Not as far as I know. I'm a little more tired than I'd like to be, but that's all."

"Are you avoiding all caffeine?"

"Mostly. When the information about caffeine and fibrocystic breasts first came out, I cut it out completely, but I only noticed a small difference. My gynecologist said further research had shown caffeine didn't really cause fibrocystic problems. So I do have coffee every once in awhile."

"When you tried avoiding caffeine strictly, did you eliminate tea, all cola drinks, chocolate, and all pain relievers with caffeine in them?"

"No. I never even thought of the pain relievers—but does caffeine elimination really make any difference?"

"Yes, but only for women who have fibrocystic disease or a tendency towards it. What the negative research found was that caffeine didn't give *all* women a problem. We can't use that to say caffeine doesn't give *anyone* a problem."

"I'll give it a try, and be much more careful this time. What else should I do?"

"It's really best to do an examination first. Could you go to the exam room please?

"Sure, but I've been checked before. It's definitely fibrocystic disease."

"I don't doubt you. Treatment can vary a bit according to the degree of the problem, though, so we should check. I know it hurts, but I'll be as careful as I can."

Unfortunately, Mrs. Bauer had a moderately severe problem. There were dozens of lumps in each breast, varying in size from approximately one-quarter inch to an inch in diameter. There was swelling in the tissue between and around the lumps, and of course both breasts were extremely tender.

"You don't have the worst case I've ever seen," I said. "But you're close."

She looked upset. "Does that mean I still have to wait for menopause?"

"That'll come anyway, but you can likely get substantial relief before then. We'll follow the procedures developed by Dr. John Myers."

"Dr. John whom?"

"Dr. John Myers. He was a pioneer in the clinical uses of minerals—starting in the 1930s and 1940s. He worked out a treatment program for fibrocystic breast disease that substantially lessens or eliminates both the cysts and the symptoms for the very large majority of women."

"In the 1940s? I been having my problem since the 1970s! So why hasn't anyone told me about Dr. Myers' treatment?"

"Partly because it doesn't involve surgery or anything patentable. Also, as far as I'm aware, Dr. Myers never published his treatment anywhere, though he lectured about it dozens of times at doctors' seminars."

"What's Dr. Myers' treatment?"

"Mostly, iodine. However, Dr. Myers applied iodine in different ways according to the severity of the fibrocystic disease. In your case, we'll follow his procedure for the more serious problems."

"What's that?"

"Dr. Myers recommended iodine swabbed into the vagina followed almost immediately by intravenous injection of magnesium."

"That's certainly an unusual way to take a treatment! Did he explain why the iodine can't just be swallowed?"

"He did. Dr. Myers did experimental work with beagles with fibrocystic breast disease. He surgically removed the ovaries from one group, left the others intact, and treated them all with iodine. Only the intact beagles improved—none of the beagles without ovaries showed any improvement at all. He then found that placing the iodine as close to the ovaries as possible got the best results."

"And swabbing it into the vaginal area is as close as we can get."

"Right."

"What about the magnesium?"

"He didn't explain why, except that his dog research had shown it helped the iodine to work."

"You've used Dr. Myers' treatment?"

"Many times."

"What about less severe cases?"

"In less severe cases—and for you, once you improve enough—we'll have you swallow the iodine, along with magnesium, vitamin E, and other supporting nutrients. Since you have your worst problem premenstrually, there'll be extra vitamin B6 at that time."

"As long as I'm here, can I start the treatment now?"

"If you want."

Mrs. Bauer stayed in the examination room after the nurse and I gave her Dr. Myers' treatment. Twenty minutes later, we went back to recheck. She looked simultaneously surprised, puzzled, and pleased.

"I've already checked myself," she said. "And I'm better! I don't hurt as much, and I think the swelling is less. I think even some of the lumpy areas are a little less. Is that possible? Does this usually happen this fast? Why didn't you tell me?"

"Would you have believed me?" I paused. "Please let me check, too."

On both sides, she had distinctly less pain with the same degree of pressure. As she'd noted, her tissue swelling was slightly less, and some of the lumps were slightly smaller.

"Dr. Myers had doctors bring volunteer patients with severe fibrocystic breast disease to his seminars. He'd have the doctors check them, treat them, and check them again a few minutes after. They'd improve, just like you did. No one could argue with results like that."

"I guess not. But you're right, I probably wouldn't have believed you. So what's next?"

"We'll repeat this treatment once or twice weekly until you're improved enough to switch to an oral treatment program entirely. However, except for the iodine and magnesium, please start the rest of the oral program now. As you said, eliminate absolutely all caffeine in anything. Continue vitamin E . . ."

"How much?"

"Considering your degree of severity, 800 IU daily. Also, extra vitamin B6, 100 milligrams daily most days, 3 times daily before your periods, and primrose or black currant oil, 2,000 milligrams daily. And if you're not taking one, a high-potency vitamin-mineral combination."

"Is that all part of Dr. Myers' program?"

"No, but since I attended his seminar in 1976, I've found that these items help the whole program go faster."

"Anything for faster. I can't wait to see if I can get rid of this thing! Could it possibly go away completely?"

"Sometimes it does. More often, the pain clears up, swelling is gone, and the cysts become considerably smaller, but they don't go away completely."

"As long as it doesn't hurt, I'd be glad to live with that."

After 6 weeks of direct iodine treatment along with magnesium injections, Mrs. Bauer was improved sufficiently to switch to the oral program. I wrote her a prescription for Lugol's iodine, 7 drops daily, and recommended she continue all her other supplements along with 200 milligrams of magnesium (in the citrate form) daily. Since she'd been treated with a substantial amount of iodine, I asked her to get a blood test for thyroid function. Like nearly every woman treated with iodine for fibrocystic breast disease, her thyroid function remained normal. Seven months later, she was back—happy and excited. "I can sleep on my front or my back, whichever I want," she said. "I haven't had any pain in 2 months now! All those lumps are a lot smaller, and I think some of them are gone. I feel generally better all over! I'd really like to thank Dr. Myers. Can I write him a letter?"

"Dr. Myers died in the early 1980s. I'm sure he'd be very happy you're better, though."

"What about all my supplements?"

"Usually, they can be tapered down, but the iodine frequently needs to be continued at a low level—a drop or two a day, indefinitely." I wrote her a new list. She read it over, and got up to go. I went with her towards the door.

"I almost forgot," she said. "I told my husband and kids I had something special to show you . . ." And she gave me a big, enthusiastic hug!

DR. GABY'S COMMENTARY

Fibrocystic breast disease is a painful condi-tion for many women. Unfortunately, conventional medicine offers little help for women suffering from this condition. But eliminating caffeine and using some nutritional supplements can offer many women significant relief from this problem.

Dietary Considerations
Effect of Caffeine

Perhaps the most important dietary factor contributing to fibrocystic breast disease is ingestion of caffeine and related compounds (these chemicals are collectively known as methylxanthines). The major sources of methylxanthines in the diet are coffee, tea, chocolate, cola beverages, some other soft drinks, and certain pain medications.

In a 1981 report from Ohio State University Hospital, 45 women with fibrocystic breast disease stopped all methylxanthine consumption. Of those 45 women, 37 (83%) had a complete resolution of breast cysts, 7 were improved, and 1 was unchanged. Another 28 women decreased methylxanthine consumption by more than half. Of those, 7 (25%) had a complete resolution of cysts, 14 were improved, and 7 were unchanged.[1] This study shows that reducing methylxanthine intake is helpful to some extent, but that completely avoiding these compounds is necessary to produce the best results.

Conflicting Study

After this important study was published, other investigators challenged the results. In an often-quoted study, 158 women with fibrocystic breast disease were randomly assigned to consume a diet free of methylxanthines or to a control group receiving no dietary advice. Four months later, the condition had improved by an average of about 25% in the women in the methylxanthine-free group, but it had become slightly worse in the women in the control group. Although the difference between the two groups was highly statistically significant, the authors of the study concluded that the improvement was minor and was probably of little clinical significance.[2]

Largely because of this report, some doctors remain skeptical about the relationship between methylxanthine intake and fibrocystic breast disease. However, a closer reading of that study reveals that the authors' conclusions were probably unwarranted. When fluid obtained from the breast cysts of women assigned to the caffeine-free diet was analyzed, substantial concentrations of caffeine were found in many cases. Apparently, many of the women who were asked to eliminate caffeine did not do so—or at least not completely. It had already been shown by the Ohio State researchers that partial elimination of methylxanthines does not work as well as complete abstinence. The 25% improvement found in the second study was, in fact, just about what would have been expected, given the degree of dietary compliance. When viewed in that light, the results of the second study actually confirm, rather than refute, the Ohio State report.

Nutritional Supplements
Effect of Vitamin E

In a 1965 study, 20 women with chronic fibrocystic breast disease were given 200 or 400 IU of vitamin E per day for 3 months. Sixteen of the 20 women experienced moderate to complete relief of breast symptoms, and in 13 of the women the cysts either became smaller or disappeared completely.[3] In another study, 12 women with fibrocystic breast disease received 600 IU of vitamin E per day for 2 months. Seven women experienced a complete resolution of the condition, while

3 others improved.[4] The beneficial effects of vitamin E could not be confirmed in a third study.[5] Interestingly, the doctor who found negative results with vitamin E was the same doctor who reported that caffeine avoidance was ineffective (see above). Since vitamin E is nontoxic and seems to be effective in clinical practice, we usually recommend it for women who have fibrocystic breast disease.

Effect of Iodine

WHEN rats were given the iodine-blocking drug perchlorate to make them deficient in iodine, they developed breast lesions that, under the microscope, resembled human fibrocystic breast disease.[6] Iodine deficiency also rendered breast tissue more susceptible to the effects of estrogen.[7]

Studies in humans treated with iodine have produced impressive results. In one study, 172 women with fibrocystic breast disease were treated with an iodine-containing solution for 4 months. Of those treated, 72% became completely symptom-free, and an additional 27.5% improved. Thus, virtually everyone receiving iodine therapy had a complete or partial response.[8, 9]

It should be noted that some commercially available products contain iodides, which are not as effective as elemental iodine. As far as we know, the only product on the market that contains elemental iodine is called Lugol's solution. The usual effective dose of Lugol's solution is 2 to 3 drops per day, dissolved in at least 4 ounces of liquid. We have occasionally used larger doses—up to 7 drops per day, in severe cases.

Large doses of iodine can, on occasion, cause either hypothyroidism or hyperthyroidism, as well as certain other toxic effects. Iodine therapy must therefore be supervised by a doctor, and individuals taking iodine should have periodic blood tests to monitor thyroid function. However, when administered with caution, iodine is fairly safe.

Kelp, a natural source of iodine, is not likely to be of value in the treatment of fibrocystic breast disease, because the amount of iodine it contains is substantially less than the amount present in a few drops of Lugol's solution.

Hormone Therapy
Thyroid Hormone

ANOTHER effective treatment for fibrocystic breast disease is thyroid hormone. The benefits of thyroid hormone appear to be unrelated to its iodine content. In one study, 19 women with painful breast cysts received 0.1 mg of levothyroxine (Synthroid, a commonly prescribed form of thyroid hormone) per day. Within 3 months, many of these women experienced softening of the breast tissue and decreased lumpiness.[10] Prior to receiving thyroid hormone, only one of the women had laboratory evidence of hypothyroidism. It is possible that some of these women had a subtle deficiency of thyroid hormone that failed to show up in a standard blood test (see chapter 4). However, it is also possible that thyroid hormone exerts a beneficial effect on breast tissue that is unrelated to correcting a deficiency of the hormone.

Other Factors

SEVERAL STUDIES HAVE suggested that consuming a diet low in saturated fat can relieve the symptoms of fibrocystic breast disease.

Supplementation with essential fatty acids in the form of evening primrose oil (EPO) has also been found to be helpful. In one study, 200 women with breast cysts were randomly assigned to receive 6 capsules (about 3 grams) of EPO per day or a placebo for 12 months. Treatment with EPO significantly reduced pain and lumpiness in the breasts, but had no effect on the recurrence rate of cysts.[11] Some doctors use black-currant-seed oil or borage-seed oil as less-expensive alternates to EPO, as they are all similar in their fatty acid composition. However, neither of these oils has been tested as a treatment for fibrocystic breast disease.

Taking B-vitamins may help the body to detoxify excess estrogen. In addition, supplementing with natural progesterone may help balance some of the unwanted effects of estrogen, including breast cysts. However, there is little research on the use of these treatments.

A number of pesticides and environmental pollutants have been shown to have estrogenic effects. Some scientists believe that these chemicals promote breast cancer, and it is possible that they also contribute to the development of fibrocystic breast disease. Women with cystic breasts might therefore benefit from consuming organically grown foods, which are relatively free of pesticides.

Conclusion

FIBROCYSTIC BREAST DISEASE is a common and often painful condition. It might be a precursor to breast cancer, although the evidence in this regard is conflicting. For some women, avoiding caffeine and related compounds (methylxanthines) is all that is needed to eliminate breast cysts. For other women, supplementing with vitamin E, iodine, and thyroid hormone have also been found to be beneficial. Most women who participate in a properly supervised nutritional program experience good results.

Summary of Recommendations for Treating Fibrocystic Breast Disease

PRIMARY RECOMMENDATIONS:

- DIET
  - ➤ Avoid all methylxanthines (caffeine, as well as related compounds found in tea and chocolate).
  - ➤ Keep saturated-fat intake to a minimum.

- SUPPLEMENTS
  - ➤ Vitamin E, 400 to 800 IU per day.
  - ➤ Iodine (under medical supervision only) in severe cases, or if other treatments are ineffective.

OTHER RECOMMENDATIONS:

- ➤ Thyroid hormone, in selected cases.
- ➤ Evening primrose oil or another source of gamma-linolenic acid (borage oil or black-currant-seed oil), providing 90 to 270 mg of gamma-linolenic acid per day.

GALLSTONES *(avoiding gallbladder surgery)*

🌿 THE GALLBLADDER IS *a digestive organ located in the right upper portion of the abdomen. It stores bile, which is made in the liver, and releases it during meals to aid in the digestion and absorption of fats and other nutrients.*

Many individuals living in Western countries develop stones in their gallbladder, which consist primarily of cholesterol, calcium, and, in some cases, bilirubin (a breakdown product of hemoglobin). In some cases, the stones are "silent," in that they produce no symptoms. Other people with gallstones experience recurrent abdominal pain, bloating, and gas. If the gallbladder becomes inflamed or infected, or if a stone gets caught in a bile duct, serious problems can result and emergency surgery may be necessary.

Doctors often recommend that patients with painful gallstones have their gallbladder removed—either to relieve symptoms or to prevent an emergency situation from arising. On the other hand, the general consensus among doctors is that silent gallstones do not require surgery.

Other than surgery, conventional medicine does not have much to offer. Most doctors advise their gallstone patients to avoid fatty foods; however, that dietary change alone often does not eliminate the symptoms. Attempts have been made to dissolve gallstones by giving patients certain bile acids, such as chenodeoxycholic acid or ursodeoxycholic acid. While these compounds do sometimes work, bile-acid therapy is expensive, frequently causes diarrhea or intestinal upset, may require years of continuous treatment, and (as suggested by animal studies) might cause cancer. Furthermore, gallstones often recur when treatment with bile acids is discontinued.

DR. WRIGHT'S CASE STUDY

"I'd rather keep my gallbladder," Laura Winston said. "My father wouldn't let them take my tonsils, I've got all my teeth, and I found a way around hemorrhoid surgery. I want to keep my gallbladder, too." She frowned. "Sure is getting harder with all the pain I've been having lately. My husband says 'just go do it', but

Dora Watkins at church said she hasn't had one speck of gallbladder pain since she went strictly on your program. She'd had trouble for years. I asked her what she did, and she said, 'Girl, you better go yourself 'cause gallbladder attacks are caused by allergies, everybody's allergies are different, and what works for me might not work for you'. I never heard of such a thing, and the doctor says he never did either. But Dora's fine, and I don't care for that knife, so here I am.

Don't know a thing about having any allergies, though."

"Why did the doctors want to take your tonsils out?"

"When I was a child, I kept getting sore throats and tonsil infections all the time. It got so bad, I was missing too much school. My father wasn't much for reading, but he hit the books and found out black people usually don't digest milk too well, so he took all the milk and cottage cheese and ice cream out of the house, and I quit having problems near as much. But I thought that was a digestion problem, not an allergy."

"Very often both," I said. "Do you drink milk now?"

"Hardly ever. Didn't want my kids getting sick like me and besides my Dad's still around. He'd get after me if I gave his grandkids any."

"How long have you had gallbladder trouble?"

"Started getting little pains here and there just after I turned 40, so about 9 years. But it wasn't too bad until about 2 years ago."

"How often does it hurt?"

"Near every day, now. 'Course it's better sometimes, worse others, but the last bad one was so bad they put me in the hospital. Wanted to take my gallbladder right then but I told 'em no, just do like the time before. So they gave me pain pills and IVs and nothing else for 3 days 'til the pain went down and they let me go."

"I'm glad the allergy treatment worked."

Mrs. Winston shifted in her chair, crossed her arms, and looked at me with an interesting combination of skepticism, surprise, and suspicion. "What allergy treatment do you have in mind? Those doctors just put me in bed and let me lay. I didn't have any allergy treatment!"

"What did they give to you eat?"

She snorted. "Eat? Nothing! That's why they gave me those IVs! I've been in the hospital 3 times with real bad gallbladder—first thing they do is not let you eat!"

"If you don't eat, you can't have an allergic reaction to food, can you?"

She looked surprised for a moment, then smiled and relaxed. "Never thought of that. Those doctors were treating me for food allergy after all and didn't even know it."

"Right. And it's been going on for years."

"Isn't that something!" She frowned again. "But they tell me the pain is due to stones, and I sure have stones on the X-ray the doctor showed me."

"Over 20 years ago, Dr. James Breneman demonstrated that the pain of 'gallbladder attacks' is triggered by food allergy, and can be eliminated by identifying and removing the offending foods. Very rarely, a gallstone gets stuck in the bile duct, causing spasm, blockage, and intense pain. But that's very unusual. A major medical journal concluded a few years back that if a person had gallstones but no pain—so-called 'silent gallstones'—it's best not to operate, as the risks of surgery are greater than the risk of blockage of the bile duct."

"Well, I sure would appreciate my gallstones being silent. In fact, I'd like them to shut up for good right now! Then all I'd be left with is all this bloating, belching, and gas."

"Tell me about that, please."

"For years . . . it goes back before this gallbladder pain . . . I've had indigestion most times when I eat. It's gotten steadily worse—sometimes the food sits in my stomach, and lots of times my stomach all bloats up after I eat. And I'm always all gassy and get heartburn sometimes. The doctor said that was my gallbladder, too, and cutting it out would fix it. But I'd rather put up with it than be carved on. I'll just keep taking antacids like I do now."

"No need to let it go on. Blaming those symptoms on the gallbladder is a common medical mistake. Bloating after meals, belching, indigestion, and heartburn are usually due to stomach malfunction, not gallbladder trouble. Years ago, a few doctors pointed out that people with gallbladder problems usually have stomach malfunction, too."

"What kind of stomach malfunction?"

"Normal stomachs make large amounts of hydrochloric acid and pepsin to digest the food we eat. The most common stomach malfunction is underproduction of acid and pepsin, so food doesn't digest, and indigestion, bloating, belching, gas and heartburn are the resulting symptoms."

"Sounds like the stomach just gets old, wore out, and tired."

"In many cases, that's exactly what happens."

"Makes sense, the rest of us gets older and slower, too. But . . ." She thought for a moment, ". . . that means those antacids are the wrong thing. They can't help my digestion any."

"No, they can't. We'll run a test to make sure, but chances are what you really need is replacement hydrochloric acid and pepsin in capsules with meals, which not only relieves symptoms, but improves digestion, and your health, too!"

Two months later, Mrs. Winston was back. She looked a lot happier and much more relaxed than on her first visit.

"Haven't had one of them gallbladder pains—not one—since I quit eating all that allergic stuff," she said enthusiastically. "I like this kind of food allergy treatment better than that one with IVs! And that hydrochloric acid and pepsin stuff—it takes care of all that indigestion and bloat! Gave me a little trouble at first, but I figured my stomach just needed to get used to it 'cause it hadn't had much hydrochloric acid around for a few years. So I went slow and now my digestion's just fine, thank you. But I got some questions . . .", she rummaged around in her purse, ". . . written down here. Your nutritionist who helped me put my diet back together—I sure was allergic to a lot of foods—explained a lot to me, but I need to ask again, 'specially cause if I'm the cook that's how we're going to eat and my husband he's wanting me to make sure.

"I've gotten rid of all the sugar and white flour products from our house. Tell me again why that's important."

"Research work in large populations has shown that the more refined and processed the food supply is, the higher the incidence of gallstones. Some populations, like pre-1950s northern Canadian Eskimos, had a record of no gallstones at all until their diets became 'civilized.' Very-low-sugar, high-fiber diets also are associated with a much lower incidence of atherosclerosis and heart attack, diverticulitis, hemorrhoids, and colon cancer, as well as less gallbladder problems."

"My husband's family is heavy on heart trouble. So this change is as good for him as it is for me."

"Avoiding sugar and emphasizing unprocessed, high-fiber food is good for everyone."

"'Long as they're not allergic to it. Which reminds me—how long do I need to avoid all those foods. I'm taking those desensitization drops . . ."

"Which work for most things, but not necessarily everything. And there are some things I don't recommend desensitizing as they're not good for us anyway."

"Like milk?"

"Like cow's milk. As the saying goes, 'mother's milk is best for little babies, and cow's milk is for little cows'. Please check back with the technician who screened you for allergy and sensitivity. She'll tell you when it looks like you've desensitized and it's safe to try those foods again. But be cautious, and try them one at a time."

"That way I can tell if any of them are still trouble, and which ones, right?"

"Right. Your own body reaction is the best test."

"The nutritionist also said you'd tell me about some vitamins and things that might cut down on making more gallstones, and maybe even help dissolve the ones I got."

"Right. Please remember, though, that as long as there's no pain, no surgery's needed to remove them."

"I remember. But now that I got 'em to shut up and be 'silent', I figure it wouldn't hurt to try to persuade 'em to go away, too."

"Makes sense. I'll write down the things that might be helpful." I gave her the pieces of paper.

"Let's see . . . vitamin C, 2 grams, twice daily. Lecithin capsules, 1,200 milligrams, 3 twice daily. Flaxseed-oil capsules, 1,000 milligrams, 2 twice daily. Vitamin E, 400 IU once daily. High-potency multiple vitamin and mineral, one of the 4-capsule-a-day varieties. And this . . . " She looked at the second piece of paper. ". . . looks like a prescription I can't read. What's it for?"

"Iodide, specifically potassium iodide. Iodide helps dissolve cholesterol in test tubes, and at least in theory it can help dissolve it in people, too. Most gallstones contain a lot of cholesterol, so it's possible—although not certain—that iodide can keep the cholesterol from precipitating into stones in the future. Unless you're allergic to iodide—and we'll test you to find out—please use 3 drops daily for now."

"Alright. Now I understand I should stay on this good diet forever, but how long do I need to take all these vitamin pills?"

"The multiple vitamin and mineral, and the vitamins C and E should be indefinite. But likely you can adjust the other things downward as time goes on."

"You said get this iodide tested in case I'm allergic. What about this other stuff?"

"Sensitivity to the other supplements is less likely, but not impossible. So while you're checking on the iodide, you might as well check those, too."

"I'll check on everything. I've gotten real fond of not being in pain. I surely want to keep all my original parts!"

It's been several years now, and except for "a rumble once in a long while when I'm not careful" Mrs. Winston has had no further gallbladder pain.

DR. GABY'S COMMENTARY

As LAURA WINSTON learned, eliminating allergenic foods, eating better, and supplementing with hydrochoric acid and pepsin can relieve the symptoms associated with gallbladder disease. When gallbladder symptoms are relieved, patients are left with "silent gallstones." In other words, the gallstones are still there, but the symptoms are not. And while some doctors recommend surgery for symptomatic gallstones, patients who suffer from silent ones can be spared the knife. Additionally, preliminary evidence suggests that certain nutritional supplements may help prevent stones from developing.

Dietary Considerations
The Food Allergy Connection

Apparently, in the majority of cases, the abdominal symptoms attributed to gallstones are in fact caused by food allergy. As mentioned in the case study, James Breneman, M.D., former chairman of the Food Allergy Committee of the American College of Allergists, studied the relationship between food allergy and gallbladder disease in 69 patients.[1] Each patient was suffering either from symptomatic gallstones or from the "post-cholecystectomy syndrome" (abdominal complaints that persisted after the gallbladder was removed). The patients followed an elimination diet consisting of beef, rye, soy, rice, cherry, peach, apricot, beet, and spinach for one week. All 69 patients experienced relief of their symptoms after one week on the diet. After that, foods were added back one at a time, to determine which ones were causing the "gallbladder symptoms."

The most common symptom-provoking foods were egg, pork, and onion, with reactions occurring in 93%, 64%, and 52% of the patients, respectively. When the offending foods were removed from the diet (the average number of allergenic foods per person was 4.4), the patients remained symptom-free.

One of the elimination diets I have used in my practice is presented in Appendix A. Some doctors use other tests for allergy and sensitivity, as well as desensitization techniques. The reliability and effectiveness of some of these methods is controversial (see chapter 3 for additional discussion).

Dr. Breneman believed that food allergy causes swelling of the bile ducts and thus restricts the flow of bile from the gallbladder. A poorly draining gallbladder becomes prone to infection and stone formation. Animal studies done 50 years ago demonstrated that the gallbladder can, indeed, be the "target organ" for allergic reactions.[2] Therefore, it is possible that identifying and avoiding allergenic foods at an early age would prevent gallstones from developing in the first place.

Other Dietary Factors

EVIDENCE shows that a diet low in refined carbohydrates (i.e., sugar and white flour) and high in fiber and unrefined carbohydrates may help prevent gallstones from developing. In one study, 13 individuals with gallstones ate a diet containing refined carbohydrates for 6 weeks, then ate a diet containing unrefined carbohydrates for an additional 6 weeks. The cholesterol-saturation index of bile (a measure of the tendency of cholesterol stones to form) was higher in 12 of the 13 people during the refined-carbohydrate period than during the unrefined-carbohydrate period.[3] High-fiber diets may also prevent gallstones by enhancing the flow of bile. It is important to note that gallstones are extremely rare in Africa and other parts of the world where the diet is high in fiber and low in refined sugars.

The Role of Stomach Acid

WHEN the stomach does not secrete enough hydrochloric acid, digestive complaints such as bloating, belching, heartburn, and gas may develop. These symptoms, which frequently occur in individuals with gallstones, are usually attributed to the gallbladder disease. However, in a study of 50 patients with gallstones, more than half (52%) had coexisting hypochlorhydria (low stomach acid).[4] In our experience, when hypochlorhydria is identified and treated with hydrochloric-acid supplements, so-called "gallbladder symptoms" often improve.

Nutritional Supplements
Vitamin C

IN theory, certain nutritional supplements might help prevent the development of gallstones. In one study, guinea pigs were fed a vitamin C-deficient diet, which resulted in gallstone formation.[5] In patients with gallbladder disease, supplementing with 500 mg of vitamin C, 4 times a day, reduced the tendency to stone formation by changing the chemical composition of the bile.[6]

Essential Fatty Acids

ESSENTIAL fatty acids (EFAs) may also be important in preventing gallstones. In one study, hamsters fed a diet deficient in EFAs developed gallstones.[7] Although the typical American diet contains a lot of fat, it is usually not the type of fat that prevents EFA deficiency. Fried foods, margarine, partially hydrogenated vegetable oils, and foods high in saturated fat can interfere with EFA utilization. Good dietary sources of EFAs include nuts, seeds, vegetable oils, fish oil, and flaxseed oil.

Many of my patients show evidence of EFA deficiency, manifesting dry, flaky skin, which returns to normal when they avoid the "bad fats" listed above and supplement with EFAs for about 6 weeks. For an EFA supplement I usually recommend 1 tablespoon of oil per day for the first 6 to 12 weeks, and lower doses thereafter. In most cases, I prefer to balance the amount of omega-3 and omega-6 fatty acids by supplementing with flaxseed oil (rich in omega-3) one day and sunflower oil (rich in omega-6) on alternate days. You should always take additional vitamin E whenever you are taking an EFA, because extra EFAs increase the requirement for vitamin E.

Lecithin

LECITHIN is found naturally in bile, where it helps keep cholesterol dissolved in the bile, rather than crystallizing to form stones. In theory, supplementing with lecithin might help prevent the development of gallstones. In one study of 8 patients with gallstones who took lecithin for 18 to 34 months, the stones decreased in size in one case and remained the same in the others.[8] The dosage of lecithin in this study was rather small: 100 mg, 3 times a day. Larger amounts might produce better results; however, no one has tested the effects of higher doses of lecithin on gallbladder patients.

Dissolving Stones

ABOUT 30 YEARS ago, Irish researchers developed a mixture of 6 naturally occurring plant-derived compounds (menthol, menthone, pinene, borneol, camphene, and cineol). This formula, named Rowachol, is remarkably free of adverse effects and will, in some cases, shrink or dissolve gallstones. Among 24 patients with gallstones who were given Rowachol (usually for 6 months), the stones disappeared in 3 cases and became smaller in another 4.[9] A longer treatment period probably would have produced better results, since bile-acid therapy usually takes 1 to 2 years to achieve maximum results.

Rowachol has also been used in combination with bile acids. Adding Rowachol allows the dosage of chenodeoxycholic acid to be lowered by about 50%, thereby reducing the expense of the treatment and the risk of diarrhea. In one study, a combination of Rowachol and lower-than-normal doses of chenodeoxycholic acid completely dissolved gallstones in 11 (37%) of 30 patients within 1 year and in 50% of the patients within 2 years.[10]

Rowachol is not commercially available in the United States. However, the compounds from which it is made are available, so the formula could be reproduced by a compounding pharmacist. Although no significant side effects have been reported with this product, we recommend that its use be supervised by a doctor.

Although nutrients such as vitamin C, essential fatty acids, and lecithin affect the stone-forming potential of bile, no one has demonstrated that taking these nutritional supplements can cause gallstones to go away. Dr. Wright prescribed potassium iodide for his patient, in an attempt to dissolve her gallstones or prevent new ones from developing. That recommendation is based on the observation that iodides can dissolve cholesterol in the test tube. However, I am not aware of any evidence that supplementing with iodides has a beneficial effect in humans with gallstones. Because large doses of iodides can, on rare occasions, alter thyroid function, patients taking iodides should have periodic blood tests to monitor thyroid function.

Conclusion

GALLSTONES ARE A common problem for which conventional medicine has little to offer except surgery. Identifying and avoiding allergenic foods will usually relieve the symptoms caused by gallbladder disease. Hypochlorhydria (low stomach acid) is also a problem in more than half of individuals with gallstones. When gastric secretion is low, supplementing with hydrochloric acid and pepsin (under medical supervision) will frequently relieve symptoms such as bloating after meals and belching. Preliminary evidence suggests that dietary modifications and certain nutritional supplements might help prevent the development of gallstones.

Summary of Recommendations for Treating Gallstones

PRIMARY RECOMMENDATIONS:

- DIET: Identify and avoid allergenic foods.
  - Avoid sugar and other refined carbohydrates.
  - Emphasize foods high in complex carbohydrates, fiber, essential fatty acids and vitamin C (such as whole grains, fruits, vegetables, nuts, seeds, and legumes).

- SUPPLEMENTS: Hydrochloric acid with pepsin (under medical supervision), if tests demonstrate hypochlorhydria.

- Vitamin C, 1,000 to 3,000 mg per day, in divided doses. Reduce dose if diarrhea or abdominal pain occurs.

OTHER RECOMMENDATIONS:

- Essential fatty acids and/or lecithin are of theoretical value for preventing the development of gallstones. Vitamin E should also be supplemented when essential fatty acids are used.

GOUT

GOUT IS A *condition that results in recurrent attacks of acute arthritis in the big toe or other joints. Individuals with gout may also develop chalky deposits of uric acid (sodium urate) around various joints. Some individuals may develop kidney stones or kidney disease. Gout is usually associated with elevated blood levels of uric acid, a normal breakdown product of metabolism. High uric-acid levels can result either from genetic abnormalities of uric-acid metabolism or from excessive dietary intake of purines (the precursor to uric acid).*

Conventional treatment of acute gouty attacks consists mainly of anti-inflammatory drugs. Preventive treatment is aimed at lowering uric-acid levels in the body, thereby reducing the tendency of this compound to crystallize in the joints or kidneys. In many cases, dietary changes can decrease uric-acid levels significantly. When diet alone does not sufficiently reduce blood levels of uric acid, doctors may prescribe drugs that either inhibit the production of uric acid or increase its excretion in the urine. Although these drugs are effective, they can sometimes cause severe side effects.

DR. WRIGHT'S CASE STUDY

Stephen Sampson had a slight limp. "Gout," he said. "Had it for several years. My father and grandfather did too. I take colchicine when it really acts up, and it helps, but it gives me a little headache and diarrhea. I know it's from a natural source, but I also know a little too much can be really toxic. I think I'm a little sensitive to it. So I thought I'd check if there was anything else in the natural way."

"Have you been following any diet plan or taking any other medicines?"

"Doctors have told me about allopurinol and probenecid to lower my uric-acid levels. I read up on them, didn't like the allopurinol. I tried the probenecid, but it didn't seem to work for me. And I didn't know there was any diet."

"Gout pain is caused by crystallized uric acid, usually in the 'ball joint' of the big toe. Uric acid is an end product of metabolism of purines, which are found in the largest quantities in sardines, organ meats such as kidney and liver, and proteins in general. For some of us, eating more fruits and vegetables and cutting back on animal protein is helpful."

"My wife's been trying to cure me of the meat-and-potatoes habit since we were married last year. I can give it more of a try."

"Also, fructose can raise blood uric acid, so read every label, and eliminate it, including 'corn syrup' and 'high fructose corn syrup.'"

"How about fruit itself?"

"Whole fruit doesn't seem to be a problem."

"And supplements?"

"Several that help over the long run—but for acute attacks, have you tried cherry juice?"

"Cherry juice? We're talking about serious pain here!"

"I know. Years ago, a Dr. Blau published an article describing relief of acute gout with cherry juice. It works often enough, so it's worth a try."

"How many years ago?"

"1950."

"Better late than never. How do I do the cherry juice?"

"At the first sign of a gout attack, start drinking it. Try to get down a quart or more—the larger the amount, the more likely it is to work."

"And this really works?"

"Usually. But remember, the goal is really to prevent gout attacks."

"So how do I do that?"

"Diet change, and supplements. Let's start with vitamin C."

Mr. Sampson rolled his eyes. "Cherry juice, vitamin C—I wouldn't believe it except my wife and her family say this stuff really works."

"In 1976, a medical journal published a warning against taking large doses of vitamin C, as it increased uric-acid excretion, and lowered blood uric acid by 1 to 3 milligrams per deciliter."

"A warning? Isn't getting rid of blood uric acid exactly what I want to do?"

"Yes."

"And isn't that how that probenecid drug works—by increasing uric-acid excretion?"

"Yes."

"So, I still don't understand: a warning? A warning against what we want to happen?"

"The authors theorized that excreting more uric acid might lead to uric-acid kidney stones. While that's a theoretical possibility, it's never been reported to happen with vitamin C."

"If that were a real worry, then no one should prescribe that probenecid either. This doesn't make sense."

"It does when you remember that probenecid was previously patented, and is still sold by drug companies."

"Of course. So how much unpatentable vitamin C should I take?"

"Start with 3 grams, twice daily. If that causes excess gas or loose bowels, cut back to 2 grams each time."

"Next, folic acid, a B-vitamin. Folic acid in large doses appears to inhibit the enzyme which produces uric acid. By itself, folic acid doesn't do much, but it's helpful when taken along with vitamin C. However, I'll need to write you a prescription . . ."

"Prescription? My wife was telling me that folic acid prevents birth defects. She said it's safe even during pregnancy."

"She's right. But large doses of folic acid can mask the laboratory diagnosis of vitamin B_{12} deficiency. The FDA assumes that doctors don't know this, so it has pronounced it illegal to sell folic acid without prescription except in tiny doses."

"That doesn't make sense."

"Government work. . . . Here's a prescription for 50 milligrams, twice daily."

"Let's go on to the last thing—lithium."

"Whoa . . . isn't that a drug for serious mental problems?"

"In large quantities, it is very useful in controlling manic-depressive psychosis. But lithium's a mineral, and like other minerals has many uses. In '83—that's 1883—the *Lancet* published an article showing that lithium can prevent the formation of uric-acid crystals. If uric acid can be kept from crystallizing . . ."

"It shouldn't settle out in my toe. I've been told the crystals are needle-point sharp, and that's what hurts."

"Right. Here's another prescription, this one for lithium carbonate, 300 milligrams, twice daily. That's actually about 60 milligrams of lithium, much less than what it takes to cause excess-lithium effects. But to make certain please also take flaxseed-oil capsules, 3,000 milligrams daily.

Essential fatty acids block the effects of excess lithium . . . and of course, 400 IU of vitamin E to go with the essential fatty acids." I wrote this all on a piece of paper, and gave it to Mr. Sampson.

"Less protein, eliminate added fructose, take cherry juice, vitamin C, folic acid, lithium, essential fatty acids, and vitamin E. This all better work."

Mr. Sampson hasn't been back since (although he's had follow-up lab monitoring), but his wife tells me that over the past 9 years, he's had no more gout attacks, and "hasn't needed that cherry juice!"

DR. GABY'S COMMENTARY

SOME SIMPLE DIETARY changes and nutritional supplements can help control gout by reducing uric-acid levels. Additionally, drinking cherry juice appears to be an effective natural remedy for acute attacks of gout.

Dietary Considerations

MOST DOCTORS ADVISE against the use of foods that are high in purines (such as meats, anchovies, sardines, seafood, beans, lentils, spinach, and peas). Alcohol (especially beer) should also be avoided, because it can increase uric-acid levels and provoke acute attacks of gout. It is not well known that ingesting refined sugars, particularly sucrose[1] and fructose,[2] can also significantly increase uric-acid levels.

Food Allergy

OCCASIONALLY, food or inhalant allergies can trigger an acute gouty attack and raise uric-acid levels.[3] Allergy does not appear to be a common trigger for gout; however, individuals with gout who have other symptoms suggestive of allergy might benefit from an allergy evaluation (see chapter 3).

Cherry Juice Can Help

IN a 1950 study, 12 patients with gout ingested one-half pound of cherries per day (or an equiva-

lent amount of cherry juice), with no other dietary restrictions. In all 12 cases, serum uric-acid levels fell to normal, and the patients had no further attacks of gout. Cherry juice appeared to be as effective as whole cherries. While most of the results were obtained with black cherries, sweet yellow and red sour cherries were also effective.[4] We have been impressed by the effectiveness of cherry juice as a treatment for acute gout. In many cases, relief of pain and inflammation is rapid, and anti-inflammatory drugs are unnecessary. However, some patients do not improve significantly unless they drink a full quart of cherry juice daily. We do not know how cherry juice works or what is the active ingredient.

Nutritional Supplements
Folic Acid

DR. Kurt Oster, a cardiologist who routinely prescribed up to 80 mg of folic acid per day for heart patients, found that this vitamin reduced serum uric-acid levels in most patients.[5] Studies in the 1940s had suggested that folic acid inhibits xanthine oxidase, the enzyme in the body that manufactures uric acid. Later studies showed that it was not folic acid itself, but a breakdown product of folic acid (pterin aldehyde) that inhibits xanthine oxidase.[6] Oster had also prescribed vitamin C for most of his patients, and it is possible that vitamin C promotes the conversion of folic acid into pterin aldehyde.

Folic acid is much safer than allopurinol, the standard drug used to inhibit xanthine oxidase. However, additional studies are needed to determine whether high-dose folic acid is an effective alternative to allopurinol.

Although folic acid is safe, large doses may interfere with some anti-epilepsy drugs and with a laboratory test used to screen for vitamin B_{12} deficiency. In addition, animal studies suggest that large doses of folic acid could promote zinc deficiency. For these reasons, high-dose folic-acid therapy should be monitored by a nutritionally oriented doctor.

Vitamin C

In a study that included healthy individuals and patients with gout, a single 4-gram dose of vitamin C increased the urinary excretion of uric acid 3-fold. In addition, when individuals ingested 8 grams of vitamin C for 3 to 7 days they experienced sustained increases in uric-acid excretion and significantly lowered serum uric-acid levels.[7]

Curiously, the authors of this study concluded that vitamin C may be dangerous for people with gout. That conclusion was based on the fact that drugs that promote uric-acid excretion can—on rare occasions—precipitate a uric-acid kidney stone or trigger a gouty attack by causing rapid migration of uric acid from the tissues. However, that concern has not stopped doctors from prescribing drugs that promote uric-acid excretion, drugs that are far more dangerous than vitamin C.

Although we are not aware of any published reports of vitamin C-related problems in people with gout, it is conceivable that abruptly starting high-dose vitamin C could trigger an acute attack of gout or dump too much stored uric acid into the kidneys. Those theoretical concerns could presumably be avoided by starting with a relatively low dose of vitamin C (such as 1,000 mg twice a day) and building up gradually over several months. With those precautions, vitamin C therapy appears to be a safe and effective method of lowering uric-acid levels and preventing recur-

rences of gout. Dr. Wright considers the theoretical risks of high-dose vitamin C to be negligible, and he has seen no adverse effects from starting with an effective uric-acid lowering dose of vitamin C (such as 6 grams per day). I prefer to start with lower doses and to increase gradually, because I have seen 2 patients experience a flare-up of gout in their big toe after taking large amounts of vitamin C.

Lithium

It was observed more than 100 years ago that lithium salts can dissolve uric-acid stones in a test tube. In addition, when patients with gout were given lithium, the number of recurrences was apparently reduced.[8] Based on that early report, Dr. Wright has prescribed lithium carbonate (usually 300 mg twice daily) to a number of patients with recurrent gouty attacks.

However, additional research is needed to determine whether lithium is an effective treatment for gout. Also, because of its potential to cause significant adverse effects, lithium should be used with caution. While the dose of lithium used by Dr. Wright is lower than the amount commonly associated with toxicity, some people are especially sensitive to the effects of lithium. One study suggested that supplementing with essential fatty acids (EFAs) can reverse lithium-induced tremor,[9] but it is not known whether other side effects of lithium (such as neurological disturbances, cardiac arrhythmias, and abnormalities of kidney function) can be prevented by EFAs. At this time, it is not clear whether the risks of lithium therapy outweigh the potential benefits in people with gout.

Copper

Rats fed a copper-deficient diet developed a 60% increase in serum uric-acid levels.[10] The relevance of this finding to humans is not clear. However, considering that the typical American diet provides only one-half of the Recommended Dietary

Allowance for copper, supplementing with 1 to 2 mg of copper per day may be worthwhile for people who have elevated uric-acid levels.

Avoid Niacin

LARGE doses of niacin (more than 1 gram per day) will raise uric-acid levels in some individuals[11] and should therefore be avoided by most patients with gout.

Summary of Recommendations for Preventing and Treating Gout

(NOTE: Treatment should be monitored by a doctor)

- Avoid refined sugar (particularly sucrose and fructose), alcohol, and foods high in purines.

- Vitamin C, 1,000 to 2,000 mg, 2 to 3 times a day if uric-acid levels are elevated.

- Folic acid, 25 mg, 2 to 3 times a day, if uric-acid levels are elevated.

- High-potency multiple vitamin/mineral that contains zinc and copper.

- Low-dose lithium has been used by Dr. Wright. Supplement with essential fatty acids (flaxseed oil or sunflower oil), 3 to 5 grams per day, when using lithium.

- Cherry juice for acute attacks.

HEPATITIS *(acute and chronic)*

> HEPATITIS IS AN *inflammation of the liver that can range in severity from mild to life-threatening. There are a number of different causes of hepatitis, the most common of which are viral infections; toxic reactions to drugs, alcohol or other chemicals; and autoimmune processes, in which the immune system attacks the liver. Typical symptoms of hepatitis include fatigue, nausea, malaise, low-grade fever, and jaundice (yellowing of the skin). Depending on the type of hepatitis, other symptoms may also occur, including joint pains, skin rashes, and eye problems. Most cases of acute hepatitis resolve after a period of weeks or months, although many people do not regain their original energy level for many months.*
>
> *In some instances, hepatitis does not resolve, but instead becomes chronic. In those cases, liver inflammation can persist for years and may eventually lead to serious problems such as cirrhosis (scarring) or cancer of the liver. Chronic hepatitis may result from a persistent viral infection (particularly the hepatitis B or hepatitis C viruses) or from an autoimmune disease. Infection with the hepatitis A virus typically does not become chronic, and alcoholic or toxic hepatitis usually resolves after the offending agent is withdrawn.*
>
> *Conventional medicine has little to offer patients with acute hepatitis. Supportive care includes a good diet and, when necessary, intravenous fluids. Interferon, an antiviral compound, is helpful for some individuals with chronic viral hepatitis. However, this medication is quite expensive and can have significant side effects. Drugs that suppress the immune system are often prescribed for autoimmune hepatitis, but these drugs rarely cure the problem.*

DR. WRIGHT'S CASE STUDY: (ACUTE HEPATITIS)

It was obvious from across the room that Shelby James had a liver problem. His face and all observable skin surfaces were a dark orangish-brown, and the former "whites of his eyes" were orange-brown also. He looked tired and a bit feverish. His wife, Molly, was with him.

"Thanks for seeing us on such short notice," she said. "Shelby just got back from a business trip when he started feeling bad. I took him to his regular doctor when he started getting a little orangey, and the blood tests confirmed hepatitis—the 'B' type—the highly infectious sort anyway. The doctor said nothing to do but go home, rest, drink lots of fluids, and if he really gets bad, we could give him prednisone, but usually that isn't necessary. The rest of the family should take the usual precautions against catching it—separate utensils, separate bathrooms if possible for the duration, and so on."

"And I'd likely be off work for a month or 2," Shelby said. "That's what convinced me to come in after Molly talked to the nurse here. She said I might get over this in a week or 2. Seems hard to believe after what my doctor said."

"I reminded Shelby about Jennifer's mononucleosis 2 years ago, when she was 17," Molly said. "He was on another business trip, and she got over it so fast he couldn't tell she'd ever been sick when he got home. She had as bad a case as I've ever heard of—raging high fever, terrible sore throat, big swollen glands—but 3 treatments at the clinic here, all those supplements at home, and she was back to school feeling fine and running around the track in a week! Some of her other friends who had 'mono' at about the same time missed 2 or 3 weeks of school, and took months to get their energy back. One of her friends missed nearly an entire quarter!"

"Fortunately, acute hepatitis and mononucleosis are 2 of the easier viral diseases to handle," I said. "And of course, the sooner we can get at them the better."

"Molly started us all on a lot of vitamin C the minute she got off the phone yesterday," Shelby said. "She's gotten 20 grams into me already. Actually, I think I am feeling a little better, but it could just be a placebo thing, too—just because I'm doing something instead of waiting for it to go away. But isn't that an awful lot of vitamin C?"

I smiled, but Molly beat me to a reply. "You ain't seen nothin' yet, darlin'! Jennifer took between 50 and 100 grams a day for several days—between IVs and swallowing the stuff. And all she did was get better in record time!"

"And it won't hurt anything?"

Molly combined a frown and a pout. "Do you think I'd have let Jennifer do it if it would hurt?"

"In short-term use, it's extremely unlikely to hurt anything but the virus. Taken by mouth, there's no hazard. . . . In fact, our bodies let us know later on with diarrhea when we're taking too much. Strangely, if we have hepatitis and diarrhea already, large amounts of vitamin C often make the diarrhea go away. There's a rare circumstance in which high-dose intravenous vitamin C might be hazardous. It's a genetic disorder called glucose-6-phosphate dehydrogenase deficiency—G6PD deficiency for short. It occurs very occasionally in certain ethnic groups: people of Jewish, Mediterranean, or black ancestry. Even in these groups, it's quite an uncommon condition, and can be tested for."

"As far as I know, I'm not at risk, then. But why use the vitamin C intravenously; won't it work if I just swallow it?"

"Intravenously, we can get higher blood levels, and it works faster."

"Let's do it, then."

"In addition to the vitamin C, we also give all the B vitamins, especially B_{12} and folic acid. They also speed the process. Of course, in between IV doses, take as much vitamin C as you can by mouth. If you get in a total of 100 grams a day or even more the first few days, that's fine. Your liver will appreciate your efforts!"

Mr. James' diarrhea stopped 36 hours after his first oral vitamin C. After 2 daily vitamin C IVs of 65 grams each (given with calcium and magnesium to prevent muscle spasm, as well as the B-complex vitamins), plus another 30 to 40 grams of vitamin C by mouth, his urine and stools had returned to normal color. He felt "reasonably well." Within 2 weeks he was back at work, feeling well, with no hepatitis symptoms remaining.

DR. WRIGHT'S CASE STUDY: (CHRONIC HEPATITIS)

"I got hepatitis about 15 years ago," Arthur Sheridan said. "It was a pretty bad case—6 weeks of bed rest and all that. My liver-enzyme tests were never completely normal, though. In the last 2 to 3 years they've been getting steadily worse again. The specialist says I definitely have chronic hepatitis, and if my condition deteriorates further maybe I should try interferon. But I've read about that, and it doesn't sound good to me. But beyond that, there doesn't seem to be much to do. That's why I'm here."

He handed me copies of his tests, which confirmed a progressive worsening of hepatitis B. "I hope it's not too far gone for natural treatments to help."

"Chronic hepatitis is hardly ever too bad to be improved, and usually substantially. In the worst cases, we usually need to give vitamin C and other nutrients intravenously for several weeks. Likely you can get the job done by swallowing them all. Of course, it is quite a bit of swallowing.

"I can handle that—I've been practicing swallowing since I was born. What should I take?"

"Before I make you a list, let's go over diet basics first. If we remember that livers are our principal 'detoxifying' organs, the rule is not to give your liver an extra, unnecessary load! Please eliminate all food additives—artificial flavors, colors, preservatives, and so on. Also eliminate sugar, caffeine, and alcohol."

Mr. Sheridan sighed. "My wife's been after me on that health-food thing for years. I guess it's time to start."

"Health food beats disease food every time."

"Good point. What about the vitamins and things?"

"Start with vitamin C. It's a very basic tool, which you'll need to take at least 3, preferably 4 times daily for years. Start with 1 gram, 4 times daily for a few days, then 2 grams, 4 times daily for another few days, then increase slowly to 3 grams and 4 grams each time until you get loose bowels or even diarrhea. At that point, back off to the maximum you can take without causing loose bowels or diarrhea. That's called the 'tolerance point' for oral vitamin C. You might

try a buffered vitamin C preparation, as many people say buffered vitamin C is easier to take."

"What's all that vitamin C do?"

"All the answers aren't in, but it's known to stimulate and improve many of the liver's biochemical functions."

"What's next?"

"Licorice."

"Really?"

"One of the active ingredients in licorice is glycyrrhizen, which has both anti-viral and anti-inflammatory effects. This component of licorice is widely used in Japan as a specific treatment for hepatitis. It's given intravenously there, but active components of licorice absorb well by mouth. Please use 2 grams of ground or powdered licorice root twice daily. However, there is a precaution—have your blood pressure checked regularly. It's not common, but licorice in large quantities can lead to sodium retention, potassium loss, and elevated blood pressure."

"That should be easy enough to track. Anything else?"

"Vitamin C and licorice root are just the beginning. There's also a beneficial effect from extra vitamin B12, folic acid, silymarin, *Phyllanthus amarus,* and even whole-liver extract." I added them to the list.

"I think I know what vitamin B12 and folic acid are. But what are silymarin and *Phyllanthus amarus?*"

"They're botanical remedies—plants used traditionally for hepatitis for hundreds of generations before Western science finally got around to studying them. Actually, there are many more botanical remedies for the liver than just these two. Many of the best-studied are from the Chinese and Ayurvedic systems of healing, but chances are we won't need them."

"And what's the whole-liver extract?"

"That one is just common sense. Everything a liver needs to heal itself is already in whole, disease-free liver, which also needs to be free of pesticides, antibiotics, and synthetic hormones."

Mr. Sheridan made a quick count. "That's

7 items. You did say there'd be a lot to swallow, though."

"And there's just 1 more—a multiple vitamin and mineral to 'back up' the individual nutrients."

In 1 month, Mr. Sheridan's rising liver-enzyme tests reversed course and began to drop toward normal. They all became normal after 10 months, and have stayed that way for 11 years. Mr. Sheridan continues to follow a healthy eating plan and to take all his supplements, although his "tolerance point" for vitamin C has dropped considerably over those years.

DR. GABY'S COMMENTARY

NATURAL MEDICINE OFFERS some promising treatments (primarily nutritional supplements and herbal remedies) for both acute and chronic hepatitis.

Nutritional Supplements
Vitamin C

VITAMIN C has been shown to protect the liver against damage induced by toxins.[1] For that reason, vitamin C supplements may be advisable for many different conditions in which the liver is under stress. Perhaps more importantly, vitamin C has an anti-viral effect, which presumably would be useful in the treatment of viral hepatitis. That action of vitamin C was demonstrated in 1975 by Japanese researchers, who found that a wide range of viruses could be inactivated in a test-tube by vitamin C. The vitamin appeared to act by disrupting the nucleic-acid strands of the viruses.[2]

The benefits of vitamin C have also been demonstrated in humans. In one study, 11 patients with viral hepatitis were given intravenous infusions of 10 grams of vitamin C daily for an average of 5 days. These patients recovered considerably more rapidly than would have been expected.[3] In another study, 63 patients with hepatitis who received a similar vitamin C treatment experienced rapid improvement and were able to leave the hospital in about half the usual time.[4]

Some practitioners of nutritional medicine have observed that larger doses of vitamin C can be even more effective. Intravenous infusions of 50 grams or more, combined with large oral doses (sometimes 100 grams per day or more) have been used with great success. Instead of lingering for many months, acute hepatitis can, in some cases, be cured in a matter of weeks with vitamin C therapy.

Vitamin B_{12}/Folic Acid

VITAMIN B_{12} and folic acid help protect the liver against damage and play a role in the regeneration of new liver cells. In one study, 88 patients with acute viral hepatitis received either conventional treatment (control group) or the same treatment supplemented with vitamin B_{12} injections (every other day for 10 days) and folic-acid tablets (5 mg, 3 times a day for 10 days). Compared with patients in the control group, those receiving the vitamins had a more rapid return of appetite and a 17% reduction in the duration of illness.[5]

Vitamin E

THIS important antioxidant vitamin has been shown to protect animals against experimentally-induced liver damage. Recent research in humans suggests that vitamin E also may be helpful in treating chronic hepatitis. In one study, 24 patients with chronic hepatitis B (19 of whom had failed to benefit from interferon treatment) were randomly assigned to receive vitamin E (300 IU twice a day) for 3 months or no treatment (control group). During a 9-month follow-up period, 5 of the 12 patients receiving vitamin E were apparently cured of their disease, compared with none of the 12 patients in the control group.[6] In a study of patients with chronic hepatitis C, treatment with 1,200 IU of vitamin E per day for 8 weeks appeared to inhibit the development of liver fibrosis (one of the complications of chronic hepatitis C).[7]

Herbal Supplements
Licorice Root

EXTRACTS of licorice root have shown great promise for individuals suffering from hepatitis. A component of licorice known as glycyrrhizin appears to have an anti-viral action, as well as a direct protective effect on the liver.

An injectable form of glycyrrhizin known as Stronger Neo-Minophagen C (SNMC) has been used widely in Japan to treat hepatitis. In one study, 133 patients with chronic hepatitis received 40 ml of SNMC or a placebo intravenously, daily for 40 days. Patients given the licorice extract improved to a significantly greater extent than those receiving the placebo.[8] In another study, orally administered glycyrrhizin was effective in the treatment of both acute and chronic hepatitis.[9] It is noteworthy that although high doses of licorice have been reported to cause side effects—including hypertension, fluid retention, and potassium deficiency—no significant problems were seen in the patients treated with glycyrrhizin.

The powerful protective effect of SNMC was demonstrated in another study of 18 patients with subacute liver failure due to viral hepatitis. Subacute liver failure is a very serious condition, typically fatal in nearly 70% of patients. However, among patients given intensive treatment with SNMC, the death rate was only 28%.[10]

The injectable form of licorice has been intermittently available in the United States, depending on how vigorously the Food and Drug Administration has chosen to enforce its opinion about what constitutes an "unapproved drug." Oral licorice root should also be helpful against hepatitis, but because of its potential to cause high blood pressure, potassium deficiency, and other problems, treatment should be monitored by a doctor.

Milk Thistle

THE common milk thistle (*Silybum marianum*) contains a substance called silymarin, which has been shown to prevent liver damage. Silymarin is used extensively in Europe to support the liver in patients with hepatitis and other liver diseases. Standardized European silymarin products have been available in the United States since the mid-1980s, and many nutrition-oriented physicians are now recommending this herb.

About 10 years ago, I saw a patient whose blood tests had for many years repeatedly shown elevated liver enzymes. Liver specialists had been unable to determine the reason for this abnormality. After taking silymarin for a month, his liver enzymes became normal, and with continued treatment the levels have never gone up again.

Phyllanthus amarus

PLANTS of the genus *Phyllanthus* have been widely used by traditional medical practitioners for the treatment of jaundice and other diseases. Their use was described in Indian Ayurvedic literature more than 2,000 years ago. Extracts of *Phyllanthus amarus* have been shown to inhibit hepatitis B virus.

In a study of 37 people who were carriers of the hepatitis B virus, treatment with *Phyllanthus amarus* for 30 days cleared the virus from the body (as documented by loss of hepatitis B surface antigen) in 59% of cases.[11] In a later study this herb was not effective. However, patients in that study had harbored the virus for a longer period of time, and it was suggested that treatment for up to a year might be necessary for patients who are long-term carriers. Additional research is needed to determine whether *Phyllanthus amarus* is effective against hepatitis B. To date, there are no studies of this herb as a treatment for hepatitis A or C.

Other Treatments

A NUMBER OF other nutrients and herbs have been used to treat acute or chronic hepatitis. These include dandelion root, lipoic acid (a B-vitamin), and catechin (a flavonoid). In patients with autoimmune hepatitis, identifying and avoiding allergenic foods and chemicals may be helpful. Recent research suggests that selenium may reduce the incidence of liver cancer in patients with chronic hepatitis B.[12]

Conclusion

A NUMBER OF nutrients and herbs have been found to be of value in treating both acute and chronic hepatitis. The natural approach can shorten the duration and reduce the severity of acute viral hepatitis, and it may provide relief for some patients with chronic hepatitis.

Summary of Recommendations for Treating Acute Hepatitis

(NOTE: Treatment should be supervised by a physician.)

- Vitamin C orally and (if possible) intravenously.
- B-vitamins (orally or by injection).
- Vitamin E, 400 to 800 IU per day.
- Milk thistle, standardized to contain 70 mg of silymarin, 3 times a day.
- High-potency multiple vitamin and mineral.

Summary of Recommendations for Treating Chronic Hepatitis

(NOTE: Treatment should be supervised by a physician.)

- Vitamin C orally and (in selected cases) intravenously.
- Vitamin E, 400 to 1,200 IU per day.
- Selenium, 200 mcg per day.
- Milk thistle, standardized to contain 70 mg of silymarin, 3 times a day.
- Licorice root extract in selected cases.
- *Phyllanthus amarus* (hepatitis B only).

HERPES SIMPLEX

HERPES SIMPLEX IS *a viral skin infection that usually affects the lips, oral mucous membranes, genital area, and occasionally other places on the body. The lesions usually last 7 to 10 days, and they typically look like a cluster of blisters, which can itch or cause pain. Once the herpes simplex virus has infected someone, it rarely goes away comletely. Rather, it remains dormant (usually in nerve cells) between attacks, and comes out again periodically to trigger an acute outbreak. Herpes infections tend to recur frequently and are quite contagious.*

Herpes infections are common in people with cancer, AIDS, and other diseases that compromise the immune system. However, more subtle immune-system deficiencies also seem to increase the risk of developing herpes simplex. For that reason, a comprehensive prevention and treatment plan should include measures that enhance immune function. These include avoiding refined sugar, eliminating allergenic foods from the diet, getting adequate amounts of sleep and exercise, and keeping stress at tolerable levels.

Conventional therapy consists mainly of anti-viral drugs, which are helpful to some extent. However, these drugs are rather expensive, and they can cause side effects.

DR. WRIGHT'S CASE STUDY

"It's this herpes thing," Jim McAllister said. "It's breaking out more and more often. Between herpes and work and kids, Judy and I haven't gotten together in months. I don't know if she's frustrated, but I am."

"I've been just as frustrated trying to get him to see you for the last several years about simply staying healthy," Judy McAllister said. "Jim just gets too many colds and flus, he's always at the maximum allowed for sick days. But this is what it took to get him here. Maybe 2 or 3 months of no sex is a blessing in disguise."

Jim made a face. "OK, I'm here. What can I do?"

"You could stop eating all that sugar," Judy said.

"Sugar doesn't cause herpes," Jim replied.

"Hold on here," I said. "Let me make sure we're all talking about the same thing." I turned to Jim. "You're sure this is herpes simplex?"

"That's what two dermatologists and my regular doctor all say. They all want me to take acyclovir, and I did for awhile, and it worked, but Judy really got upset when I was taking it more and more often."

"Of course I did," Judy declared. "I read up on that stuff and how it works, and it's scary. Over a long time it looks to me like it could really cause health problems. And besides, you're not getting herpes all the time because of an acyclovir deficiency. There's something else the matter;

193

some natural things you can do that aren't as likely to be harmful in the long run."

"OK, OK, I'm here. And my mother's backing Judy up. So what else can I do?"

"Actually, Judy's right about sugar. It significantly interferes with the immune system's ability to fight micro-organisms of all types. Eliminating all refined sugar is a basic step in stopping any kind of recurrent infections."

"Likely it'll also help him not get diabetes like 2 of his grandparents did when they were older," Judy observed.

"Likely," I agreed. "We also need to have Jim screened for food allergies."

"Food allergies? I don't have any food allergies," Jim declared. "Even if I did, what could that possibly have to do with herpes?"

"It's not just herpes in particular," I said. "'Recurrent infection, check for allergy' is a basic principle in nutritionally oriented medicine. We usually find it, too."

"No sugar, maybe eliminate food allergies—anything else I have to eliminate?" Jim grumbled.

"Maybe not sex," Judy said.

"Perhaps a few more things," I said. "For now, chocolate, peanuts and other nuts, and cut back on grains."

"That's what Judy and my mother have been telling me."

"But until now you wouldn't listen," Judy noted.

"Chocolate, peanuts, other nuts, and cereal grains are relatively high in the amino acid L-arginine, which can promote the growth of herpes. That brings us to something you can take—the amino acid L-lysine. Until you get this under control, please take 2 grams, 3 times a day. It works better if it's taken in between meals."

"Where do I get that?"

"Only any natural-food store, supermarket, drugstore, or all-night convenience store," Judy said. "I've pointed it out to you from time to time."

"I couldn't believe anything worthwhile against herpes would be in every overnight store," Jim declared. "If it's in all those places, why isn't everyone taking it? Why does anyone take acyclovir?"

"A lot of people are taking it or it wouldn't be in all those places," Judy replied. "And people only take acyclovir because they don't believe their wives could know about such a simple, inexpensive remedy!"

"Hold on again," I said. "We've got more to cover. The next thing is vitamin C. For now, use 2 grams, 3 or 4 times daily, and 'back up' the vitamin C with citrus bioflavonoids, 1 gram daily."

"With meals or not?"

"Doesn't matter. Next, a prescription, this time for a mineral, lithium."

"Lithium? Can't that have some bad side effects?" Judy asked.

"Yes, at high doses. But at lower amounts, it inhibits the herpes virus. Also, essential fatty acids prevent the bad effects of lithium, so I'll ask Jim to take a tablespoonful of flaxseed oil daily, along with some vitamin E.

"Also, please add zinc and selenium to the list. Please use 30 milligrams of zinc (as zinc picolinate), twice daily. Most of the research on zinc and herpes is on topical—rubbed in—zinc, but I've observed that it helps when we swallow it, too. For selenium, look for sodium selenite, 250 micrograms daily. For better utilization of the selenium, separate it by at least 1 hour from the vitamin C. Professor Will Taylor of the University of Georgia points out that selenium inhibits the ability of herpes and other retroviruses to reproduce themselves.

"Lastly, a good 'mega' formula multiple vitamin-mineral, to make up for some of the 'holes' I suspect Judy could point out in your diet for the last few years."

"Isn't that the truth," Judy said.

"Alright, I'll do it," Jim said. "But it'd better work."

I didn't see Jim again about his herpes. Judy later told me that after he eliminated sugar and allergens, quit the chocolate and nuts, and took his supplements, his herpes cleared up and didn't come back until he "messed up all over again." After 2 or 3 similar episodes, he settled down to a relatively sugar-free, allergen-free, almost-no-chocolate program with "some lysine, some vitamin C, zinc, selenium, a little lithium, and a multiple vitamin."

"Just amazing what frustration can do," Judy observed, at a later visit of her own.

DR. GABY'S COMMENTARY

INDIVIDUALS CAN OFTEN control herpes outbreaks with a few simple natural remedies. First, eliminating sugar from the diet and determining if there are any food allergies may be helpful. A few nutritional supplements can also help.

Nutritional Supplements
Vitamin C

VITAMIN C has been shown to inactivate a wide range of viruses[1] (including the herpes simplex virus),[2] and to enhance immune function. Bioflavonoids also have antiviral activity. In one study, patients with herpes simplex infections received daily 600 mg of vitamin C and 600 mg of bioflavonoids or a placebo for 3 days. Symptoms disappeared after an average of 4.2 days in the vitamin-treated group, compared with 9.7 days in the placebo group. Thus, treatment with vitamin C and bioflavonoids reduced the duration of herpes outbreaks by 57%. Vitamin therapy was most effective when it was started at the earliest sign of an outbreak.[3] Although these relatively low doses were effective in this study, we often prescribe larger amounts of vitamin C, because its antiviral effects seem to be more pronounced at higher doses.

L-lysine

HERPES simplex viruses require the amino acid L-arginine to replicate (multiply). Another amino acid, L-lysine, is known to oppose some of the effects of L-arginine. The possibility has therefore been considered that L-lysine could be used to prevent or treat herpes simplex infections. In one study, 45 patients with frequently recurring herpes outbreaks received L-lysine (usually 312 to 500 mg per day) for periods of 2 months to 3 years. When an outbreak occurred, the dosage was increased to 800 to 1,000 mg per day. Foods high in L-arginine (nuts, seeds, and chocolate) were also restricted. L-lysine treatment accelerated the recovery from acute outbreaks and reduced the frequency of recurrences.[4] In a double-blind study of patients with herpes simplex outbreaks, supplementing with approximately 1,200 mg of L-lysine per day significantly reduced the recurrence rate.[5]

It is possible that the benefits of L-lysine might be increased by reducing the consumption of foods that are high in L-arginine, such as peanuts, chocolate, cashews, peas, and grains. Indeed, many herpes sufferers report that eating chocolate or peanuts causes a flare-up of their skin condition. In addition, it may be helpful to avoid foods that have been stripped of their L-lysine content. Much of the L-lysine is destroyed when protein is heated in the presence of lactose (milk sugar), fructose, or the combination of sucrose and yeast (as in many baked goods). High-temperature cooking of meats will also destroy some of the L-lysine.

Vitamin E

IN one report, a gauze pad was soaked with vitamin E oil and applied directly to oral herpes lesions for 15 minutes. In nearly every case, patients experienced relief from the pain in less than 8 hours, and the lesions frequently disappeared in 12 to 24 hours. Larger or multiple lesions responded best when the treatment was administered 3 times a day for 3 days.[6] Other researchers have observed similar effects with topically applied vitamin E.[7]

Selenium

ACCORDING to studies conducted by Will Taylor, Ph.D., at the University of Georgia, selenium is active against a number of retroviruses, including herpes viruses. Although there have been no clinical studies, we consider it reasonable to include safe doses of selenium as part of the overall program for preventing and treating herpes simplex. Foods that are high in selenium include whole grains, meats, seafood, garlic, and mushrooms.

Other Natural Treatments

Adenosine

ADENOSINE monophosphate (AMP) is a compound that occurs naturally in the body. It is known to have activity against herpes viruses and to enhance immune function. In one study, 36 patients with recurrent herpes simplex infections (average, 6.3 episodes per year) received a series of intramuscular injections of AMP, given every other day for a total of 9 to 12 treatments. The dosage was 1.5 to 2.0 mg per kg of body weight. In most cases, the lesions began to dry up within 36 hours, and patients experienced pain relief within 48 hours. During follow-up periods ranging from 1 month to over 2 years, 64% of the patients remained free of recurrences, and the rest of the patients had less severe outbreaks.[8]

I have been particularly impressed with the effectiveness of AMP injections. One of my patients had suffered with at least one herpes simplex lesion on some part of her body every day for 8 years. Within 48 hours of receiving the first of a series of 10 injections, her lesions disappeared, and they did not return for more than 18 months. Although AMP does not work for everyone, I consider it one of the most effective treatments available for individuals with difficult cases of herpes simplex.

Intramuscular injections of AMP occasionally cause temporary chest pain. Although this pain is not related to the heart, it can be alarming. Chest pain can usually be prevented by giving half of the full dose, waiting 20 minutes, then giving the other half.

Lithium

LITHIUM is best known for helping to control bipolar disorder (manic-depression). It has also been shown to inhibit the replication of herpes simplex viruses.[9] Psychiatric patients receiving lithium therapy have observed a significant reduction in the frequency of herpes simplex infections.[10] In a double-blind study, application of an ointment containing 8% lithium succinate relieved symptoms and reduced viral shedding in patients with genital herpes.[11] The ointment also contained zinc and vitamin E, so it is not clear how much of the benefit was due to the lithium.

Dr. Wright has used small amounts of oral lithium, considerably less than the doses used for bipolar disorder, to treat patients with herpes. While using lower doses of lithium would greatly reduce the risk of side effects, no studies have been done to determine whether a small amount of lithium is effective against herpes.

Summary of Recommendations for Treating Herpes Simplex

PREVENTING OUTBREAKS:

- Diet: Avoid refined sugar and alcohol. Work with food allergies. Restrict foods high in L-arginine (chocolate, nuts, peanuts, grains).

- Vitamin C, 1 to 3 grams per day, or as directed by a physician.

- Citrus bioflavonoids, 500 to 1,000 mg per day.

- L-lysine, 500 to 1,000 mg per day.

- Selenium, 100 to 250 mcg per day.

- Adenosine monophosphate, series of intramuscular injections.

ACUTE TREATMENT:

- Larger doses of the nutrients listed above may be used short-term, under the supervision of a doctor.

- Topical vitamin E, 1 to 3 times per day.

- Other treatments used by Dr. Wright:

  ➤ Lithium succinate-zinc-vitamin E ointment.

  ➤ Low-dose lithium orally, with essential fatty acids to prevent side effects of lithium.

  ➤ Oral zinc, 30 to 60 mg per day, usually balanced with copper, 2 to 3 mg per day.

HYPERTENSION

HYPERTENSION IS THE *medical term for high blood pressure. Persistent hypertension affects millions of Americans, and it can eventually result in heart disease, stroke, visual impairment, or damage to the nervous system and kidneys. Hypertension can be caused by a variety of medical conditions—from kidney disease to hormonal problems. However, in the great majority of cases, a specific cause cannot be found, and the condition is labeled "essential hypertension."*

It has clearly been shown that controlling hypertension can reduce the risk of heart disease and stroke. For that reason, patients with hypertension are often advised to take blood-pressure-lowering drugs. However, many individuals experience side effects from these medications, such as fatigue, depression, or sexual dysfunction. In addition, the long-term effects of some anti-hypertensive drugs are unknown. For example, there is an ongoing debate about whether calcium-channel blockers can cause cancer. Because of these potential problems, many doctors and patients are seeking alternative ways to treat hypertension.

DR. WRIGHT'S CASE STUDY

"I'm always nervous when I see a doctor," Fred Keyser said. "So I brought my blood pressure records with me. I take my blood pressure at home. It's always lower than at the doctor's office, but without medication it's still too high. So Susan here . . ." he gestured to his wife ". . . insisted that I check in at your office. She does a lot of reading about health." He handed me several sheets of paper. A quick glance showed they covered several years of blood pressure records.

"Sure I do," Susan Keyser declared. "One of us needs to. I want to make sure we both stay relatively healthy and able to take care of ourselves until we're at least 90 or so. And I especially don't want Fred to have a stroke like his grandfather did. My reading tells me a natural-medicine approach might not get Fred off drugs completely, but it could, and at the very least he'll be healthier for it. So here we are."

I looked more closely at the blood pressure records. "Let's see—5 years ago your blood pressure was about 160 to 170 over 100 to 110 or so . . ."

"That's when I absolutely insisted Fred start taking medication," Susan said. "After all, he wasn't even 50 yet, and his blood pressure was up there! I'd already cut out all the added salt, eliminated the high-salt foods, and switched us to decaffeinated coffee. We cut out all the alcohol, too, except a little beer or wine. But his blood pressure just kept going up."

"Had you eliminated the added sugar and foods with sugar in them, too?"

Susan and Fred looked at each other skeptically. "Sugar? No one ever told us that sugar causes high blood pressure."

"It doesn't for everyone, but several small studies have shown that sugar can raise blood pressure significantly for some individuals, and that sugar can cause significant excretion of calcium and magnesium. My observation has been that eliminating sugar helps control blood pressure for individuals who have diabetes or hypoglycemia in their families."

"My grandmother, mother's mother, had diabetes when she was past 60 or so," Fred observed.

"Then restricting sugar and refined carbohydrate—that's mostly white flour and other refined-flour products—would be very important for you to try."

Susan pulled a notebook out of her purse, and started writing. "We'll give it a try," she said.

I looked at Fred's blood pressure records again. "You've had good blood pressure control for the past 3 years—130 to 140 over 80 to 90. What medications have you been using?"

"A calcium-channel blocker, I think it's called . . . a beta-blocker, which blocks adrenalin; and a diuretic. We tried several things to start . . . you can see the blood pressure control was variable . . . and this combination seems to do the best job. I have noticed it seems to tire me out more than I'd expect at my age, though."

"I've read that's common with many anti-hypertensive medications," Susan said.

"That's true," I said. "You know, the pressure within the arterial system—the blood pressure—is one of many factors in the health of the vascular system. Natural medicine can sometimes help us reduce blood pressure to normal without drugs, and sometimes it just lessens the amount of drugs necessary to achieve blood-pressure control. But natural medicine usually improves the health of the entire cardiovascular system, the strength of the blood vessels so they can with-

stand a higher blood pressure without rupturing as easily, the ability of the heart to pump at higher pressures, and the ability of blood to flow through possibly-narrowed blood vessels. Those are just some examples."

"Sounds good," Fred said. "What vitamins and minerals should I take?"

"Before we get to those, let's make sure we've covered basic diet and a few other 'natural medicine' things like exercise, acupuncture, and psychological aspects like meditation, biofeedback, and prayer."

"Where shall we start?" Susan asked.

"You've already done quite a bit with diet, so let's just finish that. Let's see—low salt, minimum alcohol, no caffeine, and you'll try eliminating all sugar and foods with sugar as well as refined carbohydrate. That leaves vegetables and allergies."

"As far as I know I don't have any allergies," Fred said.

"And there aren't any in his family, according to his mother and aunts," Susan said. "I've checked, because I read that occasionally allergies can make the blood pressure go up."

"Allergy is only a major factor in a small minority, but I always ask about it. Now, vegetables—many studies have shown that long-time vegetarians have significantly lower blood pressure than those of us who eat meat and other animal proteins. That doesn't mean that everyone with high blood pressure should—or even can—become an instant vegetarian, but gradually moving as far as comfortable in that direction is usually advisable. At the very least, substitute fish for beef and pork as much as possible. People who eat considerable fish have somewhat lower blood pressures, and definitely less heart attacks.

"What about eggs?"

"Eggs are one of very few sources—the other one is soy lecithin—of phospholipids in our diets, substances very important to nerve-cell membranes. Usually I don't recommend eliminating eggs unless they're demonstrated to cause problems." I looked at my notes. "That's all about diet for now. Please check in with our clinic nutritionist 'for further details', as the saying goes.

"Now—how much exercise are you getting?"

"I think I have that one covered. I tried a lot of things, and finally settled on one of those ski-track type indoor machines—this is Seattle, after all—and I use it every day while I watch the news—at least 30 minutes a day, and sometimes an hour if there's something interesting on after the news.

"About those other things: I tried biofeedback, but it just didn't seem to work for me. And I just can't do meditation—I'm too restless and more action-oriented. That's why the exercise comes easy. And I haven't prayed a lot since my mom made me—so that whole area of 'psychic' or 'psychological' or whatever just isn't working for me now."

"Not everything works for everyone—maybe later. Have you tried acupuncture?"

"I thought acupuncture was for pain relief. I didn't know it helped blood pressure," Susan said.

"It's another thing that's a major help only for a minority, but I've seen a few dramatic results," I said.

"We'll try it," Susan said, and made more notes.

"Now about those supplements—what are you taking now?"

"Not much—we thought we'd wait until after we came here. We do have a potassium prescription since Fred's taking a diuretic, and the doctor surprised us by recommending a multiple vitamin and vitamin E, 400 IU. She said there's enough study to convince her that vitamin E will prevent a significant proportion of heart attacks. She made sure to check that the vitamin E didn't raise Fred's blood pressure, either. Apparently it can do that?"

"Very rarely. But it can't hurt to check. And she's certainly gotten you off to a good start. What about calcium and magnesium?"

"There's a little in the multiple, but Fred's not taking extra. After all, he's taking a calcium blocker."

"Magnesium is very important for all cardio-vascular problems, including hypertension. It dilates blood vessels, which helps to lower blood pressure. It helps regulate blood fats, helps prevent and correct heart rhythm disorders, prevents 'sudden cardiac death' . . . very important. But supplemental calcium is important in hypertension, too. Paradoxically, it's been observed that both calcium-channel blockers and calcium supplements can help lower blood pressure."

"How does that work?"

"It's rather complicated, but it has to do with a recently discovered hormone made by the parathyroid gland that affects calcium channels and that is affected by calcium. When calcium is supplemented, often the amount of calcium-channel blocker can be reduced. Please take 1,000 milligrams or a little more calcium daily, and 300 to 400 milligrams of magnesium. Look for a combination preparation."

"Two other specific supplemental items can help control blood pressure—essential fatty acids and coenzyme Q_{10}. Please start with 2 table-spoons of cod-liver oil daily. We'll monitor your balance of fatty acids with a blood test in 3 to 4 months. Because you'll be getting about 2,800 IU of vitamin D per day in the cod-liver oil, we'll measure your serum calcium periodically, although problems are exceptionally unlikely. Coenzyme Q_{10} should be at least 50 milligrams, 3 times daily—more if you can afford it. Take it with the cod-liver oil—it absorbs better that way. Studies with coenzyme Q_{10} show it doesn't start to affect blood pressure for several months, so we'll need some patience."

Susan was writing rapidly. "Let's see—calcium, magnesium, continue the potassium and vitamin E, cod-liver oil, coenzyme Q_{10}, and the multiple vitamin-mineral. That should keep Fred busy."

"Actually, considering Fred's temperament, there's one other thing."

"My temperament? What do you mean?"

"You noted that you're always a bit nervous, and your blood pressure is always higher at the doctor's. You're action-oriented—doing your exercise regularly—but meditation and biofeedback-relaxation-type things don't fit so well. And part of your blood pressure program is a beta-blocker. Overall, an 'adrenaline-type' guy."

"You can say that again," Susan said.

"There's an Ayurvedic botanical that might help. It has many names—one is 'sarpaganda' (also called *Rauwolfia serpentina*), that's usually very effective in 'adrenaline-types' with hypertension. It works, among other things, by reducing the level of adrenaline at nerve endings in a natural way. Actually, decades ago, Western chemists and drug companies crystallized a single molecule from it, and sold it as a drug called reserpine. It was usually very effective, but had serious side effects for a few people, and was gradually replaced by more-recently patented drugs."

"So is the whole-plant remedy safe?"

"Much safer than the isolated, crystallized single molecule. It's been observed over and over again that whole herbal complexes of ingredients do the job and cause much less trouble. Isolated crystalline reserpine often caused depression, precisely because it was too strong, and decreased adrenaline and similar molecules too much. I've rarely had anyone tell me that sarpaganda does that, although of course you should watch for it."

Fred chose to try the diet, vitamins, and minerals for the first 10 months. He felt considerably better, and he was able to eliminate the diuretic, and cut the quantity of the beta-blocker and calcium-channel blocker by half while maintaining the same good blood-pressure control. He then started sarpaganda, and within another 6 months he was off synthetic medication entirely while maintaining normal blood pressure. Susan noted that with the use of sarpaganda,* he seems a little less tense, a little more relaxed.

DR. GABY'S COMMENTARY

A NUMBER OF non-drug approaches are available that can effectively reduce blood pressure, often eliminating the need for prescription drugs. Stress reduction, meditation, relaxation techniques, weight loss, discontinuing cigarettes, and participating in a medically supervised exercise program are each effective for some people. In addition, combination therapy is often more effective than any individual treatment alone.

Dietary Considerations

BASIC DIETARY CHANGES are frequently helpful in reducing high blood pressure. It is well known that avoiding excessive sodium-chloride (salt) intake will lower blood pressure for many patients, although in approximately 30% of individuals with hypertension, salt intake has little or no effect on blood pressure. Studies in animals show that a high-sugar diet can also raise blood pressure,[1] and this effect seems to occur in humans, as well.[2] Vegetarian or high-fiber diets may lower blood pressure in some patients.

Some evidence shows that both garlic[3] and onion[4] can lower blood pressure. These foods have also been shown to have other beneficial effects on the cardiovascular system, such as lowering serum cholesterol and inhibiting platelet aggregation. Although not all of the studies agree, including garlic and onion in the diet seems like a good idea.

Some studies have shown that ingestion of caffeine is associated with an increase in blood

---

*Because of the potential for serious side effects, even if rare, sarpaganda should only be used under medical supervision. At Tahoma Clinic, sarpaganda has been superseded by another Ayurvedic combination containing sarpaganda as one of its ingredients.

pressure,[5] but other studies have failed to confirm that finding.[6] Although the data are conflicting, our observation is that the blood pressure of some individuals is indeed affected by caffeine intake.

Drinking alcohol can cause a significant blood-pressure elevation in many people with hypertension.[7] Therefore, even though some studies have associated moderate alcohol intake with a lower risk of heart disease, we believe that most hypertensive patients should avoid alcohol.

Food Allergy

FOOD allergy can contribute to hypertension and, for some patients, allergy is the primary cause of the problem.[8, 9] Individuals who suffer from other allergy-related symptoms, such as migraines or nasal congestion, may experience a substantial reduction in blood pressure after identifying and eliminating allergenic foods.

I once saw a robust 26-year-old man who ate well, exercised regularly, and had little stress in his life. Yet, he had a long history of significant hypertension, which required 2 prescription drugs for adequate control. Based on his history of chronic nasal congestion, I asked him to try an allergy-elimination diet. He identified dairy products and eggs as the cause of his nasal congestion. By avoiding these 2 foods, he was able to discontinue both of his blood pressure medications, while maintaining a perfectly normal blood pressure (110/70 mm Hg) for the next 10 years.

Nutritional Supplements
Potassium

AT least 19 studies have examined the effect of potassium supplementation on blood pressure. An analysis of the combined results (called a meta-analysis) showed that supplementing with potassium significantly reduced both systolic (the higher number) and diastolic (the lower number) blood pressure.[10]

The best way to obtain potassium is by eating abundant amounts of fruits and vegetables. One would need to take a large handful of over-the-counter potassium tablets in order to supply the amount of potassium found in a high-potassium diet. While prescription-strength potassium supplements are more potent, they can be irritating to the stomach. However, in cases where dietary changes are not feasible, supplements may be desirable.

Calcium

NUMEROUS studies have demonstrated that supplementing with calcium can lower the blood pressure of hypertensive individuals. However, other studies found that calcium supplements had absolutely no effect on blood pressure. This discrepancy is due to the fact that hypertension has a number of different causes. One contributing factor is an elevated level of renin, an enzyme produced by the kidney that influences salt and fluid balance. Calcium supplements have been shown to reduce blood pressure in patients with low-renin hypertension, but not in those with high-renin hypertension.[11] These 2 types of hypertension can be distinguished by a lab test called the "renin profile," which measures plasma renin and urinary sodium excretion. On the other hand, one could also try supplementing with calcium (and magnesium) for a few months and see if the blood pressure changes.

Magnesium

THERE IS NO question that magnesium lowers blood pressure in certain clinical situations. In a double-blind study, patients taking magnesium-depleting diuretics for hypertension had a significant decline in blood pressure after adding a magnesium supplement to their program.[12] However, in another double-blind study, supplementing with magnesium had no significant effect on blood pressure.[13]

I recommend calcium and magnesium supplements for many of my patients, including those with hypertension. The optimal ratio of calcium to magnesium is often debated, but is not known. One might speculate that a calcium/magnesium ratio of 2 to 1 is best for people with low renin levels, whereas a 1-to-1 ratio is more appropriate for those with elevated renin. However, more research is needed before we will know for sure.

Essential Fatty Acids

ESSENTIAL-fatty-acid (EFA) deficiency can also contribute to hypertension. Both omega-6 fatty acids (from sources such as sunflower or safflower oil)[14] and omega-3 fatty acids (from fish oil)[15] have been shown to lower blood pressure. A physical sign that suggests the presence of EFA deficiency is dry, flaky skin. Avoiding margarine and fried foods may help prevent EFA deficiency. Good sources of EFAs (in addition to those listed above) include nuts, seeds, some vegetables, and oily fish (such as mackerel, salmon, tuna, halibut, and cod).

Coenzyme Q10

SUPPLEMENTING with coenzyme Q10 (CoQ10)—a compound that plays a fundamental role in human biochemistry—can produce a considerable reduction in blood pressure. In one study, 26 patients with hypertension received 50 mg of CoQ10 twice a day. After 10 weeks, the average systolic blood pressure decreased from 164.5 to 146.7 mm Hg, and the average diastolic pressure decreased from 98.1 to 86.1 mm Hg.[16] Similar results have been reported in other studies.[17]

The effect of CoQ10 on blood pressure was usually not seen until 4 to 12 weeks after the start of therapy. Therefore, it is important not to give up on this treatment too early.

The Role of Thyroid Hormone

IN ONE STUDY, the incidence of hypertension was 14.9% among patients with hypothyroidism, compared with 5.5% in healthy people. When the proper dose of thyroid hormone was given to the hypothyroid patients, their blood pressure fell significantly.[18] I have observed that many patients are "clinically hypothyroid," despite having normal thyroid blood tests (see chapter 4). When these patients were treated with thyroid hormone, some of them experienced an improvement in their high blood pressure.

Conclusions

THE RESEARCH I have discussed indicates that diet and nutrients play a complex but important role in the prevention and treatment of hypertension. As is often the case with natural medicine, a combination of treatments may be more effective than any single treatment alone. That is especially true for hypertension, since the effectiveness of the individual dietary changes and nutrients seems to vary from person to person. Of the patients we have seen who required prescription medications for high blood pressure, about 40% were able to wean themselves off of their medications and maintain a normal blood pressure with the help of nutritional and lifestyle changes. Others were able to reduce the dose of their medications, but could not discontinue them completely.

Because the nutritional treatment of hypertension involves so many different variables, it is important to consult a practitioner who is experienced in nutritional medicine.

Summary of Recommendations for Treating Hypertension

DIET AND LIFESTYLE

- Avoid refined sugar, caffeine, alcohol, fried foods, margarine, and partially hydrogenated vegetable oils.

- Consume salt (sodium chloride) in moderation.

- Emphasize fruits, vegetables, whole grains, nuts, seeds, legumes, garlic, and onions.

- Use oily fish in moderation.

- Work with food allergies, in selected cases.

- Maintain ideal body weight.

- Lifestyle interventions that may be helpful include regular exercise, meditation, relaxation and stress-reduction techniques, and biofeedback.

SUPPLEMENTS

- Calcium, 500 to 1,000 mg per day.

- Magnesium, 300 to 500 mg per day.

- Essential fatty acids, in selected cases. Because of their vitamin A and D content, doses of cod-liver oil greater than 1 tablespoon per day should be monitored by a physician.

- Coenzyme Q_{10}, 60 to 100 mg per day.

- Thyroid hormone, in selected cases.

❧ INFERTILITY AFFECTS AS *many as 15% of married couples. The inability to have children can result from abnormalities in either the husband or wife. Low sperm count, poor sperm function, failure to ovulate, and damage to the fallopian tubes due to infection are among the many causes of infertility. Some reproductive problems can be treated effectively, whereas others are irreversible. Conventional treatment of infertility includes various drugs to induce ovulation; the drugs are associated with a pregnancy rate of about 30%. However, many fertility drugs can cause serious side effects, including damage to the liver and lungs. Medical procedures such as in vitro fertilization are also available; however, such procedures are very expensive and are not always effective.*

DR. WRIGHT'S CASE STUDY: (MALE INFERTILITY)

"I never thought I'd have a problem," John Stoinen said. "In fact it's kind of embarrassing. My wife's been through every test you can imagine. She's OK, and they tell me I'm the reason she can't get pregnant. And I'm just 29—not 79 or something! Seems my sperm count is too low, and some of those little guys. . . . I guess there's girls, too, aren't there . . . aren't moving around the way they should, and some of them aren't even shaped the way they're supposed to be— they're even deformed. Can't understand it, I'm from a family of 9 kids, 4 brothers, and they all have at least 1 kid. It's just me."

Linda Stoinen had come in with her husband. She smiled encouragingly. "I told John there's no reason to be embarrassed. After all, he's been to the urologist, his physical exam is perfectly OK, it's only this sperm thing. And we've read that's

getting to be a more common problem these days, pollution or pesticides in the food or sub-optimal nutrition or something. I figure there's nothing we personally can do about the general pollution and pesticide problem in the next 2 or 3 years, but we can do something about what we eat. We've made a start in that direction, and decided to come here for a little more help."

"What have you done so far?"

"Just a few weeks ago I was reading . . . I don't remember where . . . a report on a study of or-ganic farmers, I think they were European, Danish or something. The report said that they had really good sperm counts, and the sperm were really healthy. That just clicked with me because of all the stuff you read about how a lot of herbicides and pesticides mimic estrogens, and male alligators in Florida with deformed penises. . . . I know it might not be scientific, but it occurred to me that it couldn't hurt if we used as much organically grown food as possible, with no pesticides and herbicides used on it. It's a little more expensive but better for our health, even if

I don't get pregnant. And I've started reading the labels on anything that isn't organic—which is still a lot—and only buying stuff with no added chemicals or artificial flavors or preservatives."

"That's a very good start." I turned to John. "Do you smoke anything or drink alcohol?"

"Funny thing, my Dad was alcoholic, smoked like a chimney, and there were 9 of us . . . but no, because of Dad I swore never to touch alcohol, and I haven't. Don't smoke anything, either."

"That's good; all of that can interfere with the quantity and quality of sperm. Have you ever had a thyroid problem?"

"Not that I know about, but Mom did."

"We'll check you, just in case. Are you taking any vitamins?"

"Not regularly, except vitamin Cs if I get a cold or the flu."

"Actually, vitamin C is a good place to start. Some research has shown that sperm movement is better and pregnancy rates higher with extra vitamin C. Please use 1,500 milligrams, twice daily."

"That's easy enough."

"But that's just a start. Other research has found that the amino acid L-arginine can often raise low sperm counts significantly. Use 1,500 milligrams of L-arginine twice daily, in between meals. One precaution, though—if you've ever had a herpes outbreak, it's possible that L-arginine could reactivate it. If that happens, stop, and call in about what to do."

"I don't think I've had that problem."

"Good, because L-arginine can be quite important. Next, vitamin E, 400 IU daily, and selenium, 200 micrograms daily. It's fairly well-known that selenium deficiency can cause infertility in farm animals, and testicles manufacture several selenium-containing proteins, so even though there's so far no positive human research, it's wisest to use a safe amount.

"Lastly, zinc—the picolinate type—30 milligrams daily, vitamin B_{12}, 2,000 micrograms daily, and folate—the natural-plant-concentrate liquid type—1 drop daily; that's five milligrams. Zinc, folate, and B_{12} are all very important to proper DNA division and duplication, and just might take care of that sperm-malformation problem. Linda might as well use those, too, as they're known to help prevent birth defects."

"What about a multiple vitamin and mineral?" Linda asked.

"Always best to add a general multiple when using individual supplements."

"That's a lot of stuff for a healthy 29-year-old guy," John observed.

"Along with the diet changes you're making, it at least raises your odds," I said.

Just 3 months later, Linda called in to let us know she was pregnant.

DR. WRIGHT'S CASE STUDY: (FEMALE INFERTILITY)

"I've had everything examined!" Kathy Oberholter exclaimed. "Multiple pelvic exams, air up my Fallopian tubes, ultrasound exams, temperature records, you name it, I've done it! My husband's been checked out, too, no problems—they even said his sperm count was a little higher than average. The doctor says the next step is fertility drugs, but I'm a little uneasy about that. I want to try natural treatment first, and besides, I'd prefer my kids—if I have any—one at a time."

"Seems reasonable, and you could still use fertility drugs later if a natural approach doesn't work."

"That's what I told my husband, and that's why I'm here."

"You're how old this year?"

"Thirty-three. We've actually been trying for 7 years, though."

"Any other symptoms or health problems besides not getting pregnant?"

"Maybe a little PMS, but nothing else I know about."

"Never had a thyroid problem?"

"No. By the way, they checked thyroid blood tests along with everything else and told me those were OK, too."

"It's been known for years that thyroid hormone has a major influence on menstrual and reproductive function. Sometimes just a little thyroid can regularize menstrual periods and facilitate pregnancy, even when blood tests are reported normal, and a small quantity is very unlikely to be harmful, especially in a younger person. But before any specific recommendations, some other questions. Do you drink coffee or use other sources of caffeine?"

She looked embarrassed. "I'm on the go a lot. I must drink 6 or more cups a day, and I'm a major chocolate eater."

"Even though you may have withdrawal symptoms, please stop. Caffeine is suspected to contribute to infertility."

"Guess I'll just drink lots of milk."

"Please don't. There's at least one epidemiological report linking high milk consumption with lowered fertility for women. Besides, cow's milk is best for little cows, anyway."

"OK."

"It's wisest to stop smoking if you do." She shook her head "no". "Also, cut alcohol back to no more than one glass of wine or beer a day."

"No problem. That's actually a little more alcohol than I drink usually, anyway."

"Good. Now, other general measures. Even if it makes no difference to fertility, it's best for the health of any developing baby to eliminate all food chemicals, additives, flavorings, and preservatives. They simply can't contribute anything useful to child development. Along the same lines, use as much organic produce as you can find and afford. It's just as well to minimize exposure to pesticides, herbicides, and so on. And of course eliminating sugar, white flour, and other refined and processed foods is good for anyone's health."

"I've been hearing a lot of this from my mother, too."

"Good for her. Now, specific items—first, para-aminobenzoic acid or PABA."

"Isn't that the stuff in some sunblocks?"

"Yes. However, it's also considered to be one of the B-complex vitamins, and it can safely increase the activity of steroid hormones such as estrogen. In the 1950s and 1960s, a well-known nutritionist, Carlton Fredericks, was able to help many infertile women become pregnant by having them use PABA. Please use 500 milligrams twice daily. Next, vitamin B_6, 100 milligrams twice daily. That's been reported to help infertility, particularly in women with a history of PMS.

"There's a group of nutrients that appear essential to normal DNA duplication, which is essential to preventing birth defects. The best studied is folate—folic acid. Vitamin B_{12} and zinc are also in this group. Even though there's no work showing they definitely improve fertility, they're very important should you become pregnant. Please use 30 milligrams zinc daily—the picolinate form. For folate, take 5 milligrams daily—use the plant-concentrate form—that's one drop. Also, vitamin B_{12}, 2,000 micrograms daily.

"Lastly, please get a good high-potency multiple vitamin-mineral at your natural-food store. It's always wisest to 'back up' individual nutrient supplements with a multiple."

"What about thyroid?"

"If this all doesn't help in a few months, it might be wise to try a small amount."

We received a call from Mrs. Oberholter 6 months later advising us she was pregnant. She later delivered a healthy daughter.

DR. GABY'S COMMENTARY

Because of the risk and/or high cost associated with conventional treatments for infertility, new approaches to this common problem are needed. Fortunately, natural medicine offers a number of promising alternatives that appear to be quite safe and are relatively inexpensive.

Infertility: A Modern Epidemic

DESPITE THE WORLDWIDE population explosion, evidence indicates that infertility is a problem for a growing number of couples. A review of 61 published studies revealed that sperm counts dropped by more than 50% between 1938 and 1990.[1] A recent report from a European sperm bank suggests that an epidemic of infertility may be just around the corner. Of the sperm donors tested before 1980, 5.4% were found to have reduced fertility and 1.6% were totally infertile. However, of the men tested since 1990, 45.8% had reduced fertility and 9% were totally infertile.[2] In addition, during the past decade, there have been an increasing number of reports of reproductive abnormalities among both male and female animals living in the wild.

The cause of these changes is not known; however, the most likely suspect is environmental pollution. Certain pesticides (such as DDT and dieldren), some plastics that are used in beverage containers and to wrap food, and various environmental chemicals are known to act as "hormone mimics"—i.e., compounds which either amplify or inhibit the action of the body's natural reproductive hormones.[3] Although some scientists dispute the significance of this "low-level" pollution, it seems that we are playing a big game of Russian roulette with our future. We are not the first civilization whose survival is being threatened by pollution. Some historians have attributed the fall of ancient Rome to the use of lead cookware and lead water pipes by the Roman upper class. The chronic lead poisoning that resulted apparently rendered most of the upper class infertile, "leaving the inheritance of the world to the less capable."[4]

Although cleaning up the planet will be a massive undertaking, you can take steps now to reduce your own exposure to hormone-disrupting pollutants. For example, you can purchase organically grown food and avoid drinking beverages that have been stored in soft-plastic bottles.

Dietary Considerations

DIETARY FACTORS MAY affect the health of the reproductive system. A number of studies have shown that women who were ingesting large amounts of caffeine (5 to 7 cups of coffee per day) had more difficulty becoming pregnant, compared with women who did not consume caffeine.[5] Emphasizing whole foods in the diet is also important. Research shows that a wide range of vitamins and minerals is required for normal reproductive function. Since unrefined foods provide more of these micronutrients than refined and processed foods, a whole-foods diet is likely to increase the probability of achieving pregnancy.

Nutritional Supplements
L-arginine

The amino acid L-arginine plays an important role in sperm production. In a 1942 study, male volunteers fed an arginine-deficient diet had a 90% reduction in sperm counts within 9 days. When L-arginine was returned to the diet, sperm counts again became normal after several weeks.[6] Supplementing a normal diet with L-arginine may also be beneficial. In one study, 178 men with low sperm counts or abnormal sperm function were given 4 grams of L-arginine per day for at least 2 months. A marked increase in sperm count and motility was achieved in 62% of the patients, and 28 pregnancies resulted. Men with extremely low initial sperm counts (less than 20 million per ml) did not respond as well as did men with higher counts.[7] Foods high in L-arginine include nuts, seeds, cereal grains, and peas.

Vitamin C

IN some men, infertility results from a tendency of sperm cells to agglutinate (clump together). Although the cause of sperm agglutination is not known, men with this abnormality do have sub-normal blood levels of vitamin C. In one study, 15 men with infertility due to sperm agglutination were given 500 mg of vitamin C twice daily. After 2 to 3 weeks, sperm agglutination was reduced, and the percentage of normal sperm cells increased. Pregnancy occurred in the wives of all 12 men who took vitamin C for 60 days. In contrast, no pregnancies occurred in the wives of the 8 men who were not given vitamin C.[8]

Vitamin C can also be effective in treating female infertility. In one study, 42 women who had failed to ovulate after treatment with the fertility drug clomiphene were given 400 mg of vitamin C per day—either alone or in combination with clomiphene. Combination therapy induced ovulation in more than half of the women. In a few women, vitamin C alone induced ovulation.[9]

Vitamin B6

IN one study, 14 women who had been infertile for 1.5 to 7 years were given 100 to 800 mg of vitamin B6 per day as a treatment for premenstrual syndrome (PMS). Eleven of these women became pregnant during the first 6 months of vitamin B6 therapy.[10] Whether vitamin B6 can help infertile women who do not suffer from PMS has not been investigated.

L-carnitine

SPERM cells contain high concentrations of L-carnitine. This nutrient plays an important role in

the production of energy, which is needed for the production and motility of sperm. In one study, 47 men with poorly functioning sperm cells received 1 gram of L-carnitine, 3 times per day for 3 months. Improvement was seen in 37 men (79%)—with the average sperm count increasing from 88 million to 159 million per ml and the average number of motile sperms increasing from 26.8 million to 53.5 million per ml.[11]

Zinc

THIS essential trace mineral also plays a role in sperm production and function. In one study, 11 infertile men with low sperm counts and low concentrations of zinc in their semen were treated with 55 mg of zinc per day for 6 to 12 months. During zinc treatment, there were significant increases in both sperm count and motility, and 3 pregnancies occurred.[12] In another study, the effect of zinc on infertility varied depending on the initial testosterone level. In men with low testosterone concentrations, sperm counts increased after supplementing with zinc, and 9 of 22 wives became pregnant. However, among the 15 men with initially normal testosterone levels, sperm counts did not increase, and no pregnancies occurred.[13]

Iron

IRON may be helpful in treating female infertility. In one study, 111 women with iron deficiency were treated with iron plus vitamin C (to enhance the absorption of iron). Seven previously infertile women conceived within 28 weeks of starting this therapy.[14]

PABA

IN one study, 16 women with infertility of at least 5 years' duration were given 100 mg of para-aminobenzoic acid (PABA), 4 times a day for 3 to 7 months. Pregnancies ocurred in 12 of the women (75%).[15] This B-vitamin is believed to work by enhancing the effect of some of the body's natural hormones.

Other Nutrients

OTHER nutrients that play a role in reproduction include vitamin E, vitamin A, selenium, folic acid, vitamin B_{12}, copper, and coenzyme Q_{10}. Various human and animal studies show that supplementing with each of these nutrients improves fertility.

The Role of the Thyroid Hormone

INFERTILITY IS A recognized consequence of hypothyroidism in both sexes. However, as we have argued in chapter 4, blood tests for thyroid function are often unreliable, and hypothyroidism is underdiagnosed by conventional doctors. I have seen several infertile young women who had classic signs and symptoms of hypothyroidism, but normal thyroid blood tests. After treatment with thyroid hormone, the symptoms disappeared, and each woman became pregnant in a relatively short period of time.

In a 1954 study, 42 women with unexplained infertility received either thyroid hormone or a placebo for 12 months. Pregnancy occurred in 23.8% of the women receiving thyroid hormone, compared with 10.7% of those in the placebo group.[16] Although this difference was not statistically significant, the results are consistent with the idea that some infertile women have undiagnosed hypothyroidism.

Thyroid hormone may also be helpful in treating male infertility. Thyroid hormone, in the form of triiodothyronine (T3), has been shown to increase sperm count, motility, or both. Of 45 men with reduced fertility who were treated with T3, 18 (40%) improved markedly, and could be reclassified as relatively or highly fertile. Pregnancy occurred in the wives of 8 of these 18 men.[17]

Conclusion

INFERTILITY IS A complex problem in both sexes. Infertile couples should have a thorough evaluation to identify medical or surgical problems that can be effectively treated by conventional means. Nutritional therapy is often effective, but it should be undertaken only with medical supervision, in order to assure proper dosing and the safest environment possible for the developing fetus.

Summary of Recommendations for Treating Infertility

- Diet: Avoid refined sugar, other refined and processed foods, food additives, and caffeine; restrict alcohol intake. Emphasize organically grown whole foods.

- Thyroid hormone, in selected cases.

- High-potency multiple vitamin/mineral (containing no more than 10,000 IU of vitamin A).

- Nutrients that have been reported to enhance fertility include L-arginine, vitamin C, folic acid, vitamin B_6, zinc, L-carnitine, iron, PABA, selenium, vitamin E, coenzyme Q10, vitamin A, and copper. Supplemental vitamin A should be limited to a maximum of 10,000 IU per day, because of concerns that higher amounts might increase the risk of birth defects. The nutritional treatment of infertility should be supervised by a doctor.

IRRITABLE BOWEL SYNDROME

IRRITABLE BOWEL SYNDROME *(IBS) is one of the most common conditions for which people consult doctors. Although it is not a life-threatening problem, IBS can cause severe discomfort and is an important contributor to health-care costs in the United States.*

The most common symptoms of IBS are abdominal pain, bloating, gas, constipation, diarrhea, and passage of mucus in the stools. Patients who have these symptoms may undergo a series of radiological examinations and other diagnostic tests. However, in a large proportion of these individuals, no specific disease is found. Typically, medications aimed at treating constipation, diarrhea, or intestinal spasm are prescribed in the hope of producing more symptom relief than side effects; however, these medicines do not address the cause of the symptoms. Patients are also advised to reduce their stress level or to seek psychological counseling, since excessive stress is a definite contributing factor in some cases of IBS.

Unfortunately, the conventional medical approach is unsuccessful for millions of Americans who suffer from IBS. Indeed, the vague name that we use to identify this condition is a face-saving acknowledgment of our ignorance (patients with IBS already know *that their bowels are "irritable"). And when we call IBS a "functional" disturbance, we merely restate the obvious—that the bowels are not functioning as well as they should.*

DR. WRIGHT'S CASE STUDY

"I've been told I have irritable bowel syndrome," Arthur Epstein said. "I know *I'm* certainly irritable by now. Seven years is entirely enough!"

"What symptoms do you have?"

"The usual, I suppose. Cramping, pain on and off but usually not too bad, gas, frequent diarrhea, generally loose stools—unless I take this stuff nearly every day." He showed me a prescription bottle containing a common anti-diarrhea remedy. "And I just don't feel right if I have to take very much of it."

"Do you have symptoms every day?"

"One or another symptom or several nearly every day the last 2 years."

"You said it's been 7 years altogether?"

"Yes. I had my first 'attack' while I was studying for my CPA exam. The doctor I saw then agreed with me it was probably due to stress. After I passed the exams, the symptoms went away for several months. When they came back worse the second time, they sent me to a psychiatrist who said I was the best-adjusted CPA he'd evaluated in years: 'A little compulsive, what do you expect', he said, 'but very well adjusted for a CPA'. So they put me on the first of a long string of anti-diarrhea, anti-spasm medicines, and my mother started her campaign to get me in here."

"Your mother?"

"My mother. She said, 'Arthur, I could have told you for nothing you're well adjusted, after all you're my son. Stress everyone has, but irritable bowels everyone doesn't have, so there must be something else the matter. Go see Dr. Wright.'"

"Your mother is . . . "

"Sarah, Sarah Abrams. She remarried after my father died."

"Now I remember. She talks about you whenever she's here, but didn't tell me your name."

He rolled his eyes. "I can imagine."

"So, if she's been trying to get you to come here for 5 or 6 years . . . ?"

"I know, I know, what took me so long? I was working long hours for a big firm, then even longer to build my own practice. . . . But to tell you the truth, I'm not sure I believe in this 'natural medicine' stuff."

"Why are you here now?"

"Like I said, 7 years is enough."

"And?"

"My mother told you, didn't she? I'm engaged to be married, and now my fiancee's on my case, too. She won't have mother-in-law problems, already she and my mother agree on nearly everything, especially about me."

"I guess you don't have a chance."

He smiled. "I guess not. So, what do I do? Have those tests for food allergies my mother's been telling me about?"

"Allergy and sensitivity testing and treatment is important in irritable bowel syndrome, but there are a few other basics to cover first."

Mr. Epstein made a face. "I've probably heard them from my mother, too, but go ahead. If I'm paying to come here, I'm going to give it a compulsive try—you know, like a typical CPA."

"OK. Your mother probably told you to eliminate all the sugar on or in foods, and all the white-flour products, too, didn't she?"

"She's been telling me that for years. Now Judy, my fiancee, is enforcing it. Three months ago, I came home, all my favorite snacks were

gone and replaced with health-food snacks. The Fig Newtons turned into whole-wheat versions, even the Cheerios were replaced by a no-sugar type!"

"Good! Even if it didn't help irritable bowel, which it does, removing sugar and white flour is better for everyone's health, anyway."

"I never paid that much attention to grocery shopping, anyway, just picked up whatever looked good and got out of there. But Judy's got me reading all the labels, scolding me if I buy anything with chemicals, and Mother's cheering her on."

"They must want you healthy or something."

"I guess. Even my coffee's been replaced with 'certified organic decaffeinated.'"

"Another good idea. It's best to get rid of the caffeine to reduce bowel irritability. Has all of this helped?"

"Only a little, and on a few days it even seems I'm worse. That's why they've been pushing me to come in here. Both Judy and Mother were expecting big things from the changes Judy's made and, since they haven't happened, Mother says it's allergies; she's betting on wheat. She says whole wheat can cause more allergy trouble sometimes than white flour, even if white flour has less nutrition."

"She's right again."

"So tell me how a blood test can find out what I'm allergic to? All I ever heard about were those 'scratch tests' on the skin."

"The blood test your mother's thinking about—called 'RAST'—tests for antibodies technically called 'IgG$_4$' and 'IgE', which can form when we're allergic to foods."

"So, if I have these antibodies to say, wheat, it means my body's reacting to wheat?"

"Correct."

"And if I don't have these antibodies to wheat, then wheat's not a problem?"

"Unfortunately not. That's why I don't use RAST testing as much anymore."

"I'm confused. If it tells what I'm allergic to, why not use it?"

"It's a good test as far as it goes. If it's positive, it's quite reliable, but if it's negative, there can still be problems."

"Why's that?"

"Even mainstream textbooks describe more than one way of being allergic or hypersensitive. Years ago, pioneering researchers described four basic types or 'systems' of allergy. The RAST tests for only one of those. By now, it's been observed that there are many more ways of reacting to not only foods and inhalants, which are well-known allergens, but also chemicals, odors, electromagnetic fields—many other things in our environment."

"If the RAST test only checks 1 of 4 or more systems, why does anyone use it?"

"Because clinically, in practice, it gets a lot of results, particularly for the average case of allergy. Before the more sophisticated electronically-assisted systems called 'electrodermal testing' came along, we made a lot of progress with RAST testing."

"And what about that scratch testing on the skin I've heard about?"

"Routine scratch testing is unreliable for food allergy. There is a type of skin testing, called 'provocative neutralization' and 'dilution-titration' done by doctors called clinical ecologists or environmental medicine specialists that's quite accurate. Unfortunately, it takes a lot longer and can cost considerably more than electrodermal testing."

"And this electrodermal testing is accurate?"

"No test is 100% accurate, and remember, no test makes a diagnosis—the doctor does that. But electrodermal testing is sufficiently accurate to enable us to get a lot of results. Also, it allows for testing many more items in a much shorter length of time than any other currently available system. That keeps costs down. Lastly, it helps us to find appropriate desensitization for many of a person's sensitivities, so avoidance of allergens doesn't need to be permanent."

"Does electrodermal testing check all 4 of those systems of allergy you mentioned?"

"That's never been formally researched, but it's been my observation that it can find many types of sensitivity or reactivity. Electrodermal testing combines 'Western' biofeedback technology with 'Eastern' medical observations of energy flows through acupuncture meridians and points. And it's enormously facilitated by another Western development—computerization."

"And you've seen it help obtain good results?"

"Excellent results most of the time. But remember, like any test, it must be taken in the context of a person's overall health situation."

"If you recommend it, I'm sure Mother's for it, so let's get it done and see if it works for me." He got up to go.

"We will. But hold on a bit. In addition to the diet changes you've had some help in making, there's a supplemental item that can reduce symptoms in irritable bowel syndrome."

"What's that?"

"Peppermint oil."

"You're not kidding?"

"Not at all. Peppermint oil, in capsules. Researchers found a significant reduction in symptoms in those who used it. Please try 3 enterically-coated capsules, twice daily." I wrote this for him.

"Lastly, to stay as healthy as we can in today's world, it's always a good idea to use a broad general multiple-vitamin-and-mineral supplement with a little extra vitamins C and E." I wrote these all down, then handed him the note.

"My mother and Judy will be ecstatic. Me, the hard-headed CPA, taking my vitamins and eating healthy food."

"Compulsively, I hope."

"If it works, you bet."

I've only seen Arthur Epstein once in the years since, but his mother has been in several times. She tells me he's had no irritable bowel syndrome symptoms since he re-adjusted his diet and took some desensitization, and that Arthur and Judy's "2 little ones" are being raised by a very strict "no-junk-food-allowed" father!

DR. GABY'S COMMENTARY

As we saw in Arthur's story, the "natural" approach to treating IBS does not involve taking a lot of natural medicines. Rather, it involves careful attention to and discipline in the types of foods one eats. Research shows that food allergy and intolerance may be a primary cause of IBS.

Dietary Considerations
Effectiveness of the Nutritional Approach

A NUTRITIONAL approach offers hope for many people with IBS who have failed to improve with drugs and counseling. Several research studies, confirmed by our own clinical experience, indicate that as many as two-thirds of people with IBS will improve or become symptom-free if they identify and avoid the foods to which they are intolerant.

In one study, 21 patients with IBS went on a strict elimination diet for 1 week, limiting their diet to a single meat, a single fruit, and distilled or spring water.[1] In 14 of these 21 patients, symptoms disappeared on the elimination diet. Foods were then added back, one at a time, in order to determine which ones were causing the symptoms. The offending foods were identified as follows (number of cases in parentheses): wheat (9), corn (5), dairy products (4), coffee (4), tea (3), citrus fruits (2).

Six of the patients who reacted to foods underwent double-blind food challenges. The purpose of these challenges was to determine whether the suspected foods were really causing problems or whether they were just producing imagined reactions in suggestible people. In a double-blind food challenge, patients are fed a liquefied food through a nasogastric tube (a tube that passes through the nose into the stomach). Since the food bypasses the taste buds, the patient does not know what he/she is being fed. The investigators are also kept in the dark about what the patients are receiving until after the results are tabulated. In this study, the patients were able to identify with 87.5% accuracy whether they were receiving an offending food or a tolerated food. That degree of accuracy was highly statistically significant.

Other researchers have reported similar results. In a study of 189 patients with IBS who followed an elimination diet for 3 weeks, 48.2% improved. The number of food intolerances ranged from 1 to 19 per person, with half of the patients reacting to 2 to 5 foods. The foods that most commonly caused symptoms were (percent in parentheses): dairy products (40.7), onions (35.2), wheat (29.7), chocolate (27.5), coffee (24.2), eggs (23.3), nuts (18.0), citrus (17.8), tea (17.6), rye (17.6), potatoes (15.4), barley (13.3), oats (12.1), and corn (11.1). Of 73 patients who avoided their symptom-provoking foods, all but 1 remained well for more than a year.[2]

Flaws in Negative Studies

DESPITE these impressive results, many doctors remain unconvinced that food intolerance has anything to do with IBS. Part of this skepticism is no doubt a result of the long-standing prejudice that conventional medicine has against nutritional therapy. In addition, a number of studies have concluded that food intolerance is not a common cause of IBS.[3, 4]

However, these studies had important flaws. Design problems included: 1) basing elimination diets on questionnaires, skin tests, and blood tests, all of which are unreliable; 2) failing to eliminate wheat, one of the most common triggers of IBS; and 3) testing foods by administering small amounts in a capsule—amounts that would, in many cases, be too small to trigger symptoms.

As the controversy about food intolerance and

IBS goes on, we continue to treat this common condition with a high degree of success, while conventional doctors continue to struggle. It would be amusing, were it not sad, to describe some of our patients' long journeys that included thousands of dollars spent on doctors, tests, and ineffective treatments; years of suffering; and frustration at being told their problems were purely emotional. Many of these patients, after discovering that their bowel problems could be cured simply by avoiding wheat, corn, or dairy products, experienced alternating joy and anger (at their previous doctors)— a significant improvement, one would suspect, over alternating constipation and diarrhea.

Allergy or Intolerance?

IT might seem like a useless academic exercise to consider whether food-induced IBS represents an allergic reaction or a food intolerance. After all, isn't the treatment the same (avoiding the offending food), no matter what you call it? There are, in fact, certain differences between allergy and intolerance—differences that might affect both the diagnosis and treatment.

An allergic reaction is one that is mediated by the immune system, whereas an intolerance may result from a digestive disturbance or from a druglike reaction to naturally occurring compounds in foods. For example, wheat, dairy products, and coffee contain compounds that either mimic or oppose the effects of morphine. These compounds could presumably have a significant effect on bowel function in susceptible individuals. Milk also contains lactose, a sugar that can trigger major intestinal complaints in people who are unable to digest it. Whereas some of the more reliable allergy tests might help identify food allergies, these tests would not be helpful in cases where food intolerance is the problem. In addition, small amounts of a food may be all that are needed to provoke an allergic reaction, whereas larger quantities might be necessary to trigger symptoms of food intolerance.

Diagnosing Food Intolerance

BECAUSE it may not be clear whether IBS is being caused by allergy or intolerance, I prefer to identify offending foods by means of an elimination diet, rather than through laboratory testing. The majority of my patients who have gone through the elimination-and-retesting program (described in appendix A) have had good results.

I do not have any experience with the electrodermal testing and desensitization used by Dr. Wright. This procedure does not appear to conform to the laws of physics as we know them and, as far as I am aware, has not been adequately researched with respect to reliability and effectiveness. On the other hand, during my 20-year association with Dr. Wright, I have repeatedly been impressed with his capacity to identify (or even develop) effective therapies long before the rest of us "catch on." I remain open-minded, but skeptical, about diagnostic and therapeutic tools that are purportedly based on "subtle energies" (see chapter 3 for additional discussion).

Importance of Dietary Fiber

HEALTH-CARE practitioners now accept that normal bowel function depends in part on having enough fiber in the diet. Good sources of fiber include whole grains, fruits, vegetables, legumes, nuts, and seeds. In addition, adequate amounts of water, such as 6 glasses per day, are needed in order for fiber to exert its beneficial effect on bowel function.

Several studies have shown that supplementing the diet with fiber does not relieve the symptoms of IBS. However, these studies typically used wheat bran as the fiber source, so any beneficial effect may have been negated by a worsening of symptoms in wheat-sensitive individuals.

If you have IBS and your diet is low in fiber, you might do well to increase your intake of high-fiber foods to which you are not allergic or intolerant.

Herbal Supplements
Peppermint Oil

FOR PEOPLE IN whom diet alone is not enough, peppermint oil may be useful. In a double-blind study, 16 patients with IBS received peppermint oil or a placebo for 3 weeks, followed by the other treatment for another 3 weeks. Peppermint oil was significantly more effective than the placebo in relieving abdominal symptoms.[5]

Peppermint oil is available in health-food stores in enteric-coated capsules (i.e., coated in a way that prevents it from breaking down in the acid environment of the stomach). Enteric coating is important, because when peppermint oil is released directly into the stomach, it can cause heartburn or reflux into the esophagus. Enteric-coated peppermint oil should not be taken with meals, because when the stomach acid is buffered by food, the capsule may dissolve in the stomach. For the same reason, individuals with hypochlorhydria (low stomach acid) are more likely to have side effects from peppermint oil than are people with normal gastric acidity. (See chapter 2 for more on hypochlorhydria.)

Summary of Recommendations for Treating Irritable Bowel Syndrome

- Work with food allergies and intolerances.
- Consume adequate amounts of water and dietary fiber.
- Enteric-coated peppermint oil, in selected cases.

KIDNEY STONES

❧ AS MANY AS *1 of every 15 men and probably half as many women in the United States will suffer from 1 or more kidney stones at some time in their lives. For some individuals, a kidney stone may cause no symptoms at all. For others, the passing of a stone will be one of the most painful experiences they will ever endure. In addition, kidney stones sometimes block the flow of urine, causing recurrent urinary tract infections or kidney damage.*

Most kidney stones are made of calcium oxalate, although some contain primarily calcium phosphate, uric acid, or other materials. Because calcium-oxalate stones are the most common and because most of the research has focused on that type of stone, this discussion will focus on calcium-oxalate stones.

DR. WRIGHT'S CASE STUDY

Although he had not been to Tahoma Clinic before, Dmitri Osmonovich had a thick file. "I had my records sent from everywhere I've been with this problem. I want you to see how bad it is," he said. "I've been to the university hospital, all the other hospitals and emergency rooms, the best urologists—everything. I've had regular surgery and lithotripsy. They've had me on a low-calcium diet for years—no dairy at all. I've taken diuretics and other drugs, nothing works. I just keep having kidney stones. I might have missed one or two, but last time I counted I've had at least 47—that's more stones than I have years! Anna here keeps telling me maybe changing what I eat and taking some vitamins will help, but how can that be? All the doctors—even at the university—tell me that diet has nothing to do with getting kidney stones!" He spread his arms wide. "My wife, I love her, but could she be smarter

than all those doctors?" He folded his arms across his chest and looked at me.

"Dmitri's a part-time actor. Don't mind the theatrics," Mrs. Osmonovich said. "During his last ride to the hospital . . . in the ambulance, he's too big for me to carry . . . I got him to promise to come here."

"I was in so much pain, I'd promise anything!" he exclaimed.

She continued unperturbed. "I got him to promise to come here if there was even a tiny chance of stopping or even slowing down these kidney stones. There is a tiny chance, isn't there, doctor?"

"I looked through your record earlier," I said. "The few times your kidney stones were analyzed, they were mostly calcium oxalate—the most common type. Calcium-oxalate kidney stones are usually quite preventable."

Anna smiled at Dmitri. "I'm glad we came," she said.

"Preventable? This must be something brand

new, not tested—how could all those doctors not know, even at the university?"

"Likely because they still don't think vitamins and minerals are important," I answered. "Actually, in 1974, Drs. Gershoff and Prien published an article in a major urology journal about successful prevention of calcium-oxalate kidney stones in humans using a mineral and a vitamin. And they'd been carefully establishing the basis of that work in animals for years before."

"1974? I must have had 2 dozen kidney stones since then, and no one told me I could maybe prevent them!"

"Actually, Dmitri, I have told you on and off since we were married, and that's been 10 years now."

"Oy, maybe I should keep the kidney stones so I won't have to hear forever how I should have listened to my wife! But tell me, in case it works, what vitamin and mineral I should try?"

"Before I tell you that, let's go over basic diet first. Vitamin and mineral supplements are important, but they are supplements to a basic good diet. And water, too; our bodies are 60 to 70% water. . . . Do you drink much water?"

"No, mostly coffee and tea, sometimes beer. Actually, water just tastes wrong. Not bad, but wrong."

"Not a surprise if you're drinking most 'city water'. It's treated with chlorine, medicated with fluoride, and frequently has other chemicals besides. Many of us have never tasted truly pure water. It's really quite good. If you can, install a water filtration system at your house for the water you use in cooking and drinking. If that's not possible, use distilled water or water of known composition without chemical additives and 'medications' like fluoride. Please try to drink at least a quart of really pure water daily."

"A quart? I'll float away!"

"You drink more coffee and tea than that already, dear, and you're not floating yet," his wife said.

"Actually, all that caffeine isn't so good either. Caffeine promotes calcium excretion for 2 to 3 hours, and if you're drinking coffee frequently . . ."

"I'm peeing out extra calcium all day long!" He spread his arms dramatically wide again. "So, what good will a low-calcium diet do anyway, if this is true? It just gets messed up again with the caffeine!"

"Actually, there's very little evidence that low-calcium diets do any good, anyway, caffeine or not. When we cut down on dietary calcium, our bodies start to make more parathyroid hormone, which just takes calcium off the bones, and puts it in circulation in the bloodstream."

"From where I just pee it out again! Do these doctors know nothing of nutritional science, Anna? Why didn't you tell me?"

Anna smiled and said nothing.

"So, more pure water, stay away from caffeine. What about those vitamins and minerals?"

"We'll get there, but we still have to discuss a few more things about diet. Both sugar and salt can cause excess calcium loss, as can lack of fiber in the diet. I read through the diet record you sent in . . ."

"I should have known. Anna's been after me about the sugar for years, also. I admit, I have a sweet tooth. This part may be hard."

"Just remember your first surgery and eat a piece of fruit instead, Dmitri."

"High-sugar diets are often highly processed and low in fiber. Eating more fiber than you currently have in your diet will likely cut down on calcium excretion. Remember—whole grains, more root vegetables, beans—I'm sure Anna can tell you."

"I'm sure she can, too, and she will. Is that all the diet changes? It's certainly enough—no caffeine or sugar, less salt, more fiber, lots of pure water . . . my image I'll lose, I'll be a health-food-nut! Are you sure this will work?"

"Very little is 100% certain, but combined with the right vitamins and minerals it does the job for most people."

"So, now can you tell me which vitamins and minerals? I can't take the suspense any longer!"

"Dmitri . . ."

"Sure. The main ones are vitamin B6 and magnesium. Vitamin B6 cuts down on the production of oxalate. Magnesium makes oxalate more soluble, so it doesn't precipitate and form stones so easily."

"How much should I take?"

"Since you've had a long and dramatic stone history, please start with 100 milligrams of vitamin B6, and 200 milligrams of magnesium, both twice daily."

Dmitri looked skeptical. "Isn't that a lot? I've heard you can get poisoned on vitamins, too."

"Dmitri, I'm sure the doctor knows what he's doing," Anna said.

"Thank you. I think I do, too, but questions are always fine. If the magnesium is too much, it'll give you diarrhea, and you'll know to use less. There has been talk of possible vitamin B6 excess at much higher quantities, but that's fairly easy to tell also. In very large excess, B6 might cause numbness or tingling in the fingers or toes. If that even starts to happen, please stop taking it. As long as you keep the dose of B6 at 200 milligrams per day or less, toxicity is not at all likely."

"And just this magnesium and vitamin B6 can make me quit having kidney stones? It seems unbelievable! So simple!"

"Dmitri!" Anna exclaimed. "Already you've forgotten the pure water, no sugar, no caffeine . . ."

"I haven't forgotten, I'll just let you remember for me."

"It's you with the kidney stones, though," I said.

Dmitri sighed. "You're so right about that." He got up to go.

"In addition to vitamin B6 and magnesium, take a good multiple vitamin and mineral," I paused to write these items down. "There's some evidence that low levels of vitamin A are associated with kidney-stone formation. Please make sure you have 25,000 IU of vitamin A daily for the next year or so."

"Is beta-carotene OK?" Anna asked.

"Won't hurt, but actual vitamin A is better."

"I have one question, too," Anna said. "I've read that too much vitamin C might cause oxalate kidney stones. Is this true?"

"Theoretically, it's possible. In actuality, I've only observed the possibility twice in 10 years. If it were important for Dmitri to take more than a gram or 2 a day of vitamin C, we could do a urine test to check for oxalate both before and after starting the vitamin C, to see if it might be a problem. Even then, the extra vitamin B6 will cut down on oxalate production from vitamin C, should it happen."

"So should Dmitri take extra vitamin C?"

"If we're really trying to stay healthy, at an absolute minimum it's wisest to take vitamins C and E along with that good multiple vitamin and mineral. For Dmitri, I'd suggest 1 gram of vitamin C and 400 IU of vitamin E each day."

"But this has nothing to do with preventing kidney stones?" Dmitri asked.

"Dmitri, we're here for the best of health, too, not just to prevent stones," Anna said.

"OK, OK, Anna this time I listen to you, and this doctor. Lots of water, no sugar, no caffeine, less salt, more whole food with fiber, vitamin B6, magnesium, multiple vitamin and mineral, vitamin C, vitamin E. It better do the job! Even if it just cuts them in half, it's worth it. . . ."

In the first year after his visit, Dmitri had only one kidney stone, a small one, which "hardly hurt at all." Since 1983, he's reported no further kidney stones.

Good Nutrition and Supplementation Are Never "Out of Date"

I SAW Dmitri Osmonovich in 1983. That's a long time ago. Isn't this case and the nutritional treatment recommended obsolete nearly 20 years later? If we were writing about a patented drug used in 1983, it probably *would* have been declared obsolete by now, replaced with a "new, improved" drug (often shortly after the patent for the older drug has expired). But even though drugs change, human biochemistry has been the same (with individual variations on the same theme) for as long as humans have been around. This simple fact makes it likely that, if (from the chapter on benign prostatic hyperplasia, for example) men's prostate glands could be helped by essential fatty acids in 1941 and by zinc in 1974, these nutrients will still help in 1999 and any year in the future.

Dr. Wright's Book of Nutritional Therapy (published in 1979 and still available "online" and in used-book stores) describes the successful use of zinc and essential fatty acids for the prostate, as well as magnesium and vitamin B6 to prevent calcium-oxalate kidney stones. So why do we write the same things over again? Fortunately, many more people are now interested in preventing and treating disease with good diet, vitamins, minerals, and herbs, than were interested in the mid-1970s when we got started. Secondly, new information about diet, supplements, and herbs

is being published at an ever-greater rate. Our universities have decided to "take over from the health-food nuts," and they are discovering that much of what those "health-food nuts" had to say is true. Just as importantly, research is increasing on "folk remedies." We're finding that our ancestors were frequently very good observers. For example, using saw palmetto for the prostate was taught by native Americans to colonists along the eastern coasts of Georgia and South Carolina 2 to 3 centuries ago, and it was probably known to local native Americans for centuries before then. But it's just now being "confirmed," so (along with *Pygeum africanum, Urtica dioica,* and other items), we've added it to the essential fatty acids and zinc written about in 1979.

The same applies to calcium-oxalate kidney-stone prevention. As the biochemical problem leading to these stones is the same, the basic biochemical remedies will remain the same, no matter what the year.

DR. GABY'S COMMENTARY

THE BASIC STRATEGY for preventing kidney stones from forming is to keep calcium and oxalate dissolved in the urine, rather than allowing these molecules to crystallize. One way to keep calcium and oxalate in solution is to reduce their concentration in the urine. That can be accomplished in part by drinking more water, which will increase the volume of urine and thereby dilute the urine's constituents. The concentration of calcium and oxalate can also be influenced by what you eat and by taking certain nutritional supplements.

A second way to prevent calcium oxalate from crystallizing is to increase the urinary concentration of so-called "inhibitors" (compounds that increase the solubility of calcium oxalate), such as citrate and magnesium, as described in the following section.

Dietary Considerations
Dietary Factors

OXALATE occurs naturally in a number of foods, and is also a byproduct of normal metabolism. The amount of oxalate in the urine can be reduced by minimizing the intake of foods high in oxalate, such as spinach, collards, eggplant, beets, celery, summer squash, sweet potatoes, peanuts, blueberries, blackberries, Concord grapes, rhubarb, parsley, and cocoa. While black tea contains a large amount of oxalate, most herbal teas are low in oxalate and are therefore acceptable.

Diets high in refined sugar may promote kidney stones by increasing the amount of calcium in the urine. An individual's susceptibility to sugar is inherited to some extent. In one study, for example, patients with kidney stones and their relatives had a much greater increase in urinary calcium after ingesting 100 g of sugar than did healthy individuals.[1] This means that eating sweets is more likely to cause problems if kidney stones run in your family than if they do not.

Eating large amounts of animal protein (meat, chicken, fish, and eggs) tends to increase the amount of calcium and oxalate in the urine.[2] In addition, eating animal foods increases urinary excretion of uric acid,[3] a compound that promotes calcium-oxalate crystal formation. Consequently, individuals who have a tendency to form stones may be able to reduce their risk of recurrences by leaning more towards a vegetarian diet.

Excess salt intake may also promote kidney stones. In a study of 282 individuals with kidney stones, the amount of calcium in the urine increased with increasing sodium intake.[4] It is therefore a good idea for individuals who have a tendency to form stones to "go easy" on the salt.

Caffeine ingestion also increases urinary calcium excretion,[5] and it may be another risk factor for kidney stones.

Dietary Fiber Beneficial

INCREASING the amount of fiber in the diet may also be helpful for individuals who have a tendency to form stones. In one study, patients with kidney stones were given 24 grams of unprocessed wheat bran daily for 2 months. There was a significant reduction in urinary calcium excretion in 86% of the patients.[6]

Rice bran may be even more effective than wheat bran. In a study of 164 patients with kidney stones who excreted excessive amounts of calcium, treatment with 10 grams of rice bran twice a day significantly reduced the amount of calcium in the urine. More important, rice-bran treatment reduced the number of kidney stone recurrences by more than 78%.[7]

Dietary fiber is believed to decrease urinary calcium excretion by reducing the amount of calcium absorbed. It might seem that inhibiting calcium absorption is not such a good idea, particularly since many kidney-stone patients already have thinner-than-normal bones. However, there is no evidence that increasing dietary fiber intake makes the bones thinner. To be on the safe side, individuals who are at risk of developing osteoporosis should have their bone mineral density monitored by a doctor, regardless of whether they are taking a fiber supplement.

Cola Drinks Harmful

DRINKING certain soft drinks may also promote kidney stones through an effect that is unrelated to their sugar content. In 1 study, 1,009 men with a history of kidney stones who drank at least 1 quart of soft drinks per week were divided into 2 groups. One group was advised to discontinue all soft drinks, while the other was given no dietary advice (control group). After 3 years, the men in the no-soft-drink group developed significantly fewer new stones than the men in the control group. However, the improvement occurred only in men whose usual soft drinks contained phosphoric acid (primarily cola beverages). Among those who consumed soft drinks other than colas, discontinuing them did not reduce the risk of stones. The results of this study suggest that completely avoiding colas and other phosphoric acid-containing soft drinks can reduce the risk of kidney stone recurrences by as much as 36%.[8]

Citrate Inhibits Stone Formation

CITRATE (citric acid), a compound present in citrus fruits, has been shown to inhibit the formation of calcium-oxalate crystals in urine. In fact, potassium citrate, a prescription drug that is used to increase urinary citrate excretion, has been shown to reduce the recurrence rate of calcium-oxalate stones by as much as 80%.[9] However, potassium citrate is somewhat expensive and frequently causes gastrointestinal side effects. Another way to increase the concentration of citrate in the urine is to ingest foods that contain citric acid. Lemons are the richest source of citric acid, containing about 5 times as much as oranges. In one study, 12 patients with a history of kidney stones and low urinary citrate levels ingested 2 liters of lemonade per day. Urinary citrate excretion more than doubled and became normal in 7 of the 12 patients.[10] Ingesting 1.2 liters of orange juice per day also has been shown to increase urinary citrate excretion. Al-though oxalate levels also increased, overall there was an apparent reduction in the stone-forming potential of the urine.[11]

While it may not be feasible to consume that much lemonade or orange juice every day, it is possible that ingesting smaller amounts would still be beneficial. In addition, individuals with kidney stones who take supplemental calcium, magnesium, or zinc could consider using these minerals in the citrate form. Urinary citrate can be mea-sured by most laboratories, and this test may help identify those individuals who are most likely to benefit from an increase in dietary citrate.

Nutritional Supplements
Magnesium

LIKE citrate, magnesium inhibits the formation of calcium-oxalate crystals in urine. As early as the seventeenth century, magnesium was being recommended to prevent kidney stones, and modern research has confirmed the value of that old folk remedy. In one study, 55 patients with recurrent kidney stones were given 500 mg of magnesium per day, in the form of magnesium hydroxide, for up to 4 years. Urinary magnesium excretion increased promptly and remained elevated during the entire study. The average number of stone recurrences fell by 90%, and 85% of the patients remained stone-free (compared to only 41% of similar patients who did not receive magnesium).[12]

Vitamin B6

VITAMIN B6 also plays a role in kidney-stone prevention, primarily through its effect on oxalate metabolism. In addition to being absorbed from food, oxalate is manufactured in the body from the amino acid glycine and from other compounds. Many individuals who have a tendency to form stones produce excessive amounts of oxalate—an abnormality that can be corrected (at least partly) by supplementing with vitamin B6.

Lab tests show that some individuals with kidney stones have subtle deficiencies of vitamin B6.[13] When as little as 10 mg of this vitamin was given daily to patients with kidney stones, the amount of oxalate in their urine declined gradually but progressively, reaching a 45% decline after 120 days.[14]

The combined effect of vitamin B6 and magnesium was tested in a landmark study performed 25 years ago. Some 149 recurrent stone formers were given 300 mg of magnesium oxide (equivalent to 180 mg of magnesium) and 10 mg of vitamin B6 daily for 4.5 to 6 years. Before receiving this treatment, these patients suffered an average of 1.3 stones per person per year. During therapy with magnesium and vitamin B6, the stone-formation rate fell to 0.1 per person per year, an improvement of 92.3%.[15]

Moderate doses of vitamin B6 (10 to 50 mg per day) will effectively lower oxalate levels for most people. However, some individuals have a rare genetic disorder, known as primary hyperoxaluria, in which the metabolism of oxalate is defective. Individuals with this condition excrete massive amounts of oxalate and develop frequent and severe kidney stones, which can lead to kidney failure. Large doses of vitamin B6, such as 1,000 mg per day, have been shown to prevent further stone formation in these individuals.[16] Such large doses of vitamin B6 (more than 200 mg per day) can cause nerve damage and should be monitored by a doctor. Fortunately, most stone patients do not need to take large amounts of vitamin B6 in order to decrease the amount of oxalate in their urine.

Effect of Vitamin A

ANIMAL studies have shown that vitamin A deficiency increases the risk of kidney stones. In India, vitamin A deficiency is seen frequently, and it is a risk factor for kidney-stone formation.[17] Vitamin A deficiency is uncommon in the United States, but it may occur in strict vegans or in individuals with malabsorption.

Nutritional Questions About Kidney Stones

Should Calcium Be Restricted?

SOME doctors recommend restricting the amount of calcium in the diet, in order to reduce urinary calcium. However, recent research suggests that calcium restriction is not a good idea and may, in fact, make things worse. Calcium binds oxalate in the intestinal tract, thereby preventing the oxalate that is naturally present in food from being absorbed. It turns out that urinary oxalate influences stone formation to a greater extent than does urinary calcium. Consequently, a high-calcium diet may actually prevent stone formation by reducing the urinary concentration of oxalate, even though such a diet might increase calcium excretion.[18]

In one study, the risk of developing kidney stones fell as the amount of calcium in the diet increased.[19] However, while dietary calcium appears to be protective, the effect of calcium supplements on stone formation is more complex. The available evidence suggests that taking calcium with meals that contain oxalate would reduce stone formation by preventing the oxalate from being absorbed. However, taking calcium between meals (when there is no oxalate to bind) or with meals that contain little or no oxalate would increase the incidence of stones, because urinary calcium would increase while oxalate levels would not change.[20] Thus, calcium supplements are best taken with meals. And for individuals whose diets are low in oxalate, taking extra magnesium (300 to 500 mg per day) would probably prevent any potential adverse effect of supplemental calcium.

Is Vitamin C Dangerous?

THERE has been a good deal of controversy about whether vitamin C causes kidney stones. Since this vitamin can be converted to oxalate, taking large amounts could theoretically cause a stone to develop. One study showed that the average person can take up to 4,000 mg of vitamin C per day without producing a statistically significant increase in urinary oxalate.[21]

While larger doses of vitamin C (such as 8 grams per day) may increase the amount of oxalate in the urine, even in these large amounts, vitamin C does not seem to cause stones. In fact, nutrition-oriented doctors who routinely prescribe megadoses of vitamin C have been impressed by the relative rarity of kidney stones among their patients. Vitamin C is capable of binding calcium in the urine, which would leave fewer calcium ions available to combine with oxalate. Any tendency of vitamin C to increase oxalate levels is probably counterbalanced by this calcium-binding effect. In a study of more than 45,000 men, the incidence of kidney stones was 22% lower in those who ingested 1,500 mg or more of vitamin C per day than in those who consumed less than 250 mg per day.[22]

Although vitamin C does not seem to promote kidney stones in the average person, a rare individual (perhaps one in several hundred) will develop extremely high oxalate levels when taking vitamin C supplements. This unusual reaction to vitamin C, which is probably inherited, can be detected by measuring urinary oxalate before and after beginning vitamin C therapy. Individuals with a personal or family history of kidney stones who wish to take large doses of vitamin C should have such testing done. Fortunately, a vitamin C-induced rise in oxalate excretion can often be corrected by supplementing with vitamin B_6.[23]

Summary of Recommendations for Preventing Calcium-Oxalate Kidney Stones

PRIMARY RECOMMENDATIONS:

- DIET
  - ➤ Drink 1 to 2 quarts of water per day.
  - ➤ Emphasize foods high in fiber.
  - ➤ Avoid refined sugar, caffeine, alcohol, and colas.
  - ➤ Restrict foods that are high in oxalate.
  - ➤ Consume animal foods and salt in moderation.
  - ➤ Do not restrict dietary calcium.

- SUPPLEMENTS
  - ➤ Magnesium, 200 to 600 mg per day. Reduce dose if diarrhea occurs.

  - ➤ Vitamin B$_6$, 10 to 100 mg per day. Larger doses may be needed (with medical supervision), if urinary oxalate remains elevated.

OTHER RECOMMENDATIONS:

- If calcium supplements are being used, take them with meals, rather than on an empty stomach.

- Wheat bran or rice bran, in selected cases.

- Lemonade or orange juice for individuals with low urinary citrate.

- Vitamin A, 25,000 IU per day, if evidence of a deficiency. Reduce to every other day after 3 months.

- Measure urinary oxalate excretion if taking large amounts of vitamin C.

SYSTEMIC LUPUS ERYTHEMATOSUS *is a serious and sometimes fatal autoimmune disease in which the body's immune system attacks its own tissues. The disease affects an estimated 60,000 to 740,000 Americans. The word "lupus" is Latin for "wolf," and "erythematosus" means "redness." Together these terms refer to the reddened lesions resembling a wolf bite that appear on the face of lupus patients.*

Lupus can attack many different organs and tissues. Common manifestations include fever, weight loss, arthritis, hives, light sensitivity, nervous-system problems, and in some patients, heart damage. Although the disease can come and go unpredictably, some individuals suffer progressive and eventually fatal complications, often from kidney failure.

Conventional treatment includes prednisone (a drug similar to cortisone) and other powerful drugs that suppress the immune system. These medications may reduce the damage from lupus, but they do not cure the disease or even adequately control it for many patients. In addition, drugs used to treat lupus can have significant side effects.

DR. WRIGHT'S CASE STUDY

"I've got to stop this lupus before it stops me," Angela Boynton said. "I made this appointment the day I left the hospital. I've been in 3 times, and it's always the same—prednisone, anti-inflammatories, prednisone, more prednisone. And they're saying the only options left if prednisone stops working are cyclosporin and other really tough drugs that would suppress my immune system! I looked all that stuff up, and it's poison! It'll kill me if lupus doesn't! I'm determined that there isn't going to be any 'next time', so here I am!"

She crossed her arms, and looked determined.

After a moment, she smiled and relaxed. "I can beat this lupus, can't I?"

"Sounds like you've already taken the most important step—deciding that you're going to do whatever it takes to get yourself better. Is that what I heard?"

"You bet. I made the appointment here 3 months ago. I've already been reading your books and other stuff. I've completely restocked my kitchen. I have only whole foods, whole grains, no refined flour, no foods with artificial flavor, color, or preservatives, in fact, as much organically-raised stuff as I can find. Absolutely no sugar, no artificial sweeteners, no hydrogenated or partially hydrogenated oils, practically no canned stuff—just real food like it's supposed to be! And you know what, I've gotten to like it better. That organic stuff is tastier, and I've been able to taper down this prednisone faster than after the other 2 times I was hospitalized. 'Course I've been using a bunch of buffered vitamin C, too—do you think that helped?"

"What's a 'bunch'?"

"I read somewhere that at high amounts, vitamin C is anti-inflammatory, which I need. So I worked up to my 'bowel tolerance', which . . ." she took a deep breath ". . . for me right now is 24 grams total, 6 grams, 4 times a day! I hope that was OK."

"Is there any history of kidney stones in your family?"

"No."

"Good. Just to be on the safe side, we'll check a 24-hour urine test for excess oxalate, which is occasionally associated with taking large amounts of vitamin C. Too much oxalate could contribute to stone formation, and possibly damage your kidneys. As you know, kidneys are a potential weak point in lupus."

"Oh, dear, I hope I haven't caused any problems."

"Probably not. Since 1973, I've only seen oxalate kidney stones associated with high-quantity vitamin C twice. You're likely correct—large amounts of vitamin C can probably help in tapering prednisone more rapidly. The diet changes you made were just as important, though. Permanently eliminating non-foods is an absolutely necessary step for optimal health. Congratulations!"

"Thank you. But once I made the decision to get myself well, it wasn't so hard."

"The next steps might be harder. Before we even go on to vitamins and other things, there's more diet rearrangement for you to do—total elimination of wheat, oats, barley, and rye. These grains contain proteins called gluten and gliadin. Fortunately, there's no gluten or gliadin in corn and rice."

"So corn and rice are OK?"

"Don't know yet, but if you test sensitive to them, we'll desensitize you, so that elimination will be only temporary."

"I'm getting confused here. Sounds like you're saying that allergy may be part of the cause of lupus, but some allergy is permanent, and some is temporary, 'cause you can desensitize it. Why don't you just desensitize it all?"

"It's been pointed out that many autoimmune diseases such as lupus, ulcerative colitis, Grave's disease (hyperthyroidism), juvenile diabetes, vitiligo, and several others, frequently share tissue types (similar to blood types)—technically called HLA types—B8, DR3, and DR4. Those are also common to celiac disease—that's the disease caused by gluten and gliadin. When we eliminate gluten and gliadin in celiac disease, it's cured, so it just makes sense that eliminating grains containing these proteins might help other diseases, such as lupus, that share the same tissue types. The folks with lupus I've worked with have found gluten and gliadin elimination very important, along with permanent elimination of cow's milk and dairy products."

"Those, too? Lead me to your nutritionist. If I need to permanently eliminate all that gluten-gliadin stuff plus milk and dairy, then work around allergies—even temporary ones—I'm going to need help!" She wrote a few more notes on a pad. "What's next? No other tests besides allergies?"

"Can't escape tests. Folks with lupus—or any autoimmune disease—almost all seem to have a problem assimilating a whole variety of nutrients. Usually stomach function is very poor. I can't remember the last time someone with lupus had a normal stomach test. They usually have no stomach acid at all, or very little. They almost always need replacement hydrochloric acid and pepsin capsules. Frequently, pancreas function isn't so sharp either, and supplemental digestive enzymes are needed."

"Those things fix the assimilation problem?"

"Partially. But for lupus and other autoimmune problems, it's usually necessary to inject many of the nutrients, too, especially B-vitamins and minerals. Even with the replacement of hydrochloric acid and pepsin, and digestive enzymes, you still might have assimilation problems we can't identify."

She wrote rapidly for a moment. "This is getting complicated. We haven't even gotten to taking vitamins and minerals yet!"

"Hormones, too. But we'll leave those for last. First, the nutrients. Start with vitamin B$_6$, 500 milligrams, 3 times daily."

"Why so much?"

"Almost all the drugs that can cause lupus and lupus-like symptoms severely inhibit enzymes that depend on vitamin B$_6$. So I've asked folks with lupus to try it, and nearly everyone says they feel better with larger quantities like this. So far, no one who has lupus has developed signs of too much B$_6$, which would be numbness or loss of sensation in the extremities, particularly the fingers or toes. As an added bonus, vitamin B$_6$ inhibits overproduction of oxalate."

"Oh, I remember, that's the stuff that can cause kidney stones."

"Right. And any single B-vitamin should always be taken along with a 'background' of the entire B-complex."

She wrote rapidly. "B$_6$ and B-complex. What's next?"

"Essential fatty acids are very important. Please take at least 1 tablespoonful of flaxseed oil daily, along with an oil containing gamma-linolenic acid, also called GLA. Evening primrose, black currant, and borage oils are all good sources. Make sure there's a total of 240 milligrams of GLA daily.

"Anytime we take supplemental essential fatty acids, extra vitamin E is necessary. Please use 800 IU daily. And to help the metabolism of the essential fatty acids, take zinc (picolinate), 30 milligrams daily."

"You know, I tried some vitamin E along with my vitamin C. I thought it gave me a reaction, so I quit."

"People with lupus or any autoimmune disease can be sensitive to practically anything—foods, vitamins, minerals, anything! So even if we recommend it here, we'll make sure to screen you for allergy or sensitivity to it. Sometimes it's a particular form of a nutrient that causes problems, and sometimes it's all forms. So, we either find a form you're not sensitive to, or we desensitize you. If desensitization is needed first, it does slow things down a little, but you'll still get the job done—just a little more slowly."

"It's a good thing your receptionist told me to bring a note pad, or I couldn't keep track of all this stuff! Now you mentioned hormones? But I'm only 34 and still having my menstrual cycle. I don't need hormones, do I?"

"Not 'female' hormones like estrogens and progesterone. In fact, estrogens actually aggravate lupus and some other autoimmune diseases."

"They do? That doesn't seem fair, especially since there's not a whole lot I can do to avoid having female hormones!"

"And your husband and children wouldn't want you to avoid having them, either. But you can rebalance your hormones. In your reading, did you notice that the incidence of lupus in women is 8 or 9 times higher than in men?"

"That was one of the first things I read."

"Women normally have small quantities of testosterone and larger quantities of another androgen called DHEA. Both women and men with lupus almost always have lower-than-usual levels of these 2 hormones for their respective sexes. So we have them take enough to bring them up to 'high normal' for their sex, and it often is a big help in lessening lupus symptoms."

"I won't start getting big muscles or a beard?"

"No. DHEA won't do that anyway. Besides, we do careful testing before and after to make sure that levels of these hormones go to 'high normal', *not* higher than normal."

She wrote a few more lines, then paused to review. "No gluten-gliadin-containing grains and no milk and dairy ever. Temporarily avoid, then desensitize other food sensitivities, very likely hydrochloric acid and pepsin capsules, digestive-enzyme capsules, vitamin and mineral injections, vitamin B$_6$ and B-complex, essential fatty acids, vitamin E, zinc, and DHEA and testosterone if my levels are not high enough. And I assume I continue my vitamin C and general multiple vitamin and mineral?"

"And real food only—no chemicals or other non-food."

"Well, I've decided to get better, so here we go. What are my chances?"

"Very good, actually. I'm working with several individuals who've had their lupus completely under control—no symptoms, for several years. Of course, they've all been very strict."

"Strict beats having lupus." She got up to go. "By the way, is there anywhere I can do any reading about all of this?"

"Some of the concepts and details are covered in a book by Dr. Christopher Reading, *Your Family Tree Connection* (Keats Publishing, New Caanan, Connecticut, 1988). It's out of print right now, but you might be able to find it used at a store or on the Internet. Good reading!"

It's been nearly 7 years since Mrs. Boynton's first visit. Although it took her over a year and a half to get all these factors under control and working for her, she's been symptom-free for the last 5 years.

DR. GABY'S COMMENTARY

WHILE CONVENTIONAL MEDICINE has struggled to find a safe and effective treatment for lupus, several "alternative" approaches have shown great promise and, sometimes produced dramatic successes. These include both dietary modifications and nutritional supplements.

Dietary Considerations
Role of Food Allergy

FOOD allergy is one of the first places to look when evaluating someone with an autoimmune disease. We know that individuals with autoimmune diseases such as lupus manufacture proteins called antibodies, which attack the body's tissues and organs. Ingestion of an allergenic food is one reason—though certainly not the only reason—that people produce antibodies. If a person has a certain genetic makeup, these antibodies can cross-react with "target organs" in the body. For example, if a milk-allergic person drinks a glass of milk, he will produce antibodies to milk which might attack the joints, kidneys, or other tissues.

Although there has not been much research on the role of food allergies in lupus, 2 studies point to a connection. In 1 report, a child with symptoms and laboratory tests suggestive of lupus was found to have antibodies to milk in his bloodstream. The child's symptoms resolved after milk was eliminated from the diet, but they returned on 2 occasions when he drank milk.[1] In a study from Australia, 4 patients with lupus had a marked improvement in symptoms after following a program that included nutritional supplements and avoiding allergenic foods. In addition, their antinuclear antibody (ANA) tests (used to diagnose and monitor lupus) became normal.[2] Our own clinical experience supports the view that food allergy is a factor in some patients with lupus.

The Yeast Connection

DR. William Crook has suggested that chronic intestinal yeast infections are a contributing factor to a wide range of illnesses, ranging from fatigue, depression, and bloating to more serious diseases such as multiple sclerosis and lupus.[3] The common yeast germ known as *Candida albicans* is thought to produce toxins which are absorbed from the gastrointestinal tract into the body. These toxins could theoretically provoke either autoimmune reactions or other adverse effects. Treatment for the "yeast syndrome" includes a diet low in refined sugars, avoidance of allergenic foods, and use of drugs or herbs that kill candida.

Although the relationship between candida and chronic illness remains controversial, I have seen several patients with lupus whose symptoms resolved and whose laboratory tests became normal after they went on an "anti-candida" program. In one such patient, symptoms returned and the ANA test again became abnormal shortly after she stopped her anti-yeast medication (nystatin). However, when she resumed the medication her symptoms again cleared up and the ANA became negative.

Hormone Therapy

IN RECENT YEARS, doctors have been investigating the possibility that hormone therapy with dehydroepiandrosterone (DHEA) and/or testosterone may be helpful for lupus patients. There are several reasons to believe that these hormones might have therapeutic value. Both DHEA and testosterone play a role in promoting healthy immune function. They may therefore help bring "back into line" the "out of control" immune system that is seen in patients with lupus. In addition, low blood levels of DHEA and/or testosterone are commonly seen in women (and possibly in men) with lupus.[4] Moreover, in a genetic strain of mouse that spontaneously develops a disease resembling lupus, supplementing with DHEA reduced the severity of the disease.[5]

In a study from Stanford University Medical Center, 10 women with mild or moderately severe lupus received 200 mg of DHEA per day for 3 to 6 months. Eight of the 10 women reported improvements in overall well-being, fatigue, energy, or other subjective symptoms. In addition, the physicians' overall assessment of disease activity showed significant improvement. Of 3 women who had excessive protein in their urine (a sign of kidney damage), 2 had a marked reduction in protein excretion and 1 showed modest improvement.[6]

In a follow-up double-blind study from Stanford, 28 women with lupus received either DHEA (100 mg per day) or a placebo for 3 months. On average, the condition worsened in the placebo group, but it improved in the women receiving DHEA. The difference between the two groups was statistically significant. In addition, disease flare-ups occurred in only 3 women receiving DHEA, compared with 8 women in the placebo group.[7] Side effects in these 2 studies were limited mainly to acne (occurring in about one-third of the women) and a slight increase in hair growth (occurring in a few of the women).

The doses of DHEA used in these studies are considerably greater than the amounts normally produced by the body. We have found that lower doses of DHEA are helpful for some patients, when used as part of a comprehensive nutritional program.

It should be pointed out that yam-based products that are purported to contain "DHEA-precursors" do not contain DHEA, are not converted by the body into DHEA, and are not recommended as a substitute for DHEA. Although DHEA is available without a prescription, the purity and potency of some of these over-the-counter products is questionable. We therefore advise our patients to obtain their DHEA from a compounding pharmacist or from a reputable distributor. In addition, because DHEA is a powerful steroid hormone with the potential for adverse effects with long-term use (see chapter 4), DHEA therapy should be monitored by a doctor.

Testosterone is usually thought of as a "male" hormone, but it is produced by both women and men. Women with active lupus were found to have abnormally low levels of testosterone, apparently because their bodies break down this hormone with unusual rapidity.[8] Several case reports published in medical journals demonstrated an improvement in lupus after treatment with testosterone[9] or related synthetic hormones.

Nutritional Supplements

ESSENTIAL FATTY ACIDS have anti-inflammatory effects, and they might therefore help reduce some of the inflammation that characterizes autoimmune disease. In a genetic strain of mouse that spontaneously develops a lupus-like disease, supplementing the diet with omega-3 fatty acids derived from fish oil or flaxseed oil reduced the severity of the disease. Although it has not been studied specifically as a treatment for lupus, gamma-linolenic acid, an omega-6 fatty acid found in evening primrose oil, borage oil, or black-currant-seed oil, has also been used with some success against autoimmune disorders.

Whenever essential fatty acids are used, additional vitamin E is required to prevent the conversion of the fatty acids into toxic free radicals. Vitamin E may also exert its own beneficial effect on autoimmune disease, possibly through a mild anti-inflammatory effect.[10]

Other nutrients that are of theoretical value against autoimmune disease include zinc, copper, selenium, and vitamin C. However, there are no studies on the effect of these nutrients in individuals with lupus.

Dr. Wright has observed that administering large doses of vitamin B6 will often improve overall well-being in patients with lupus. Although the reason for this is not clear, vitamin B6 is known to block the toxic effects of certain drugs and chemicals that cause lupus.[11] Doses of vitamin B6 greater than 200 mg per day can cause nerve damage and should be medically supervised.

Conclusion

ALTHOUGH LUPUS CAN be a serious disease, a number of natural treatments have been found to help. Not everyone responds to the natural approach, but many patients have improved, and in some cases the disease has cleared up completely.

Summary of Recommendations for Treating Lupus

PRIMARY RECOMMENDATIONS:

- Work with food allergies.
- DHEA and/or testosterone, in selected cases.
- Essential fatty acids (omega-3 and gamma-linolenic acid [GLA]). Sources of omega-3 fatty acids include flaxseed oil and fish oil. Sources of GLA include evening primrose oil, borage oil, and black-currant-seed oil.

OTHER RECOMMENDATIONS:

- Vitamin E, 400 to 800 IU per day.
- High-potency multiple vitamin/mineral.
- Treat "candida", in selected cases.
- Assess digestion and absorption, and use appropriate digestive aids when indicated.

Macular Degeneration

❧ AGE-RELATED MACULAR *degeneration (AMD) is the leading cause of blindness in the United States and other developed countries. At least 10% of Americans over the age of 65 have suffered some visual loss as a result of AMD; among those over age 75, as many as 30% are affected.*

AMD begins with a deterioration of a portion of the retina called the retinal pigment epithelium, followed by degeneration of the rods and cones (the light and color sensors of the retina, respectively), and it culminates in the death of visual cells. The macula is the central portion of the retina, which provides the greatest degree of visual acuity; as a result, degeneration of the macula can cause significant problems with vision.

Approximately 90% of individuals with AMD have what is known as atrophic (or "dry") macular degeneration, in which the macular tissue slowly deteriorates. Less common is the "wet" form of AMD, characterized by swelling, hemorrhage, and proliferation of new blood vessels. This latter form is more likely to result in significant visual loss. Because individuals with "wet" macular degeneration may benefit from laser therapy, AMD should always be diagnosed and monitored by an ophthalmologist. Conventional recommendations for preventing or slowing the progression of AMD include smoking cessation, controlling elevated blood pressure and cholesterol levels, and wearing sunglasses in bright sunlight.

DR. WRIGHT'S CASE STUDY

Elaine and Tom MacDonald walked to my office, Tom guiding Elaine as unobtrusively as he could. He showed her a chair, and they both sat down.

"As you may have guessed, I'm not seeing as well as I'd like to," Elaine began. "My eye doctor tells me it's macular degeneration in both eyes, though the left is worse than the right. I've been taking those vitamins that eye doctors are starting to use these days, but they don't seem to be helping at all, and my vision is slowly getting worse."

"We've heard you have a treatment that can help macular degeneration sometimes," Tom said. "We're hoping it's not to late to help Elaine."

"As it is now, I can read an interstate highway sign if I'm standing right in front of it," Elaine said. "And that's with my glasses on. I was a teacher before I retired, and I so miss being able to read my books and newspapers."

"Of course, she can't drive anywhere either," Tom added.

"How's your health otherwise?" I asked.

"As far as I can tell, it's OK. I don't have the energy I'd like, but then I'm 67, so I guess that's to be expected."

"No other bothersome symptoms?"

"None that I can think of."

I asked about her health history, family health history, diet, and exercise. Then we went to an examination room for a physical exam. All appeared OK until we got to her fingers. Her nails bent very easily.

"Excuse me, but your fingernails aren't very strong, are they?"

"They've been that way all my life. Never have been able to grow nice nails like some women do. Mine, they cracked, peeled, and chipped. I took gallons of gelatin when I was younger, but it never helped. The last few years I've been taking a lot of calcium—it helps a little. They're stronger for awhile, but then they get bad again. Can't really put it together with anything."

"Do you get cramps in your legs?"

"Yes."

"How often?"

"Oh, 2 or 3 times a week, especially at night, but occasionally when I've been doing a lot of walking. But there's nothing unusual about that, is there? Tom gets them, too, and so do some of our friends. We thought it just went with our time of life, like this gray hair." She touched her head.

"You're right—those of us past 50 do get more leg cramps than younger people, but those cramps aren't an inevitable part of aging. They're a correctable malfunction." I made a few notes. We finished her exam, and went back to my office.

"What shall I do first about my eyes?" Elaine asked. "I'm anxious to get started right away."

"First, have your stomach tested . . ."

"My stomach? How will that help my eyes?"

"As we get older, an increasing number of symptoms and health problems need to be approached by checking the stomach and the rest of the digestion first. By the time we're 60, at least half of us who have symptoms or health problems have problems with digestion and nutrient assimilation. The leg cramps that you

and many over-50 people have are usually a symptom of inadequate digestion and assimilation of calcium, magnesium, potassium, and other minerals.

"In your particular case, it's likely you've had digestion/assimilation problems for years. If we don't 'patch up' these problems as best we can, we won't have as much of a chance to help your eyes, since all the nutrients our eyes need enter our bodies through the digestive tract."

"Maybe that's why these vitamins the eye doctor gave me aren't working?"

"Likely that's part of it. But they don't have all the necessary nutrients, and the few they do contain are in very small quantities."

"Why do you think I've had digestion problems for years? I don't have any digestive symptoms, as far as I can tell."

"Your fingernails are one good sign. A large majority of women who have cracking, peeling, and chipping fingernails also have poor stomach and digestive function."

"Really? You're saying I could have had glamorous fingernails all these years had I only known?"

"Don't know about glamorous, but at least a lot stronger. But getting back to tests—along with the stomach test, we need to check further on your digestion through a stool analysis. We'll be looking at mineral levels, amino acids, and hormones—particularly testosterone."

"So far, I think I understand checking my digestion and the minerals—even these nails you say are weak have minerals. But I don't understand the need to check amino acids and testosterone."

"Amino acids are the building blocks of protein. If we hope to rebuild cells and tissues, we need to make sure your amino acids are adequate. Yours have a higher probability of being low."

"Because of poor digestion and assimilation."

"Exactly."

"But what about testosterone?" Tom asked. "What does that have to do with eyes?"

"It's certainly not the most important factor, but vision is so important that we want to 'cover all the bases' right away. Testosterone is the most powerful anabolic steroid that our bodies make naturally. Anabolic steroids do much more than stimulate the growth of muscles. They stimulate repair and regrowth of many damaged body tissues. I've observed that correcting abnormally low levels of testosterone can help tissue repair in either sex."

"How long will it take to get the tests done, so I can get started?"

"The tests are important, but I recommend you start treatment today or tomorrow—as soon as your tests are turned in. Over the years, I've found that if we give key nutrients intravenously—particularly zinc and selenium—twice weekly, we make much faster progress. We make sure the quantities are safe of course, but also sufficient to do the job."

"Just zinc and selenium?"

"Those are the most important minerals, but we make sure to 'back them up' with a variety of minerals and other nutrients. And of course, I'll ask you to start with oral supplementation, too."

"But what about digesting and assimilating them properly?"

"Your stomach test will be completed and we'll know the results today. The remaining tests on your digestion will be completed in just 2 or 3 days."

"What about the rest of the tests? Shouldn't we wait for them?" Tom asked.

"We'll adjust or add to what we're doing as soon as they become available, but since we know many of the major items of importance, we can start them right away."

"How often does this work?" Elaine asked.

"Not every time, but definitely more than half the time."

"How long before I know one way or another?"

"In my experience, if we use the IVs, digestive aids, all the oral supplements, and hormones if necessary, you can see—literally—results starting in 4 to 6 weeks. If there's been no improvement in 6 to 8 weeks, then it's not likely this will help."

"I hope it works for me. In addition to the IVs, what supplements should I take?"

"Very likely the list will start with betaine hydrochloride with pepsin with meals, to replace what your stomach likely isn't doing, and pancreatic enzymes after meals. Together, these should restore a large part of weak digestive function."

"We've already covered zinc and selenium—the two most important minerals. Vitamin E and taurine are very important, too. Bilberry and ginkgo, herbal medications, contain flavonoids and other substances important to the retina. Vitamin A and copper . . ."

"Hold on," Elaine said. "I can't remember all of this."

"You don't need to. There are several 'combination formulas' available in natural-food stores that contain most or all of these ingredients."

"IVs, digestive aids, and a combination formula with the nutrients you've recommended. Anything else?" Tom asked.

"The tests will tell us if amino acids, testosterone, and possibly other hormones are advisable."

"When I start seeing results, how long will I need to continue having IVs?" Elaine asked. "I certainly can't get those done for years and years."

"You won't need to. Remember, much of the problem is due to poor digestion and assimilation. You'll be taking care of that so that oral supplementation has a better chance to do the job. But just for 'insurance', when the IVs are discontinued, we'll ask you to use some of the key nutrients dissolved in DMSO (dimethylsulfoxide, a natural extract of wood-pulp). When applied topically, this solution carries the nutrients in through the skin. But don't worry about that now, we'll cover it when the time comes.

"Also, please remember that this treatment doesn't work every time. I've observed it helping a majority of cases; unfortunately that's not 100%."

"At least all these nutrients won't hurt me," Elaine said.

"And we'll pray that Elaine's in that majority," Tom added.

"Please do! That'll help, too."

In 4 weeks, Elaine's vision started to improve.

After 8 months of treatment, she reported that instead of just being able to read interstate highway signs, she could read books and newspapers again. She's continued her treatment, and 11 years later has maintained her vision at that level.

DR. GABY'S COMMENTARY

ALTHOUGH SOME CONSIDER AMD to be a natural consequence of the aging process, evidence shows that certain nutrients can delay or inhibit age-related retinal damage. In other words, it may not be necessary to fall apart, just because you are getting older. If individuals who are at risk could delay this visual deterioration by 10 or 15 years, then their eyes would last as long as the rest of their body.

We still have a lot to learn about AMD. However, research that has already been published suggests that we can delay the vision loss or even improve eyesight by supplementing with certain nutrients. Antioxidants such as vitamins C and E, selenium, and carotenoids are of particular importance, since they can inhibit the damaging effects of oxygen and ultraviolet light on the retina. In addition, nutrients such as zinc, taurine, and certain plant-derived flavonoids play an important role in the normal metabolism of retinal tissue. Since nutrients work in the body as a team, it is likely that a combination of nutrients would perform better than any single nutrient by itself. Elderly individuals often have weak digestive systems, and many older people consume diets of questionable nutritional value. As a result, multiple nutritional deficiencies are common in this age group. A comprehensive nutritional program might, therefore, be of great value for individuals with AMD. While we have not seen any studies documenting the effect of such a program, our patients with AMD frequently tell us they

can see better within a month or 2 of starting treatment.

Nutritional Supplements
Zinc

ZINC is present in high concentrations in healthy eyes, and it plays a key role in maintaining normal vision. When rats were fed a zinc-deficient diet, they developed impaired retinal function and loss of visual acuity.[1] Since the concentration of zinc in human retinal tissue declines with age,[2] it is possible that zinc deficiency contributes to the development of AMD. In a double-blind study, 155 patients with AMD received 45 mg of zinc per day or a placebo for 1 to 2 years. Compared with the placebo, zinc significantly slowed the rate of visual loss.[3] Supplementing with zinc seems to be especially important for the elderly, whose daily intake of this mineral is usually well below the Recommended Dietary Allowance.[4] Because taking large amounts of zinc can cause a deficiency of copper, we typically advise patients to balance their zinc supplement with additional copper.

Taurine

HIGH levels of the amino acid taurine are also found in the retina. Taurine is believed to act as a "cellular buffer," protecting retinal cells from the harmful effects of ultraviolet light and toxic substances. When animals were fed a diet low in taurine, their retinal tissue degenerated and their visual acuity declined.

In the past, taurine has been considered a "non-essential" amino acid, because the human body is capable of synthesizing it from methionine (another amino acid). However, the capacity of humans to manufacture taurine is limited,[5] and deficiencies of this amino acid are known to occur in certain circumstances. For example, children receiving long-term intravenous nutrition were found to have subnormal levels of taurine, and this deficiency was associated with abnormal retinal function. After the children were supplemented with taurine, their vision returned to normal.[6] Taurine deficiency is also common in diabetes, a condition associated with severe retinal damage.[7] Elderly individuals often fail to consume enough protein (the body's source of amino acids) and many do not digest their protein adequately. As a result, some older people may be deficient in either taurine or the amino acid from which it is produced.

Antioxidants (vitamins C and E, selenium)

One of the causes of progressive retinal deterioration is a lifetime of bombardment by tissue-damaging oxygen free radicals and ultraviolet light. Because the eye is highly susceptible to this type of injury, antioxidant nutrients are especially important for maintaining eye health. For example, vitamin C is naturally present in high concentrations in the eye, and it has been shown to prevent retinal damage in animals that are exposed to excessive amounts of light.[8]

Vitamin E is another key antioxidant for the retina. Monkeys that were fed a vitamin E-deficient diet developed macular degeneration, apparently as a result of increased oxidation damage to the retina.[9] In a study of 39 patients with AMD, supplementing with vitamin E improved vision in 28 patients (72%).[10]

Selenium is also present in high concentrations

in the eye, where it plays a role in one of the body's main antioxidant defense systems. Dr. Wright has seen several patients with AMD whose visual acuity improved after taking supplements of selenium and vitamin E.[11]

Carotenoids

POPULATION studies have shown that the risk of developing AMD is significantly reduced in individuals whose diet contains large amounts of fruits and vegetables rich in beta-carotene.[12] Other carotenoids (compounds similar to beta-carotene) such as lutein and zeaxanthin may be even more important than beta-carotene. A survey of 876 elderly individuals revealed that those whose intake of lutein plus zeaxanthin was high (top 20 percentile) were 56% less likely to have AMD, compared with those whose intake of these carotenoids was low (bottom 20 percentile).[13] Lutein has been shown to accumulate in the macula, where it protects against the damaging effects of certain light wavelengths.[14] The main dietary sources of lutein and zeaxanthin are dark green vegetables, particularly spinach and collard greens.

Herbal Supplements
Ginkgo biloba

EXTRACTS from the leaves of the *Ginkgo biloba* tree have been shown to prevent or reverse some of the manifestations of aging, including memory loss, depression, impotence, and atherosclerosis. AMD is another age-related disorder that appears to respond to ginkgo. In a double-blind study of 10 patients with AMD, ginkgo was significantly more effective than a placebo, as demonstrated by improvement in long-distance visual acuity.[15]

Flavonoids

A GROUP of chemically-related substances known as flavonoids are found in a wide variety of plants. The most beneficial flavonoids for the eyes are the anthocyanosides, which are found in high concentrations in blueberries (especially the European blueberry, also called bilberry), grapes, and other fruits and vegetables. In addition to being powerful antioxidants, these compounds are thought to act as biochemical amplifiers in retinal photoconduction (in other words, they help us see better).[16] In one study, administration of anthocyanosides to healthy individuals improved dark adaptation (night vision), macular sensitivity, and other aspects of visual function.[17]

How Our Patients Have Responded

WE HAVE GIVEN intravenous injections of selenium and zinc, sometimes combined with other trace minerals, to more than 80 patients with AMD (the more-common type known as "dry" macular degeneration). Most of these patients also took oral supplements containing the nutrients listed above. More than half of the patients had a sustained improvement in visual acuity. Among those who took only oral nutrients, the results were usually slower and not as dramatic. Nevertheless, many of these patients improved or at least showed no further progression. Individuals whose AMD was treated within the first year or 2 after the diagnosis was made responded better than those with more-chronic disease.

Conclusion

AMD IS THE most common cause of visual decline. Published research and our own clinical experience strongly suggest that the loss of vision associated with this condition can be delayed or arrested and, in some patients, can actually be reversed.

Summary of Recommendations for Treating Macular Degeneration

- Diet: Consume a wide variety of fruits and vegetables, particularly spinach, collards, blueberries and grapes.

- Intravenous injections of zinc, selenium, and other trace minerals, in selected cases.

- Vitamin E, 400 to 800 IU per day.

- Vitamin C, 1,000 to 3,000 mg per day.

- Zinc, 30 to 50 mg per day. Balance with copper, 2 to 3 mg per day.

- Selenium, 200 mcg per day.

- Taurine, 500 to 1,500 mg per day.

- *Ginkgo biloba* extract (standardized to contain 24% ginkgo heterosides), 40 to 120 mg per day.

- Bilberry (standardized to contain 25% anthocyanosides), 40 to 120 mg per day.

- Lutein, 5 to 20 mg per day.

- Assess digestion and absorption; use appropriate digestive aids when indicated.

MEMORY LOSS AND DEPRESSION
(age related)

AGE-RELATED DECLINE *in brain function is a common and sometimes serious problem. Often referred to as dementia, senile dementia, or cognitive decline, mental deterioration can manifest in many ways, including loss of intellectual capacity, memory impairment, poor judgment, and personality change. Psychological depression is frequently associated with dementia. In some patients, it is difficult to determine whether the dementia is a sign of depression or a separate entity. Doctors sometimes prescribe antidepressant medication for patients with dementia, in the hope that other aspects of their mental function will improve.*

Some physicians are reluctant to conduct a thorough investigation of patients with dementia, possibly because they feel that senility is an inevitable and untreatable consequence of the aging process. However, even in conventional medicine, a careful search will occasionally reveal a treatable problem. Elderly individuals are often taking a wide array of prescription and over-the-counter medications, some of which can adversely affect mental function. If the dosages of these drugs can be reduced or if other treatments can be given instead, dementia may improve. Hypothyroidism (underactive thyroid gland) and vitamin and mineral deficiencies are also treatable causes of dementia. Unfortunately, the vast majority of people suffering from dementia are not helped significantly by the conventional medical approach.

DR. WRIGHT'S CASE STUDY

"I'm 76 this year, and my wife Theresa here thinks I'm losing it," Vincent Parnelli said. "I was just passing it off, but now I think she's right. Last week, I drove off and left the boat at the launch for the second time in a month—with the dog in it, too. Had the fish in the car; don't know how I thought I caught 'em. Had to drive all the way back to get the boat and the dog."

His wife reached over to pat his arm. "You're not 'losing it', dear, you've just been a little more absent-minded these last couple of years."

"Theresa's always putting a good face on things," he said, smiling at her. "But if I can't even remember the boat and the dog, 'losing it' is more accurate. After I did that, I decided to have a good look at how I'm doing. Theresa's been trying to get me to come in here for the last 5 years, and here I am."

I made a note. "Besides your memory, have you noticed anything else about your health that doesn't seem right?"

"I asked Theresa to come along so she could tell you what she's seeing. Like I said, I've been passing things off—probably too much." He turned to his wife.

"Well," she hesitated. "Vinnie has been more forgetful for several years now. I mean, we all are now and again, but it's been more than that. I've been finding a lot more socks in the refrigerator, car keys in the laundry, unmailed letters in the car—things like that. To begin with, I just took care of it, but then I stopped because I wanted him to notice, too. When he didn't, I was surprised, so I started pointing things out—but until he forgot the boat and the dog twice, it didn't make any difference."

"Anything else?"

She looked at her husband. "Vinnie, I'm not being critical. It's because the doctor asked."

This time, he reached over and touched her arm. "It's OK, I want you to tell the doctor everything. I'd probably forget most of it anyway."

"That's another thing, doctor. Vinnie's just been more 'down' the last 2 or 3 years. I wouldn't call it depressed, exactly. He's not just sitting around staring at the wall or anything, but he's not smiling or laughing the way he has in the past."

"With the politicians we got now, it's enough to depress anyone," Mr. Parnelli said.

"It's more than just politicians—you could even laugh at Roosevelt, Vinnie." She turned to me and smiled. "We've been married a long time."

"Theresa's right. I haven't seen as much humor in life in the last few years. Maybe it's because I'm not sleeping as well as I did when I was younger."

"That too, doctor," Mrs. Parnelli said. "I was reading about depression, just in case, you know, and it said that insomnia and sleeplessness are classic symptoms of depression. Is that true?"

"Depends on your point of view. Depression, insomnia, and forgetfulness could all be symptoms of something else, too," I answered. "I'll explain later on. Any other symptoms or things you've noticed?"

"Let's see," Mrs. Parnelli said. "More forgetful, maybe a little depressed, not sleeping well—and maybe tiring more easily than usual, what do you think, Vinnie?"

"I was just blaming it on being older. I am 76, but Theresa reminded me about my father. He was zipping around doing things until he was over 90. Especially when I try to work hard—chopping wood or whatever—I get tired out and my muscles just physically get more tired. Like I said, I just put it down to age and not sleeping so good, but with this forgetful thing . . ."

We finished Mr. Parnelli's health history, and went to the examination room. Everything appeared relatively OK until we got to checking his stomach and abdomen.

"Quite a bit of gassiness," I remarked.

"That's been with me for years. Most of my friends, too. Sometimes we even call ourselves the 'gassy grandpas'. Could be worse. A few years before I retired I had a bad stretch of heartburn. The doctor told me no ulcer; just take antacids, it'd pass—and it did."

"With this, your symptoms are forming a fairly typical pattern."

Mr. Parnelli sat up abruptly. "What's a lot of belching and gas have to do with forgetting the boat and the dog?" he demanded.

"Now, Vinnie, let the doctor finish. I'm sure he'll tell us," Mrs. Parnelli soothed. Mr. Parnelli looked doubtful, but lay back down, and we finished his examination.

"So what disease are you finding in whatever pattern you're talking about?" Mr. Parnelli asked. He put his shirt on and sat down, arms crossed.

"No disease, just a frequently occurring pattern of wear-and-tear," I replied.

"Wear and tear? Is that just a polite way of telling me I'm just getting older like I thought—nothing I can do?"

"We're all getting older, but if we pay attention, there's a lot we can do to stay healthy at the same time. Please remember that what I'm going to explain is just a theory until we do the tests and try the treatments, but this same pattern happens to so many of us."

"Gas, belching, and forgetting the dog makes a pattern. Wait'll I tell this to Bill . . . "

"Vinnie . . ."

"OK, Theresa, I'll be good and listen."

"As we get older, many of us lose digestive capacity—some of us sooner than others. By age 60, at least half of us have significant digestive slowdown. Usually, our stomachs aren't making as much acid and pepsin as when we were younger, so our food—especially the protein—isn't as well-digested as it might be. And inefficient digestion is very often accompanied by considerable gas. It's very likely that the 'stretch of heartburn' and increasing gas you had before you retired was a signal of progressive stomach failure."

"So if my stomach was making less acid and pepsin than necessary, why did the doctor tell me to take antacids?"

I sighed. "Habit, lack of understanding, inadequate testing—really hard to say. But when we carefully test people over age 40 who're having heartburn, indigestion, and gas, over 90% of the time we find inadequate acid (and presumably pepsin) production by the stomach. Hydrochloric acid and pepsin supplementation relieves the symptoms, further proving the point. That's likely part of what you'll need . . . but let's get back to forgetting the dog.

"Hydrochloric acid and pepsin are what the stomach uses to digest protein. The ultimate products of protein digestion are amino acids and short chains of amino acids called peptides. When we test people who have seriously inadequate stomach function, or who have had inadequate stomach function for a long time, we usually find a pattern of lower-than-average to much lower-than-average amino acids in the bloodstream. Now, most neurotransmitters are made from amino acids . . ."

"Neurotransmitters?"

"You remember, Vinnie, I was telling you neurotransmitters are the little molecules the brain cells use for sending messages to each other," Mrs. Parnelli said. "So, if Vinnie's stomach isn't working, he might not have been digesting enough protein into amino acids for his brain to use to make enough neurotrans-

mitters, so he might get forgetful?"

"Exactly. It could also account for a lot of his sleeplessness and insomnia. Those very often get a lot better when we get people on the right combination of amino acids."

"Isn't muscle made out of amino acids, too?" Mrs. Parnelli asked.

"All proteins are, and muscle is mostly protein."

"So if my stomach doesn't work right, and I'm not getting enough amino acids, then my muscles might get weak, too?" Mr. Parnelli leaned forward, uncrossed his arms, and looked much more interested. "Let's see—gas, belching, poor digestion, low amino acids, weak muscles, low neurotransmitters, sleeplessness, insomnia, depression, and forgetting the boat and dog. Damn! It all makes sense after all!"

I smiled. "One of the common patterns as we get older, if we're not careful. There are a few more details, too. If the digestion isn't working well, injections of vitamin B_{12} and other B-vitamins can be very helpful for the function of the brain and nervous system, and can be especially helpful against fatigue. Over the years, many people with poor stomach function have told me that intravenous injections of essential minerals are very helpful in restoring strength, stamina, and endurance. Also, the large majority of us at age 76 are quite low on the hormone DHEA, and many of us men are low on testosterone. Supplementing with small quantities of one or both of these hormones in an identical-to-natural form can be very useful—even reinvigorating, and can help to rebuild healthy tissue all around the body. Most people notice improvement in mental function, too."

"So when do I get started on all this stuff?"

"Remember, this is all just theory until we get the right tests done. But given the overall pattern, tests will probably show that hydrochloric acid/pepsin replacement, amino acids, B_{12} injections, essential minerals, DHEA, and possibly testosterone will be the items recommended."

"So I may not be 'losing it'; I'm just low on things that belong in my body anyway. It's more like patching and repairing an old house than treating some disease."

"Right."

Mr. and Mrs. Parnelli began to get up, but she sat down with another question. "Aren't there some vitamins and herbs that can help memory and depression, too, doctor?"

"Sure. Ginkgo, acetyl-L-carnitine, and phosphatidylserine all have had impressive studies showing their ability to improve memory and depression, especially when we're older. Let's wait to see how Mr. Parnelli does on the 'home repair' items first, then we can consider using one or more of those."

As expected, Mr. Parnelli's tests disclosed weak digestive function, low amino acids, many low minerals, and low DHEA. With the help of the appropriate amino acids, vitamin B_{12} injections (with other B vitamins), minerals, DHEA, and digestive correction, his memory, low-grade depression, and other symptoms were much improved within 8 months. At that point, we added in ginkgo to try to sharpen memory fur-

ther, as well as for its action in improving small-blood-vessel circulation and erectile function. One year later, Mrs. Parnelli told me she hadn't found anymore socks in the refrigerator, only "the occasional memory lapse like the rest of us," and Mr. Parnelli hadn't forgotten the boat or the dog since.

Make Sure the "Essentials" Are Being Taken *and* Absorbed

AS NOTED AT the end of the chapter on benign prostatic hyperplasia, it's always wise to make sure that essential nutrients are adequately supplied to our bodies before proceeding with other natural remedies or with patentable-drug therapy. When we're older, we not only need to make sure we're eating (or supplementing) all the essential nutrients, but that we're digesting and absorbing them well. So, before (or at least at the same time as) you start on St. John's wort against depression or ginkgo to aid memory, make sure all the essential nutrients are not only being ingested, but absorbed, as well.

DR. GABY'S COMMENTARY

AS DR. WRIGHT pointed out, factors that improve overall health may also enhance mental function. These include eating healthful foods, avoiding excessive alcohol intake, dealing with digestion and absorption problems, exercising regularly, taking a high-quality vitamin and mineral supplement, and maintaining a positive attitude.

"Alternative" practitioners are not universally successful in helping people suffering from dementia, but many patients do respond to certain treatments that are still being overlooked by many doctors.

Nutritional Supplements
Vitamin B_{12}

ALTHOUGH it is well known that vitamin B_{12} deficiency can cause mental decline, most doctors are unaware of how common this deficiency may be. The usual test for vitamin B_{12} status (blood levels of the vitamin) is not always sensitive enough to detect a mild deficiency. A more sensitive indicator is a urine test showing elevated levels of a compound called methylmalonic acid.[1]

However, even that test may fail to identify many patients who are likely to respond to vitamin B_{12} treatment. That is because most tests used to assess vitamin B_{12} status measure what is going on outside the brain. Conceivably, a vitamin B_{12} deficiency could be present in brain tissue, even though levels might be normal elsewhere in the body. That possibility was supported by a study of 16 elderly patients with dementia. Of those 16 patients, 12 were found to have low levels of vitamin B_{12} in their cerebrospinal fluid (CSF the fluid that bathes the brain). These patients showed improvement in mental function after receiving vitamin B_{12} injections. However, 9 of the 12 patients with low CSF concentrations of vitamin B_{12} had normal levels in their blood.[2] This study suggests that many individuals with dementia have a deficiency of vitamin B_{12} that cannot be diagnosed by standard laboratory tests, because the deficiency is localized to the brain.

Because obtaining spinal fluid for vitamin B_{12} testing is an invasive procedure, and because vitamin B_{12} treatment is safe and inexpensive, we usually forego the test in favor of a therapeutic trial of vitamin B_{12} injections. If the patient improves after a series of 4 to 8 injections, we recommend continuing the injections on an as-needed basis (typically every 1 to 4 weeks). While vitamin B_{12} injections are often beneficial, other methods of administering the vitamin—such as orally, sublingually, or intranasally—are usually ineffective.

Other B-vitamins

THIAMIN, niacinamide, folic acid, and other B-vitamins also play an important role in mental function. In a study of 228 individuals between the ages of 73 and 102, 39% had low blood levels of one or more B-vitamins. These deficiencies occurred even though food intake was adequate and everyone was taking a daily vitamin supplement.[3] This study suggests that absorption of B-vitamins is impaired in a large proportion of elderly individuals. For that reason, we frequently inject other B-vitamins along with vitamin B_{12}.

Hormone Therapy: DHEA, Testosterone, and Estrogen

DEHYDROEPIANDROSTERONE (DHEA) is a steroid hormone manufactured by the adrenal glands and sex organs that appears to have beneficial effects on the aging process. In humans, serum levels of DHEA decline with age; the levels in 70-year-old individuals are only about 20% as high as the levels in young adults. Animals treated with DHEA look younger, have glossier coats, and have less gray hair than animals not receiving DHEA.[4] Administering DHEA has also been shown to improve memory in mice.[5]

In my experience, many patients suffering from age-related physical and mental deterioration have blood levels of DHEA (measured as DHEA-sulfate) that are either below normal or near the bottom of the normal range. After taking small amounts of DHEA (usually 5 to15 mg per day for women, 10 to 30 mg per day for men), patients seem to become younger in many different ways—sometimes in a matter of weeks. Patients experience improvements in both psychological well-being and, in some cases, memory. Although DHEA supplements are available without a prescription, this hormone has the potential to cause adverse effects, and it should therefore be used only under medical supervision.

Testosterone, a hormone related to DHEA, is also low in some elderly individuals. In one study, 32 men aged 50 or older were randomly assigned to receive testosterone or a placebo. Those given the testosterone had a significant improvement in muscle strength and better performance on memory tests.[6]

In a study of 8,877 women living in a retirement community, those who had taken postmenopausal estrogen-replacement therapy (ERT) were 35% less likely to develop dementia than those who had not used ERT.[7] Other studies have shown that ERT improves cognitive function—at least in the short term—in women with dementia.[8, 9] Although additional research is needed to determine what the long-term effects are, ERT shows promise as a way of preventing or treating memory loss in postmenopausal women.

For reasons that are explained in chapter 4, we prefer using human estrogens in the approximate proportions produced by the ovaries, rather than horse estrogens (Premarin) or "unbalanced" human-estrogen preparations, such as pure estradiol (Estrace). Although no controlled studies have been done, Dr. Wright has observed that administering estrogen in this way (combined with natural progesterone) often improves mental function in older women.

Herbal Supplements
Ginkgo biloba *extract*

THIS popular herb, obtained from the leaves of the ginkgo tree, is known to increase blood flow to the brain and to improve cellular metabolism in brain tissue. In one study, 112 elderly individuals with chronic "cerebral insufficiency" received 120 mg of *Ginkgo biloba* extract daily for 1 year. Significant improvements were noted in short-term memory, vigilance, and mood.[10] Numerous other studies have found similar results.[11, 12, 13, 14] In most cases, improvements occurred after 3 months of treatment. Most of the studies with ginkgo used a commercially available product that is standardized to contain 24% ginkgo heterosides.

Other Natural Treatments
Phosphatidylserine

PHOSPHATIDYLSERINE (PS) is a compound that occurs naturally in the brain, and has been shown to enhance mental function. Administering this compound to mice prevented age-related degeneration of brain tissue.[15] In a study in humans, 40 individuals with senile dementia received 300 mg of PS daily for 60 days. Improvements were noted in memory and in various psychological symptoms.[16] Other studies have produced similar results.[17]

The PS used in these studies was extracted from bovine (cow) brain. However, bovine-brain PS is not sold in the United States, because of the fear that it could be contaminated with the organism that causes "mad cow" disease. A PS product manufactured from soybean lecithin is available in this country, but the chemical structure differs from that of bovine-brain PS. Preliminary (unpublished) research using the soy product has failed to demonstrate any benefit in a group of elderly individuals with mild impairment of memory.[18] Consequently, we cannot recommend soy-derived PS as a treatment for dementia at this time.

Acetyl-L-carnitine

ANOTHER naturally occurring substance that plays a role in brain function is acetyl-L-carnitine. In a single-blind study, 279 individuals with mild-to-moderately severe mental decline received 1,500 mg of acetyl-L-carnitine daily for 3 months and a placebo for an additional 2 months. Compared with the placebo, acetyl-L-carnitine significantly improved cognitive function, emotional status, and behavior.[19] However, in a double-blind study of 355 patients with probable Alzheimer's disease, those who received acetyl-L-carnitine (1 gram, 3 times a day for 12 months) showed the same rate of mental decline as those given a placebo.[20] Additional studies are therefore needed to clarify the role of acetyl-L-carnitine in the treatment of memory loss. Occasional side effects have been reported with this compound, including nausea, vomiting, increased aggression, and confusion. In addition, acetyl-L-carnitine is relatively expensive.

Conclusion

AGE-RELATED MENTAL decline is often a frustrating condition for the patient, the family, and the doctor. Alzheimer's disease is especially difficult to treat. However, research over the past 15 years has provided us with a number of promising new treatment options. While not everyone improves, many elderly individuals have obtained gratifying results from various combinations of the treatments described above.

Although it is possible to purchase some of these products without a prescription, the treatment of dementia can be rather complicated and should be undertaken with professional supervision.

Summary of Recommendations for Treating Age-Related Memory Loss and Depression

Primary Recommendations:

- Intramuscular injections of vitamin B_{12} (often combined with folic acid and other B-vitamins).

- Dehydroepiandrosterone (DHEA) and/or testosterone (for both men and women), if levels are low. Estrogen therapy (balanced with progesterone), for selected women.

- *Gingko biloba* extract (standardized to contain 24% ginkgo heterosides), 40 mg, 3 times a day.

- High-potency multiple vitamin/mineral.

- Assess digestion and absorption; use appropriate digestive aids when indicated.

Other Recommendations:

- Acetyl-L-carnitine, 500 mg, 3 times a day.

MENOPAUSE

✣ MENOPAUSE IS A *natural process that typically occurs in women between the ages of 45 and 55. At that time, the reduced secretion of estrogen and possibly other hormones is no longer sufficient to produce menstrual cycles. As estrogen production by the ovaries slows down, the adrenal glands compensate by manufacturing steroid molecules (estrogen precursors) that are converted elsewhere in the body into estrogen. During the first several years after menopause, this contribution from the adrenal glands is usually enough to maintain normal structure and function of secondary sex tissues such as breasts, urethra, vagina, and vulva. With increasing age, however, secretion of adrenal estrogen precursors also declines and estrogen-dependent tissues begin to atrophy.*

The most common symptoms associated with menopause are hot flashes—those uncomfortable sensations of intense body heat accompanied by flushing of the skin and sometimes by profuse perspiration. For most women, hot flashes occur for about 1 to 2 years after menopause, although for some women they may last as long as 5 years. Depression is also a frequent symptom of menopause. Post-menopausal depression is caused partly by hormonal deficiency, but it may also be related to the perceived loss of sexuality and youth in a society that places great emphasis on these qualities.

As estrogen deficiency becomes more severe, atrophy of the vaginal tissues may occur, leading to itching or inflammation, pain on intercourse, and narrowing of the vaginal opening. Thinning or inflammation of the urethra (the urinary-tract opening) may also occur, and women may experience pain on urination or a tendency to leak urine.

Estrogen replacement therapy (ERT) is nearly always successful in relieving the symptoms of menopause. However, the main reasons that ERT is promoted by doctors are its alleged protective effects against osteoporosis and heart disease. While ERT does help prevent osteoporosis during the early years of its use, the benefits decrease with time. By age 75, more than 70% of the improvement in bone density resulting from continuous ERT is lost.[1] Moreover, bone loss can be minimized in other ways.[2] ERT is also said to prevent heart disease, because women who use ERT develop heart disease less often than women who do not. However, the reduction in the incidence of heart disease may be attributable entirely to the fact that women who take hormones are healthier and more motivated before they start the treatment. Randomized, double-blind studies have failed to demonstrate even a slight protective effect of ERT on the heart.[3, 4]

While the benefits of ERT appear to have been exaggerated, there are real concerns about the safety of this treatment. Research suggests that ERT as it is used in this country (typically horse estrogens [Premarin] plus medroxyprogesterone acetate [Provera]) may increase the incidence of breast and ovarian cancer (although the studies on breast cancer have been conflicting). ERT also has been shown to increase the risk of thrombophlebitis (blood clots). In addition, women who take ERT often experience unpleasant side effects. For these reasons, many women are seeking alternatives to ERT.

DR. WRIGHT'S CASE STUDY

"I'm confused," Samantha Brennan said. "I've been having hot flashes, I'm not sleeping well, my husband says I'm a lot more short-tempered than usual. I've been feeling more depressed and moody than I have in years. My menstrual periods just stopped a few months ago, so I'm sure it's all just menopause."

"And you're confused about . . . ?"

"What to do. When my periods first started to get lighter, and I had just a few hot flashes, I added 400 units of vitamin E daily to my multiple vitamin, and that seemed to take them away. After a few months, though, I started skipping periods, and the hot flashes came back and I just felt . . . well, just sort of anxious and unwell. I started waking up at night. I increased my vitamin E to 800 units, which reduced the 'flashes' a little, but that's all. So I did some reading, went to the natural-food store, and got some Vitex. I think that's called 'chaste berry'. I also got some Dong quai, along with a combination 'women's herbal' with black cohosh that the clerk told me about, and those really helped for over a year. My periods acted like they were coming back—they got a little heavier, the hot flashes disappeared, and all the 'nerve' symptoms got better. But now I haven't had any menstrual bleeding for about 6 months, and all the symptoms are back. My sister, she's 7 years older, is just laughing at me. She doesn't believe in vitamins or herbs or anything. She says they weren't really doing anything for me at all, I just talked myself into it, and I should just take Premarin and Provera like she does. She says our mother and her sisters—our aunts—all had a terrible time with menopause, and I will too, and all the vitamins and herbs in the world won't help."

"Many women do very well with a bit of diet change as well as vitamins and herbs. In case it would help you to know, there are perfectly good scientific studies confirming the efficacy of the herbs you mentioned for menopausal symptoms. Black cohosh is particularly well studied for helping with the psychological symptoms of menopause—those 'nerve' symptoms you mentioned. Remember, though, that modern science has just recently started serious research on herbal or botanical remedies. And where do scientific researchers get their ideas about which herbs to research for which conditions? From so-called 'folk' or 'ethnic' medicine—in effect from the experiments of thousands of generations of grandmothers! Don't let your sister get to you. It's actually sad that she's cut herself off from thousands of years of accumulated knowledge."

Mrs. Brennan sat up straighter in her chair. "When you put it that way, I should be feeling sorry for her, right? But I still have all these symptoms. My gynecologist says I should take Premarin and Provera, too, or maybe try the estrogen patch. But I've done some reading about those, too, and there's a lot of debate. Most of the experts say that this kind of hormone replacement therapy—they call it 'HRT'—raises the risk of cancer. Some say it's a slight added risk, some say it's more than that. My gynecologist says that when Provera—he calls it progesterone—is part of HRT, then the risk is lessened again."

"Does your family have any history of heart attack or perhaps osteoporosis?"

"Both. That's another reason I'm thinking that the vitamins and herbs might not be enough. Mother had a heart attack when she was 68, and another at 73. The doctors said they weren't too bad, and she's made a good recovery, but I'd rather avoid that. On the other side, 2 of my father's sisters have broken their hips. So I guess I don't have the lowest odds, do I?"

"No, you don't. Are you watching your diet closely, taking some calcium and magnesium, and so on?"

"Oh, yes. I don't eat any processed or refined foods, except on trips when I can't avoid it. I read all the labels to eliminate added chemicals, and eat as many fresh fruits and vegetables as I can. I've cut down on beef and pork, too, and eat lots more fish. Also, I take cod-liver oil for both my heart and arteries, and calcium, magnesium, and other minerals. And I take some extra vitamin C."

"Along with your multiple vitamin-mineral and the extra vitamin E, you're doing well."

"Thank you." She paused. "Did I hear you say something about diet change for menopause a little while ago?"

"Yes, you did. Soy products contain 'plant estrogen' compounds that can help ease menopausal symptoms. Also, many fruits and some vegetables contain the flavonoids you mentioned, which can help a little, too."

"I'm already doing the fruits and vegetables as well as extra flavonoids. But I hardly ever eat soy. I'll add that in. But that won't take care of all these symptoms, will it?"

"Probably not."

"So I'm stuck with HRT even with the added risk of cancer?"

"If you mean stuck with Premarin or Provera or the so-called 'estrogen patch'—not at all! Actually, Premarin and Provera aren't really 'hormone replacement therapy.'"

Mrs. Brennan looked puzzled. "They're not? My gynecologist . . . and magazines I've read, and . . . everyone says they are! Now I'm really confused!"

"Premarin is excellent estrogen replacement—for a horse! Even the name says that—'Pre' for 'pregnant', and 'marin' for 'mare', Premarin is a concentrated extract of pregnant-horse urine!"

She sat back in her chair obviously very surprised. "My sister's swallowing a concentrate of horse urine?"

"Along with millions of other women. It's the most commonly written prescription in the United States at this time."

"Is pregnant-horse estrogen the same as human estrogen?"

"Human bodies contain very specific types of estrogen—estrone, estradiol, and estriol. Only two of the dozen or so types of molecules in

Premarin are substantially similar. All the rest aren't."

"So why not replace human hormones with human hormones?"

"Exactly! In natural medicine, that's the only logical thing to do. Instead of Premarin, we recommend a combination of estrone, estradiol, and estriol in proportions similar to those found in the body. Instead of Provera, we recommend progesterone—the molecule found in human bodies."

"So what is Provera then?"

"Medroxyprogesterone—a molecule synthesized in a test tube and never found in human, horse, or any other animal bodies."

"So what's it good for?"

"It can be patented."

"Wait a minute. You're telling me that millions of women have taken millions—probably billions—of doses of Provera for probably 40 years because it was patentable, while the exact natural-replacement hormone—progesterone—was available all along?"

I just looked at her, but she scarcely noticed.

"And the same for Premarin?" She was visibly angry.

I nodded.

"So all that controversy about 'does hormone replacement therapy cause cancer' and all that research is actually just an argument about the safety of giving women horse hormones and synthetic patentable hormone substitutes? That's just ridiculous!"

"And tragic. We've wasted nearly 50 years of research energy and dollars, and likely caused needless suffering and death to at least a few women with these patent medicines. It's been scientifically sloppy and inexcusably negligent. Nearly all of so-called 'hormone-replacement therapy' research is irrelevant to real human hormone replacement. But let's get back to you." I started to write a prescription for 'triple estrogen', a precisely measured combination of estrone, estradiol, and estriol, and another prescription for progesterone.

"But . . . are these natural human hormones safe?" she asked.

I couldn't resist a big grin.

"What's so funny?" She hesitated, then smiled. "I think I get it. I'm asking if the very hormones that have been circulating in my body since I was 13 years old are safe! My husband will get a real laugh from that. I didn't tell you—he's a pastor, and he's always saying, 'If God made it that way, it must be right; there must be a reason.'"

"Likely he's right. But as we both know, not even everything in the 'original creation' is 100% safe for us humans. Even natural hormones produced by a woman's own body can cause a few problems. For example, estrogen has been associated with a higher risk of thrombophlebitis—blood clotting in the veins—especially during pregnancy. Also, estrogen can sometimes induce depression, especially if there isn't enough vitamin B_6 in the body. If we were all eating 100% organic, nutrient-rich food that was grown on well-mineralized soil, there wouldn't be much hazard. But we're not, so a few supplements are called for even when using identical-to-natural hormones."

"Which ones are those?"

"Probably you're taking them all, but let's go over them just to be sure. Vitamin E and a source of essential fatty acids will reduce the risk of blood clotting. Both of these act as 'platelet anti-aggregants', which make the blood platelets more slippery so they don't stick together abnormally and cause a clot. Please continue the same amount of vitamin E and use 1 tablespoonful of cod-liver oil daily."

"Oh, I'm already doing that to protect my bones."

"Good. It'll protect your heart and arteries too, right along with the human, not horse, hormone replacement. Lastly, make sure to use a good daily multiple vitamin with at least 25 milligrams of vitamin B_6."

"I'm pretty sure I'm doing that already, but I'll check. Is that all?"

"Actually, we've only partly covered the topic of human hormone-replacement therapy, but before we consider testosterone and DHEA, your levels should be tested. Even though they're most likely low, too, they're androgenic—that means male-like. It's not wise to replace them for women without careful measurement."

Mrs. Brennan thought for a moment. "That's right—ovaries make testosterone, don't they? My sex drive has been down—isn't testosterone responsible for that? I hadn't thought of that. I just attributed it to nerves and general upset. But you're right, let's check that carefully. I don't want to grow whiskers!" She went to the lab to have the testing done.

Within a few days, Mrs. Brennan's hot flashes, moodiness, depression, and "nerves" were gone. She was sleeping well again, and her husband said she was back to her old self. The chances are excellent that she's reduced her risk of atherosclerosis, osteoporosis, and senile dementia, without incurring as much cancer risk as she would with horse hormones.*

---

*For further information, readers might look for *Natural Hormone Replacement for Women Over 45,* by Jonathan V. Wright, M.D. and John Morgenthaler (120 pages; Smart Publications, Petaluma, California, 1997, $9.95) available at compounding pharmacies and natural-food stores.

DR. GABY'S COMMENTARY

THE COVENTIONAL USE of ERT to relieve the symptoms of menopause is quite controversial, as there are some significant risks associated with these treatments. In contrast, natural treatments can be quite effective and are probably safer. Women should gather all the information available and make an educated choice about which route they want to take to relieve the symptoms of menopause.

Nutritional Supplements

VITAMIN E HAS been reported in a few studies to relieve menopausal hot flashes.[5, 6, 7] However, none of these studies included a control group, so the possibility of a placebo effect cannot be ruled out. In the only placebo-controlled trial that has been done, a small dose of vitamin E (50 to 100 IU per day) was no more effective than the placebo.[8] We usually advise women entering menopause to take vitamin E—if only for its protective effect against heart disease. Some women experience an improvement in their hot flashes with vitamin E, although most women do not find it to be effective.

In a double-blind study, the combination of vitamin C and food-derived flavonoids (hesperidin complex and hesperidin methylchalcone) was found to relieve hot flashes. The women in that study received 1,200 mg of vitamin C, 900 mg of hesperidin complex, and 300 mg of hesperidin methylchalcone daily.[9] The only side effect of the vitamin C/flavonoid preparation was a slightly offensive odor to the perspiration, and a tendency for it to discolor the clothing. It is not known how this treatment works, although the chemical structure of hesperidin is similar to that of estradiol (a form of estrogen).

Soybeans contain two flavonoid compounds—genistein and daidzein—which have mild estrogenic activity. Consumption of large amounts of soy products by Japanese women may account for the rarity of menopausal symptoms in Japan.[10] In a recent study, 104 postmenopausal women were randomly assigned to consume 60 grams (about 2 ounces) of isolated soy protein per day or a placebo for 12 weeks. The frequency of hot flashes was reduced by 45% in the soy group, compared with 30% in the placebo group (a statistically significant difference).[11] Eating soy products also reduces serum cholesterol[12] and may help prevent cancer.[13] For these reasons, adding soy to your diet is probably a good idea.

Herbal Treatments

HERBAL REMEDIES, INCLUDING dong quai (*Angelica sinensis*), black cohosh (*Cimicifuga racemosa*), alfalfa (*Medicago sativa*), licorice root (*Glycyrrhiza glabra*), and ginseng (*Panax ginseng*), have been used for many years in treating menopausal symptoms, and they are frequently effective. As far as we are aware, black cohosh is the only herb that has been demonstrated by clinical research to relieve menopausal symptoms,[14] although the other herbs mentioned have been shown to have estrogen-like effects in animal studies.[15, 16, 17, 18] In a double-blind study, dong quai was no more effective than a placebo at relieving menopausal symptoms.[19] However, most herbalists use dong quai in combination with other herbs, rather than by itself, as in that study. On rare occasions, ginseng has caused vaginal bleeding in postmenopausal women, apparently because of its estrogenic activity.

Herbalists may recommend different combinations of herbs for different women, depending on their particular clinical picture. To maximize safety and effectiveness, women who wish to treat their menopausal symptoms with herbs should consult a practitioner who is trained in their use.

Hormone Therapy
"Alternative" Hormone Therapies

IN addition to estrogen, the ovary also produces progesterone, dehydroepiandrosterone (DHEA), and testosterone. We have found that, for some patients, a combination of progesterone and DHEA will relieve menopausal symptoms, thereby eliminating the need for estrogen therapy. The effectiveness of these hormones may be due to their partial conversion to estrogen, although they may also have direct effects of their own. In addition, DHEA enhances the functioning of the immune system in postmenopausal women, and it may help prevent some types of cancer (see chapter 4).

Testosterone deficiency is less common in post-menopausal women, unless their ovaries have been surgically removed. However, when testosterone deficiency does occur, it can result in fatigue, depression, and reduced libido. In those cases, treatment with low doses of the natural hormone is extremely effective.

"Natural" Estrogen Therapy

ESTROGEN therapy may be desirable in cases in which other treatments are ineffective, or for its possible protective effect against memory loss (see previous chapter). However, logic suggests that when estrogen is used, it should be administered in a way that mimics normal human physiology (instead of using horse estrogens, which have a different chemical structure than human estrogens).

Three different forms of estrogen are normally found in the human body—estrone, estradiol, and estriol. Whereas estrone and estradiol promote the development of cancer, some evidence (though conflicting) indicates that estriol may actually have an anti-cancer effect. In one study, treatment with estriol resulted in regression of bone metastases in some women with breast cancer.[20] On the other hand, estriol has also been found to promote the growth of breast-cancer cells in a test tube.[21]

Another possible advantage of using estriol relates to its effect on the uterus. Whereas conventional ERT frequently causes uterine hyperplasia (abnormal cellular proliferation of the uterus, a pre-cancerous change), several reports indicate that estriol does not cause this problem.[22] However, that observation, too, has been challenged in some studies.[23]

Doses of 2 to 6 mg per day of estriol will sometimes relieve menopausal symptoms. This hormone is frequently prescribed in Europe and by some natural-medicine doctors in the United States. However, estriol is a rather weak estrogen, and it does not always relieve menopausal symptoms effectively. Although higher doses may be more effective, some women experience nausea when the dosage is increased.

An alternative to estriol is "triple-estrogen," a formula developed in 1982 by Dr. Wright. Triple-estrogen contains estrone (10%), estradiol (10%), and estriol (80%). For relief of menopausal symptoms, triple-estrogen is frequently as effective as Premarin and other standard forms of estrogen. Triple-estrogen also appears to cause fewer side effects than conventional estrogen regimens. Dr. Wright has been using this combination for the past 17 years, and he has not seen any cases of estrogen-induced uterine cancer. In the few cases in which vaginal bleeding occurred, uterine biopsies were done and no evidence of uterine hyperplasia was found. My own experience and that of other doctors who use triple-estrogen has been similar.

Of course, large-scale studies must be done before we can be sure of the long-term safety of these "alternative" hormone regimens. In addition, there is very little research on whether administering triple-estrogen or estriol by itself will prevent osteoporosis, heart disease, or other problems.

Triple-estrogen is typically administered for 25 consecutive days each month, with natural progesterone (not Provera) added on days 14 to 25. Clinical observations suggest that 2.5 mg of triple-estrogen is similar in potency to 0.625 mg of Premarin. For additional information about estrogen therapy, please see *Natural Hormone Replacement for Women Over 45,* by Dr. Wright.[24]

Combining Premarin and Progesterone

NATURAL progesterone is available over the counter, in the form of creams for topical application. A typical over-the-counter preparation contains about 20 mg of progesterone per quarter-teaspoon. Higher concentrations of progesterone for topical use can be obtained by prescription through compounding pharmacists. Progesterone for oral administration is also available by prescription. Although both routes of administration are effective, many doctors prefer the topical route, because a large proportion of orally administered progesterone is broken down in the liver before it reaches the bloodstream.

When estriol or triple-estrogen is used, small doses of natural progesterone (such as 25 to 50 mg per day, on days 14 to 25) appear to be adequate to balance the estrogen. However, larger doses of progesterone are needed to prevent Premarin from causing uterine hyperplasia. Fortunately, a high dose of natural progesterone (200 mg per day by mouth, taken 12 days per month) has been shown to prevent Premarin-induced uterine changes as effectively as does Provera.[4]

Although natural progesterone is available over the counter, self-treatment with hormones can be dangerous. Hormone-replacement therapy should always be supervised by a trained health-care practitioner.

Conclusion

SYMPTOMS ASSOCIATED WITH menopause can in some cases be controlled by dietary changes, nutritional supplements, and herbs. If symptoms persist, estrogen-replacement therapy (ERT) or treatment with other ovarian hormones (progesterone, DHEA, or testosterone) may be necessary. Since ERT as it is commonly prescribed in this country may cause cancer and other side effects, doctors of natural medicine are exploring other ways of prescribing estrogen. Although we still have a great deal to learn about hormone-replacement therapy, the use of identical-to-natural hormones may eventually be accepted as a major advance. However, this approach can be quite complicated. It is therefore important that you seek professional advice, rather than attempting to treat yourself.

Summary of Recommendations for Menopause

THE TREATMENTS DISCUSSED in this chapter should be monitored by a doctor. While we advise most women entering menopause to incorporate soy into their diet and to take 400 IU of vitamin E and a high-potency multiple vitamin/mineral each day, other recommendations are usually tailored according to a woman's individual needs.

MENORRHAGIA AND CERVICAL DYSPLASIA

THE PATIENT DESCRIBED *in this chapter has 2 fairly common gynecologic problems: menorrhagia (the medical term for excessive menstrual bleeding—pronounced "men-oh-rajah") and cervical dysplasia (abnormal cells lining the cervix).*

Menorrhagia should always be evaluated by a physician to rule out medical conditions that might be causing the problem. Common causes of menorrhagia include uterine fibroids and hormonal imbalances. If a specific medical problem is identified, appropriate treatment will often restore menstruation to normal. In many cases, however, the gynecologist is unable to determine why a woman experiences heavy menstrual bleeding.

Cervical dysplasia is a term used to describe abnormal cervical cells. Because cancer of the cervix is a fairly common and sometimes fatal disease, women are advised to have periodic Pap smears. This test checks the health of the cells that line the cervix. Pap smears allow the doctor to detect and effectively treat pre-cancerous changes before they become more serious. Cervical dysplasia is usually graded according to its severity, which can range from mild inflammation to pre-cancerous to localized cancer.

DR. WRIGHT'S CASE STUDY

"I thought I had enough problems with these terribly heavy menstrual periods," Jill Langston said. "They've kept me miserable for nearly a week every month for years! I get cramps and fatigue, and have a hard time going anywhere with all the bleeding. But now I've turned up with an abnormal Pap smear, too. They told me not to worry—it's not cancer, but I'd better have my cervix frozen or operated on so it won't get worse. That's when I decided to pay attention to Jan—that's my older sister—and come over here.

She's been into raw carrot juice, organic liver, lots of spinach and broccoli, and nuts and berries for years. She's on my case all the time. I've got to admit, she's a lot healthier than I am." She paused.

"When was the abnormal Pap smear done?"

"Just 3 weeks ago. Someone canceled, and I got in here really fast. Jan said she was praying for me, too."

"That might help in more ways than one. Let's see—how old are you this year?"

"I'm 27."

"How long have you had heavy menstrual bleeding?"

"Seems like forever—since sophomore year in high school."

"You've seen doctors about it?"

"Several. The first one tried me on birth control pills, but after 2 or 3 months on different brands, I kept getting sick, so I gave that up. One doctor did a D & C operation, and my periods were better for 2 months, then they were just as heavy as ever. When she suggested another one, I passed. I've been on iron continuously for years, otherwise I get anemic from all the bleeding. Even with the iron, my blood count barely stays normal."

"Do you know about your ferritin?"

"What's that?"

"It's the best measurement of body-iron storage, except in very unusual circumstances."

"Guess I don't."

"You've been checked for fibroid tumors, polyps, and other physical abnormalities?"

"Lots of times. They never find any of that."

"Are you a smoker?"

"No. Tried it once or twice in high school, but that's all."

"Good. Smoking would just raise your risk of cervical cancer. Are your periods regular?"

"Regularly awful."

"Take any prescription medication?"

"Not routinely."

"Please tell me what you're eating every day."

She blushed. "Jan told me I'd better be straight with you or I might mess up my chances of improvement, but I guess I'm still embarrassed. She's been after me for years to change, but it's like I'm so busy I don't have the time to make a plan. I just grab anything available and run."

"Breakfast?"

"Most of the time I don't have any. At work, I usually do a doughnut and coffee, or some 'Danish' or something like that."

"Do you eat lunch?"

"Yeah, we all usually go to a fast-food place, for Chinese food, or something like that."

"What do you eat?"

"Hamburger, taco, chicken nuggets, pork fried rice—something like that."

"Do you eat between breakfast and lunch or lunch and dinner?"

"Yeah. Usually a pastry and a cola or something like that."

"Dinner?"

"Depends. Quite a bit of pizza, chicken, beef, and potato—and a salad. But sometimes it's ice cream and cookies, or a couple of slices of bread and jelly. Jan really gets after me for that, so I usually don't tell her. But sometimes she's at my apartment, and she noses around my shelves and refrigerator."

"You're not married—no roommate?"

"Guess it's obvious, isn't it? Got tired of the roommate thing a couple of years ago. It's just me and the cat. She probably eats better than I do! And I really don't like cooking much."

"Do you eat any fruit or vegetables?"

"I keep apples around."

"How about broccoli, brussels sprouts, spinach, celery, carrots?"

"Well, occasionally. Never did like vegetables much. Mom forced me to eat them when I was little though, but when I got older I stopped."

"Fish?"

She made a face.

"Nuts—peanuts, cashews, walnuts, and almonds, that kind of thing? They don't require cooking."

"No, I never got in the habit."

"Eggs?"

"I did learn to fry an egg, so I do that every few days."

"You drink any water?"

"Not much—mostly coffee and Pepsi."

"Take any vitamins or minerals?"

"Jan did talk me into taking vitamin C in the wintertime. She was right—I don't get as many colds."

"No other vitamins or minerals?"

"That's why I'm here."

"We'd really best start with food, first. Since you haven't been eating with good health in mind for quite awhile, it'll definitely be necessary to add in a number of supplemental items. But let's start with the foods, first, and relate them to your current problems."

She nodded and I continued.

"Over 2 decades ago, researchers found that very heavy menstrual periods could be normalized in over 50% of women, and lessened in nearly all of the rest, with extra quantities of vitamin A. Vitamin A itself is found in relatively few places in our diets—liver is the best source, and cod-liver oil is good, too."

"Aren't carrots high in vitamin A?"

"Not exactly. Carrots, sweet potato, yams, spinach, cantaloupe, kale, and broccoli are some of the best food sources of beta-carotene, which our bodies can convert to vitamin A. But beta-carotene and vitamin A aren't exactly identical, and beta-carotene isn't nearly as effective in normalizing very heavy menstrual bleeding."

"Why is that—if our bodies just turn beta-carotene into vitamin A anyway?"

"Only a limited amount of beta-carotene can be converted into vitamin A, so if you need 'therapeutic doses' of vitamin A, beta-carotene will not do much good. If your thyroid gland is weak, this conversion would be impaired even more. Vitamin A itself is also a key nutrient in helping to revert an abnormal Pap smear to normal."

"Whoa . . . are you saying that enough vitamin A might stop my heavy periods and improve my abnormal Pap smear—both?"

"I'm saying that if you'd been eating enough foods with vitamin A and beta-carotene, you might have prevented those problems in the first place."

"Maybe Jan's onto something with that organic liver, carrot juice, and spinach. But it can't be that simple, can it?"

"Certainly a lot simpler than a D & C operation or freezing your cervix, no? Jan's onto more than just vitamin A. Liver, broccoli, spinach, and many other green leafy vegetables—and fresh-squeezed orange juice, too—are excellent sources of folic acid, also called folate. Researchers have found folate to be another key nutrient for reverting abnormal Pap smears. Also, liver is an excellent source of iron and vitamin B_{12}. Vitamin B_{12} can help with that Pap smear. Iron not only helps make up for blood loss, it also helps prevent overly heavy menstrual bleeding in the first place. Other nutrients that help slow overly heavy bleeding include flavonoids—those are found in all those berries that you said Jan eats."

"I'm getting the picture. I'd better start with the liver, then go take some lessons from Jan."

"Liver's a very good idea, but make sure it's an organically raised source. 'Regular' liver is much too likely to contain residues of antibiotics, pesticides, herbicides, and even synthetic hormones. Please do go talk to your sister. It's never too late to start again with a wide variety of whole, unprocessed foods, vegetables, fruits, whole grains, eggs, fish, and other animal proteins. Get rid of the doughnuts, pastries, other white-flour and sugar products, the Pepsi and other soft drinks. Drop out of the 'Pepsi de-generation!'"

"How about drinking milk?"

"In general, cow's milk should be reserved for little cows. If you like 'milk-type' products, there are many types and flavors of soy milk, rice milk, and almond milk available in all the natural-food stores and now in most grocery stores.

"But even if you change your entire diet by tomorrow—and please start working on it—you'll still need a few vitamin supplements for quite awhile if you're going to try to normalize both your Pap smear and your heavy menstrual periods. I'll make you a list."

The list read:

- Vitamin A—75,000 IU daily
- Folic acid (folate)—25 milligrams, twice daily
- Vitamin C with citrus flavonoids—500 milligrams of each, twice daily
- Iron—30 milligrams daily
- Vitamin B_{12}—1,000 micrograms daily
- High-potency multiple vitamin-mineral

"Also, I'd recommend testing and possibly a trial of a small quantity of thyroid hormone. Even a very slightly weak thyroid can contribute to heavy menstrual bleeding."

"Is that because the thyroid helps convert beta-carotene into vitamin A, and vitamin A can stop heavy menstrual bleeding?"

"Quite possibly. You're catching on already."

"I've heard that a lot of vitamin A can be dangerous."

"With both an abnormal Pap smear and heavy menstrual bleeding, you need a lot for several months. Early warning signs of vitamin A overdose include fatigue, headache, joint pain, muscle aches, bone pain, and hair loss. These side effects disappear if the vitamin is discontinued. However, it would take much longer than a few months to cause vitamin A toxicity with the dose recommended. The only important precaution would be any possibility of pregnancy, since high doses of vitamin A have been associated with an increased risk of some birth defects."

She laughed. "No chance of that anytime soon. Jan's not only eating right, but she's got enough children for both of us, for now."

She got up to go. "I guess I'll get Jan off my case now. Organic liver, carrot juice, spinach, and all those vitamins, here I come! Sure beats freezing my poor cervix to death."

Three months later, Jill's Pap smear had improved from class 3 to class 2. Her next Pap smear in another 4 months was normal—class 1. By then, her menstrual bleeding was "average, just like Jan's," and she reported that "with the occasional lapse for old times' sake, I'm eating just as well as Jan!"

DR. GABY'S COMMENTARY

Many patients with "unexplained" menorrhagia can be successfully treated by natural means. Three effective treatments that are overlooked by most conventional doctors are vitamin A, iron, and thyroid hormone. Some natural treatments have also been shown to be effective in treating cervical dysplasia. These include vitamin A and folic acid.

Nutritional Supplements for Menorrhagia

Vitamin A

In a 1977 study from South Africa, vitamin A levels in the blood serum were significantly lower in 71 women with menorrhagia than in healthy women. Of those women, 40 were treated with vitamin A, 25,000 IU twice a day for 15 days. Menstruation returned to normal in 57.5% of the women, and an additional 35% experienced substantial improvement. Overall, 92.5% of the women who received vitamin A experienced either complete relief or significant improvement.[1] Since there was no control group in this study, some of the benefit may have been due to a placebo effect. However, many of our patients have appeared to benefit from vitamin A therapy, so we continue to recommend it.

It is not known exactly how vitamin A normalizes excessive menstrual flow. The beneficial effects may have something to do with estrogen levels, which were found to increase after vitamin A therapy.

We often advise our patients to take a therapeutic dose of vitamin A (such as 50,000 to 75,000 IU per day) for 6 weeks, rather than just 15 days, because we believe that building up tissue stores of vitamin A may produce a longer-lasting effect. In addition, we typically recommend maintenance doses of vitamin A (usually 10,000 to 25,000 IU per day) to help prevent a recurrence.

It should be noted that prolonged use of more

than 25,000 IU of vitamin A per day can cause toxic effects, and that taking more than 10,000 IU of vitamin A per day during pregnancy may increase the risk of birth defects. Vitamin A therapy should therefore be monitored by a health-care professional. Early-warning signs of vitamin A excess include fatigue, headache, joint pain, muscle aches, bone pain, and hair loss. These side effects disappear if the vitamin is discontinued.

Iron Therapy

ALTHOUGH we know that heavy menstrual bleeding can result in iron-deficiency anemia, few doctors are aware that iron deficiency is itself a cause of menorrhagia. A vicious cycle can develop, in which heavy bleeding results in iron deficiency, which, in turn, makes the bleeding even worse.

When the uterine lining sheds at the end of each cycle, exposed blood vessels begin to leak blood, resulting in the menstrual flow. Normally, this bleeding is halted by the contraction of uterine muscles, which clamp down on the bleeding vessels. Iron is a component of a key enzyme involved in muscle contraction. When iron supplies are inadequate, uterine-muscle contraction is impaired. As a result, the uterus of an iron-deficient woman may be unable to "clamp down" on excessive menstrual bleeding.

Several studies have shown that iron therapy often cures menorrhagia in women who have iron deficiency.[2, 3] However, higher-than-normal doses of iron may be necessary to restore body-iron reserves in a woman who is bleeding heavily. In some cases, iron must be given by injection to break the vicious cycle. Since large doses of iron can cause gastrointestinal side effects or other problems, iron therapy for a woman with menorrhagia should be monitored by a health-care practitioner.

Vitamin C and Flavonoids

IN a 1960 study, 16 women with menorrhagia were treated with vitamin C and citrus flavonoids (also known as "bioflavonoids"), 600 mg of each per day. During the first 3 months, 14 of the 16 women showed improvement, ranging from 50 to 100%.[4] Vitamin C and flavonoids are believed to help control excessive bleeding by improving the integrity of capillaries.

As with the vitamin A study described previously, it is possible that some of the improvement attributed to vitamin C and flavonoids was due to a placebo effect. Nevertheless, since these nutrients are safe, inexpensive, and beneficial to the body in a number of ways, it is reasonable to include vitamin C and flavonoids in any treatment plan for menorrhagia.

Hormone Therapy for Menorrhagia

MANY DIFFERENT TYPES of menstrual problems, including menorrhagia, can result from hypothyroidism (an underactive thyroid). Other symptoms of hypothyroidism include fatigue, depression, cold extremities, constipation, dry skin, and hair loss. Conventional doctors rely on blood tests to diagnose thyroid underactivity. However, many nutrition-oriented physicians have observed that these tests are unreliable (see chapter 4). In the 1970s, Dr. Broda Barnes popularized the still-controversial idea that individuals with signs and symptoms of hypothyroidism can often benefit from treatment with thyroid hormone, even if their blood tests are normal.[5] Other doctors have also reported that standard blood tests, including the more sensitive thyroid-stimulating-hormone (TSH) test, may fail to detect hypothyroidism in women with menstrual abnormalities.[6] In our experience, treatment with thyroid hormone (based on clinical evidence of hypothyroidism, despite normal blood tests) will sometimes provide relief for women with menorrhagia or other menstrual disorders.

Nutritional Supplements for Cervical Dysplasia

Antioxidant Vitamins

A NUMBER of studies suggest that women with cervical dysplasia may need additional amounts of antioxidant nutrients, including vitamin E, vitamin C, beta-carotene, and selenium. In one study, the concentrations of beta-carotene and vitamin E in blood plasma were significantly lower in women with cervical dysplasia than in healthy women. The levels of these nutrients decreased with increasing severity of the dysplasia.[7] Low levels of selenium have also been found in women with cervical dysplasia.[8] In another study, low levels of vitamin C in the diet were associated with an increased risk of cervical dysplasia.[9]

Although there is no direct proof that these deficiencies actually cause cervical dysplasia, there is ample evidence that each of these nutrients has an anti-cancer effect. We therefore advise women with cervical dysplasia to increase their intake of vitamin E, vitamin C, beta-carotene, and selenium.

Vitamin A

VITAMIN A promotes the health and integrity of many different tissues in the body, including the cervix. Vitamin A is also an important anti-cancer nutrient. Low dietary intake of vitamin A is associated with a nearly 3-fold increase in the risk of cervical dysplasia.[10] Although there have been no studies showing that vitamin A reverses cervical dysplasia, our clinical experience suggests that it can help. In more severe cases, Dr. Wright has injected vitamin A directly into cervical tissue, and has seen good results.

Folic Acid

PERHAPS the most important nutrient for women with cervical dysplasia is folic acid. Abnormal Pap smears are common among women who take oral contraceptives, which are known to deplete folic acid. In one study, 47 women with cervical dysplasia took 10 mg of folic acid per day or a placebo for 3 months. All of the women were on birth control pills both before and during the study. After treatment, Pap-smear results were significantly improved in the folic-acid group, but they were unchanged in the placebo group.[11] Our experience suggests that folic acid may also help improve Pap smears in women who are not taking birth control pills.

Folic acid also has been shown to have an intriguing relationship with the human papilloma virus (HPV), the virus that causes genital warts. Infection with HPV is known to increase a woman's risk of developing cervical dysplasia. However, the effect of this virus on a woman's cervix appears to depend on her folic-acid status. According to one study, women with HPV infection did not have an increased risk of cervical dysplasia if their folic-acid level was in the top 30 percentile (approximately the top one-third). However, HPV-infected women whose red-blood-cell folic-acid levels were lower than that were 5 times more likely than normal to have cervical dysplasia.[12] Although this study does not prove a cause-effect relationship, it suggests that maintaining adequate folic-acid levels may eliminate the capacity of HPV to promote cervical dysplasia.

Maintaining adequate folic-acid levels does not require massive doses of folic acid. Most women can probably achieve adequate folic-acid status by eating a few helpings of vegetables and taking a multiple vitamin every day. Women who already have cervical dysplasia might need larger amounts of folic acid. Because of potential interactions between vitamin B_{12} and folic acid, high-dose folic-acid therapy (more than 400 mcg per day) should be medically supervised.

Summary of Recommendations for Menorrhagia

NOTE: Treatment should be supervised by a doctor.

- Vitamin A, 50,000 to 75,000 IU per day for 15 to 30 days, then 10,000 to 25,000 IU per day for maintenance. (Warning: Supplementation with large doses of vitamin A during pregnancy may increase the risk of birth defects.)

- Iron supplements, if iron deficiency is present (dosage as recommended by a doctor).

- Vitamin C and citrus flavonoids, 500 to 1,000 mg of each per day.

- Thyroid hormone, in selected cases.

Summary of Recommendations for Cervical Dysplasia

NOTE: Treatment should be supervised by a doctor.

- Folic acid, 0.4 to 1.0 mg per day for prevention, 10 to 50 mg per day for treatment. Supplemental vitamin B_{12} may enhance the effect of folic acid. (Warning: Supplementing with more than 0.4 mg of folic acid per day can interfere with the laboratory diagnosis of vitamin B_{12} deficiency; doses of folic acid greater than 0.4 mg per day should therefore be supervised by a doctor.)

- Antioxidant nutrients: Vitamin A, beta-carotene, vitamin C, vitamin E, and selenium (dosages as recommended by a nutritionally oriented doctor).

- High-potency multiple vitamin and mineral (adjust doses of other nutrients as needed).

MIGRAINE HEADACHE

> ❧ MORE THAN 20% *of Americans experience migraine headaches at some time during their lives, with women being affected more often than men. Migraines are sometimes described as "sick headaches." They can cause intense and throbbing pain and are often associated with nausea, vomiting, diarrhea, visual changes (auras), and sensitivity to light.*
>
> *Despite decades of research, scientists still have an incomplete understanding of how and why people get migraines. Nor has conventional medicine found any consistently effective treatment. Although drugs such as beta-blockers and calcium-channel blockers may reduce the recurrence rate, they rarely eliminate migraines completely. In addition, these drugs have side effects. Sumatriptan (Imitrex), a drug which acts on specific serotonin receptors, can relieve acute migraines in many cases. However, sumatriptan is not only expensive, it also has been associated with serious and sometimes fatal cardiovascular side effects.*

DR. WRIGHT'S CASE STUDY

Shelley Richardson looked pale and weak. "I almost didn't come in today, this migraine is so bad," she said. "But then I thought, that's what I want to see you about, anyway, so I may as well come in. I suppose I could have taken a shot of that Imitrex stuff. It usually helps, but it costs about $36 a shot if I do it myself. And I get 2 or 3 migraines a week! Besides, I've been reading about natural medicine, and to change a quote a little, migraine headache isn't caused by an Imitrex deficiency."

I couldn't help but smile. "My apologies, a migraine headache isn't funny, but you're right. We definitely need to look for the causes of your migraines, and deal with them, so you won't get them in the first place. Before I start asking you a long list of questions, would you like to try a mineral and vitamin injection that frequently relieves migraine in a few minutes?"

"In a few minutes? Lead me to it!" She paused. "Are there side effects possible?"

"Practically none if the injection is given properly. Of course, it's possible to be allergic or sensitive to anything, so we'll make sure to screen you first."

Thirty minutes later we were back in my office. Her weakness and pallor had vanished. "I still can't believe it," she said. "Three minutes into that IV, I felt warm, and the pain started to fade. At 8 minutes—I was watching the clock—the headache was completely gone! The nurse said it doesn't work every single time, but it usually does, so she really enjoys giving those 'migraine IVs'. And she said the shot itself—needle, syringe, and contents—would cost me less than $5! The charge for her time is more than that."

"I'm glad it did the job. Now let's go over your health history."

"Before we do, tell me again what was in that shot. The nurse said magnesium and vitamin B_6. Is that all?"

"That's all. Magnesium appears to do most of the work in relieving migraine. Vitamin B_6 helps magnesium do its job. In general, relatively rapid intravenous injection of magnesium quickly re-regulates and relieves acute muscle contraction/relaxation disorders—for example, bronchial spasm in asthma, coronary-artery spasm in angina, esophagus spasm, back-muscle spasms, severe menstrual cramps, and migraine. And that's only part of the list."

"But magnesium and vitamin B_6 don't actually cure all these problems, do they?"

"Not by themselves, although they're part of the overall solution. I wish it were that simple, but we still need to look for the cause or causes of the problem. In all the problems I mentioned, including migraine, IV magnesium can relieve the acute situation. But what triggered that acute situation must still be found and dealt with. So back to your health history. How long have you had migraines?"

"Forever! I'm 29, and I started getting them the first year I had menstrual periods. That's 15 years of migraines now—more than half my life!"

"As far as you're aware, do you have allergies, or are there allergies in your family?"

"I have a light case of hay fever in the springtime, but what does that have to do with migraines? I have headaches all year 'round."

"Allergy, particularly food allergy, is the number one trigger for migraine. We'll make sure to screen you for allergy to foods, as well as allergy in general. But allergy certainly isn't the only possible trigger. Do you notice any relationship between migraines and your menstrual cycle?"

Ms. Richardson managed to look skeptical and amused at the same time. "You have to ask? Doesn't everybody notice that? Everybody female, that is? I always get my worst ones at the exact same time every month! I schedule my work and social life around them. A few years ago, I just started marking those days on my calendar in advance, so I wouldn't make any important plans. Especially plans involving men."

I smiled again. "Speaking of that, are you taking birth control pills?"

She grinned. "I must be a slow learner; I tried birth control pills twice, and both times I got some of the worst migraines ever. Nausea, vomiting, my head exploding, trips to the emergency room. I haven't gone near those things since I was 21. Don't get me wrong. I like guys, but there's no man in this world worth that kind of grief!"

"Do you smoke?"

"Never have."

"Do you wake up around 3 to 6 A.M. with migraines? Do you get them if you go too long without eating, or if you get very hungry?"

"I must say you're original—no one ever asked me those questions together before. Yes, to both. Sometimes I can just tell I'm going to get a bad one unless I get some food in me. But I never thought that was important, because other times I get them right after I eat, and sometimes they're not related to meal time at all."

I made some more notes. "Is anyone in your family diabetic?"

"Grandma, mother's mother, but she didn't get it until she was in her 70s. And she doesn't need insulin or anything."

"Combined with some of your symptoms, that makes hypoglycemia—low blood sugar—another thing we should screen you for. Low-blood-sugar episodes are another common trigger for migraines."

"That's what my chiropractor's been saying for years, but I haven't been able to get any of the dozens of doctors I've seen to pay any attention. The most any of them have said about it is that hypoglycemia's a rare condition. Then they tell me to take the pain pills."

"Does chiropractic treatment help?"

"Sometimes, especially if I've been working hard and not exercising, but other times it doesn't do a thing. I keep trying—my chiropractor listens to me. She's the one who told me to come here, too; it just took me awhile."

"You've tried biofeedback?"

"My chiropractor got me to do that right after the first time she saw me several years ago. The first 2 months, I thought it was the answer, the headaches practically went away, but then they came roaring back. I still get some help from the relaxation techniques I learned, but it mostly 'takes the edge off' rather than getting rid of them entirely." She looked wistful. "I met some people who got totally rid of their headaches that way."

"Don't give up yet." After we finished her health history and did her check-up, I wrote her a summary note that went as follows:

- Please have food allergy and sensitivity screening done.

- Also, screen for allergy and sensitivity to hormones, foods, and other possibilities.

- Please take desensitization for any allergies/ sensitivities that are found.

- Test for hypoglycemia (low blood sugar).

- After allergy/sensitivity screening and hypoglycemia test, please see nutritionist to make a diet plan.

- Use the following supplements for now (after screening them for allergy and sensitivity):

  ➤ magnesium (citrate), 200 mg, twice daily

  ➤ vitamin B$_6$, 200 mg, twice daily

  ➤ riboflavin (vitamin B$_2$), 200 mg, twice daily

  ➤ feverf ew, 2 capsules, twice daily

  ➤ hypoallergenic multiple vitamin-mineral

I gave her a copy of the note. She looked it over and sat back. "Well, mother always said life isn't easy. Are you sure I'm going to need to do all this stuff? How come I never heard of 99% of it before? All I'm ever told is 'we don't know what causes migraines dear, have some nice expensive Imitrex and go away'?"

"Expensive might have a little something to do with it," I observed. "Expensive and heavily advertised and promoted to doctors. Also, medical students are required to take courses in drugs and pharmacology, but they are rarely required to take any courses in nutrition and the uses of nutrients."

"I have some questions about these recommendations. What's the riboflavin for? And what's feverfew? Sounds like maybe an aspirin."

"Recently, researchers reported that large quantities of riboflavin—vitamin B$_2$—can prevent a significant proportion of migraines; better than half. Feverfew is an herb—a botanical that has also been found to prevent migraines."

"So what's this about screening them and the other supplements, if they're supposed to help relieve migraine? Could they cause migraines, too?"

"Anything you're allergic to can trigger a migraine—even if it's something that usually helps."

"OK." She got up to go. "If I can survive 15 years of migraines, I can do this."

Three months later, she was back. "If it weren't for the fact that I haven't had a migraine in 6 weeks, I'd forget this whole thing!" she declared. "Do you know how difficult it is to entirely eliminate almost half the foods I ordinarily eat, as well as all the sugar and refined carbohydrate? Not to mention taking all those desensitization drops 3 times a day, and 20 or so supplement capsules!"

"I'm glad you're feeling better," I said. "Haven't you been able to add some of the foods back to your diet yet? If you've been taking desensitization faithfully you should be able to."

"Yes, I have. It was the first 6 weeks that were really tough. It's easier to follow the diet program now, especially since I can tell the difference if I eat the wrong thing. And I can hardly believe that hormone desensitization. The first month, my regular monthly migraine was a lot less, and I haven't had one of those since. Some other things have happened, too. For the last few years I had sort of a nagging fatigue and that's disappeared.

I have no trouble getting to sleep. I've discovered that was mostly due to food allergy, too. And I can go a lot longer without eating, without worrying about getting a headache. My work output's much improved—it's easier to do a good job when my head isn't in the toilet! Even my social life's gotten better—although . . ." she grinned, ". . . with some men, a migraine would still come in handy every once in awhile!"

DR. GABY'S COMMENTARY

THE CONVENTIONAL APPROACH to preventing and treating migraines leaves a lot to be desired, in terms of both safety and effectiveness. Fortunately, a number of safe and effective treatments exist within the realm of natural medicine which can control and often cure migraines.

Dietary Considerations
The Role of Diet

FOR some patients, taking measures to control fluctuations in the blood-sugar level is all that is needed to eliminate migraines. Individuals with headaches caused by so-called "reactive hypoglycemia" usually improve when they remove all the refined sugar, caffeine, and alcohol from their diet; eat more frequently (such as 6 times a day); and increase their intake of complex carbohydrates and/or protein. As early as 1949, doctors at the University of Michigan Medical School described 11 patients with "hypoglycemic headaches" who improved after they changed their diet.[1] More recently, one holistic doctor wrote, "More than 90% of all teenage headaches [only some of these were migraines] will disappear within two weeks if they totally eliminate refined carbohydrates and caffeine from their diet."[2]

The Role of Food Allergy

FOOD allergy is an even more common migraine trigger than hypoglycemia. This observation has been made repeatedly in the medical literature for more than 60 years,[3] but for some unexplainable reason, the medical profession has largely ignored the allergy-migraine connection. Conventional doctors do prescribe a diet free of tyramine (a chemical found in chocolate, citrus fruits, some wines, and aged cheeses that may precipitate migraines), but avoiding tyramine-containing foods is helpful for only a small proportion of migraine patients.

On the other hand, an elimination diet designed to identify all offending foods is successful much more often. In a landmark 1979 study, British physician Ellen Grant treated 60 patients who had been suffering recurrent migraines for an average of 18 to 22 years.[4] For 5 days, each patient consumed only 2 "low risk" foods (usually lamb and pears) and drank only spring water. Each patient then tested 1 to 3 common foods per day, looking for reactions. Foods most frequently causing symptoms were wheat, orange, egg, tea, coffee, chocolate, milk, beef, corn, cane sugar, yeast, mushrooms, and peas. The average number of foods causing symptoms was 10 per patient. When the symptom-provoking foods were removed from the diet, all 60 patients improved. The number of headaches in the group fell from 402 to 6 per month, with 85% of the patients becoming headache free. Interestingly, all 15 patients who had had high blood pressure at the start of the study saw their blood pressure return to normal.

One of the elimination diets I have used to identify food allergies is presented in appendix A. Some doctors use other tests for allergy and sensitivity, as well as desensitization techniques. The reliability and effectiveness of some of these methods is controversial (see chapter 3 for additional discussion).

Nutritional Supplements
Magnesium Therapy

MAGNESIUM deficiency appears to be one of the factors that promotes migraines. Certain situations known to provoke migraine attacks (such as pregnancy, use of diuretics, and ingestion of alcohol) are also associated with a loss of magnesium. In addition, most drugs used to prevent or treat migraines have some of the same physiological effects as magnesium.

Magnesium levels have been shown to be low during a migraine attack. In one study, 41% of 32 patients with an acute migraine had low serum magnesium.[5] In another report, magnesium levels in the brain, measured by NMR spectroscopy, were significantly lower in patients during an acute migraine than in healthy individuals.

Magnesium has been used with some success, both to prevent and to treat migraines. One doctor has used magnesium to prevent migraines in more than 3,000 patients (almost all women), with a success rate of 80%. The usual dose was 200 mg per day.[6] In a double-blind study, 20 women who suffered from migraines around the time of menstruation received 360 mg of magnesium per day or a placebo, starting on the fifteenth day of the menstrual cycle and continuing until menstruation. After 2 months of treatment, the number of days on which headaches occurred was reduced in the magnesium group, but not in the placebo group.

The duration and intensity of migraines were also significantly lower in the magnesium group than in the placebo group.[7] The preventative effect of magnesium was confirmed in another double-blind study.[8] Although one group of researchers failed to find magnesium helpful, the criteria they used to label a patient "improved" were unusually strict. Some drugs that are *known* to be effective against migraines have also failed to show any benefit when those criteria were used.[9]

For the treatment of acute migraines, intravenous injections of magnesium have been reported to produce rapid and dramatic results. In one study, 40 patients with an acute migraine were given 1 gram of magnesium sulfate intravenously over a 5-minute period. Fifteen minutes after the infusion, 35 patients (87.5%) had at least a 50% reduction of pain and 9 patients (22.5%) experienced complete relief. In 21 of the 35 patients who improved, the beneficial effect of magnesium persisted for at least 24 hours.[10]

In my experience, a combination of magnesium, calcium, B-vitamins, and vitamin C given intravenously will often relieve a migraine attack within 1 or 2 minutes (see appendix B). Dr. Wright has seen good results using intravenous magnesium and vitamin B_6. Although magnesium appears to be the most important nutrient for knocking out an acute migraine, one of my patients has a better response when calcium is included in her injection.

Riboflavin

IN one study, 49 individuals with recurrent migraines were given 400 mg of riboflavin (vitamin B_2) daily for at least 3 months. The average number of migraine attacks fell by 67%, and migraine severity was reduced by 68%. One patient had to stop treatment because of stomach pains, but no other side effects were seen.[11] The beneficial effect of riboflavin was subsequently confirmed in a double-blind study.[12] It is not known how riboflavin prevents migraines. One theory is that migraine sufferers have a biochemical defect in energy production that might be corrected by taking riboflavin.

While riboflavin is generally considered nontoxic, there are no long-term studies demonstrating the safety of doses as large as 400 mg per day (an amount more than 200 times the Recommended Dietary Allowance). Therefore, we usually advise our patients to try reducing the dose of riboflavin after their migraines improve. We have found that some patients will obtain benefit from doses of nutrients that are lower than those used in research studies, particularly if they work on their diet and take other nutrients at the same time.

Herbal Therapy: Feverfew

FEVERFEW IS A medicinal herb that has a long history as a treatment for migraines and arthritis. In a survey of 270 individuals with migraines who had taken feverfew every day for prolonged periods of time, more than 70% believed the herb decreased the frequency and/or severity of their attacks. Seventeen of those who had seen a positive response to feverfew participated in a double-blind study, in which they were either continued on feverfew or given a placebo. Individuals taking the placebo became significantly worse, with increases in the frequency and severity of headaches, nausea, and vomiting. In contrast, those who continued on feverfew maintained their previous improvement.[13]

In another double-blind study, 59 patients with migraines were randomly assigned to receive 1 capsule of dried feverfew leaves per day or a placebo for 4 months. Each patient then received the alternate treatment for an additional 4 months. The number of migraine attacks was significantly reduced by 24% during the feverfew period, compared with the placebo period.[14]

Other Factors

OTHER FACTORS THAT may trigger or aggravate migraines include cigarette smoking, use of oral contraceptives, emotional stress, and spinal misalignments. In addition, excessive use of ergotamine (a drug used to treat acute migraines) may actually increase the recurrence rate of migraines.

Conclusion

NATURAL MEDICINE OFFERS many safe and effective alternatives for the treatment of this common and often disabling condition. At least two-thirds of our chronic migraine patients have found significant relief using the natural approach, and they are no longer dependent on potentially dangerous prescription medications. Even though conventional medicine continues to ignore these effective treatments, more and more practitioners are "jumping ship" from traditional medical approaches in search of safer and more effective remedies.

Summary of Recommendations for Treating Migraine Headaches

PRIMARY RECOMMENDATIONS:

- DIET
  ➤ Avoid refined sugar, caffeine, and alcohol. Work with food allergies.

  ➤ Avoid foods that contain tyramine, such as chocolate, citrus fruits, some wines, and aged cheeses.

- SUPPLEMENTS:

  ➤ Magnesium, 100 to 300 mg twice a day. For acute treatment, intravenous administration of magnesium (plus other nutrients including B-vitamins, vitamin C, and calcium) may be effective.

  ➤ Riboflavin, 100 to 400 mg per day.

  ➤ Feverfew, in selected cases; dosage varies according to the preparation used.

OTHER RECOMMENDATIONS:

- Avoid cigarettes and birth-control pills.

MULTIPLE SCLEROSIS

MULTIPLE SCLEROSIS (MS) *is one of the most common neurological conditions. The disease is so-named because of the presence of numerous sclerotic (hardened) lesions in certain areas of the brain or spinal cord. Examination of these lesions under the microscope reveals a loss of myelin, the fatty substance that forms a sheath around nerve cells.*

MS can cause a wide array of symptoms, depending on where in the brain and spinal cord the lesions occur. The most frequent symptoms include: numbness, impaired vision, loss of balance, weakness, bladder dysfunction, and psychological changes. In many cases, the symptoms remit and recur over a period of 20 to 30 years or more. However, in up to half of all cases, the disease steadily progresses, sometimes resulting in severe disability or death.

One of the tests used to diagnose MS is called an MRI (magnetic resonance imaging), which can detect lesions of the myelin sheath. However, MS is also diagnosed clinically (i.e., on the basis of symptoms and physical signs), because an MRI may fail to demonstrate any abnormalities early in the course of the disease.

Conventional medicine has little to offer patients with MS. In recent years, beta-interferon (an antiviral drug similar to the body's own interferon) has been shown to reduce the number of symptom recurrences of MS. However, the benefits of beta-interferon are modest at best. In addition, the drug is quite expensive and can cause side effects, including flu-like symptoms, muscle aches, and possibly seizures. For those reasons, many MS patients have chosen not to use this drug.

DR. WRIGHT'S CASE STUDY

"I know there's no cure for multiple sclerosis," Rachel Herndon said. "But I'm not going to give in. There's just got to be more I can do than that interferon stuff my friend tried. It made her so sick she had to quit. I know it's supposed to be 'natural', but most of what I've read about it doesn't look good to me. My mother's been coming here for natural-medicine advice for 20 years or so. She finally convinced me to do the same

thing. It's a little easier for her since she lives here. I live in El Paso."

"Are you here for long?"

"Three weeks. Visiting mom with the kids and checking in here."

"Should be enough time to get well started. Tell me about the multiple sclerosis."

"Looking back, I had the first symptoms when I was 28 or 29. Vague numbness and tingling, mostly in my legs, but some in my arms and hands. It came and went for no particular reason. The children were small, and I was busy, so I ignored it all until I was 33 and I had the first real problem symptom."

"What was that?"

"I'm told it's not unusual for MS—I had optic neuritis in my right eye. That was really scary—I couldn't see. They gave me really big doses of prednisone. It got mostly better, but my vision still isn't as good in that eye as it was before the first attack."

"Sorry to hear that. You're not still on prednisone, are you?"

"No, I've only agreed to use it twice—the second time when my eye was acting up again. From what I read, I decided I'd better save that treatment for really serious stuff, like rescuing my vision. I haven't taken prednisone for 4 years now."

"Good idea. What symptoms do you have now?"

"For the last year or so, it's been mostly my legs. I've had the usual numb areas—mostly in my legs but some in my arms, too. I can put up with those, but it's the weakness in my legs that's getting to me. Some days my muscles get so tired I really have to push myself to keep going."

"So what are you doing about it so far?"

"Coming here. In El Paso, they tell me it's that interferon or prednisone or just wait for the MS to get worse."

"Have you heard of Dr. Roy Swank's diet program for MS?"

"No. Is that something new?"

"It's been around since the 1940s. In the early 1990s, Dr. Swank published the results of a 40-year follow-up study. Individuals with MS who had followed his diet plan for 40 years were compared with individuals with MS who'd been offered the diet plan at roughly the same time, but hadn't followed it."

"What happened?"

"The large majority of those who'd followed Dr. Swank's program were still alive. The large majority of those who had had the opportunity, but hadn't done it, were no longer with us."

"Fairly clear results. Who is this Dr. Swank? Where do I find his book?"

"Dr. Roy Swank is Professor Emeritus and former Chair of the Department of Neurology at Oregon Health Sciences University. His book is in nearly every natural-food store."

"I'm surprised no one ever told me about him."

"Particularly when the basics of his plan are so popular today for other reasons. He advises very low saturated fat and relatively high quantities of unsaturated fats. Actually, that brings us to the next thing—supplements of unsaturated oils containing essential fatty acids. Studies have shown that adding these as supplements results in longer remissions of MS symptoms, and when symptoms do recur, they're not as bad."

"So specifically what should I do?"

"Temporarily, please use one tablespoonful of flaxseed oil twice daily, along with 400 IU of vitamin E. A longer-term recommendation will follow on the results of a blood test for red-cell-membrane fatty acids."

"Is that everything?"

"Not at all. In the 1930s, a prominent physician at the Mayo Clinic linked food allergy and MS. In the late 1940s and early 1950s, St. Joseph's hospital near here in Tacoma, Washington, had an entire treatment wing for MS patients run by Dr. Jonez. His program, mostly allergy testing and treatment, was so successful that people came from all over the U.S."

"What happened to his program?"

"Dr. Jonez died. Since the rest of the medical staff disliked his program, it was shut down, even though it was helping many people, not hurting anyone, and there wasn't a better alternative at that time. But the idea never died out. You'll find books about allergy and MS in libraries and natural-food stores."

"Food allergies don't cause MS, do they?"

"No, but controlling them certainly helps many people with MS feel better. I know many people who tell me the wrong food or foods brings back or worsens symptoms."

"Mother tells me I had mild eczema when I was 2 or 3. That's allergy-related, isn't it?"

"Yes. A history of allergy makes it more likely that allergy testing and treatment will be helpful for your MS symptoms. In addition to food allergy, there's another problem common to the majority of people with MS: poor digestion and assimilation of nutrients. Most have poor stomach function, with inadequate acid and pepsin production. Some have inadequate digestive enzymes, and quite a few have both."

"Is that why my mother takes those hydrochloric acid with pepsin capsules with her meals?"

"Yes, though she doesn't have MS. Many of us also develop that problem as part of getting older."

"It's certainly helped her feel stronger, along with those vitamin B$_{12}$ shots."

"Now that you mention those, since MS is a disease of the nervous system, and B-vitamins are crucial to nervous-system function, we have MS patients try a series of injections containing vitamin B$_{12}$, folic acid, and the rest of the B-complex. Most people with MS say they can tell a difference when they take the injections and when they don't."

"A series of injections? But I have to go back to El Paso eventually."

"No problem. B-vitamin injections are quite safe, and you'll learn to give them to yourself. And while we're on the topic of self-injections—years ago, a researcher found that injections of adenosine monophosphate improved many of the symptoms of MS. Two symptoms which improved significantly were bowel and bladder control, and fatigue."

"I'm certainly fatigued. So what's this adenosine whatever?"

"Adenosine monophosphate—AMP—is a molecule produced in every cell in our bodies. It turns into adenosine triphosphate or ATP—the 'energy molecule'. Apparently, those with MS can use a few additional molecules or more of AMP."

"No hazards?"

"Not when given IM—in the muscle. When it's given too rapidly intravenously, it can cause shortness of breath and even fainting."

"You sure I can give it to myself?"

"I've worked with dozens of individuals with MS who've given their own AMP shots. Most have reported increased energy, and none have had unwanted effects."

"OK. Now what about this thing about mercury in dental fillings that my mother keeps telling me about?"

"These days, there's absolutely no excuse for inserting a toxic material like mercury into our bodies permanently or semi-permanently and calling it health care. The continued use of mercury in dental amalgams is inexcusable—it's a political and legal maneuver. . . . But excuse me, that doesn't pertain particularly to you. Our problem is that we can't predict exactly which people will have considerable and noticeable improvement after removing their amalgams and those who won't notice anything right away but will have the long-term benefits of removing toxic waste from the body."

"My mother has a book by a Dr. Huggins . . ."

"Dr. Huggins is a dentist who's led the fight against the use of mercury in our bodies. He reports many cases of successful reversal of MS symptoms with mercury-amalgam removal."

"What have you observed?"

"A few people with MS have done much better after removal of mercury amalgams. A few haven't had any change, and most find it somewhat helpful. If you can afford it, I'd recommend it."

"I only have a few; they've been there since I was a teenager. As long as I'm going to do everything possible, I'll do that, too. Maybe I'll be one of the lucky ones."

"Make sure to find a dentist who knows how to determine what dental materials are safest for you. Here's a number to call to find one."

"Thank you. Let's see if I understand everything. Dr. Swank's diet combined with a food-allergy program after testing, flaxseed oil for now with vitamin E, testing for good digestion, vitamin B$_{12}$, folic acid, and B-complex injections, AMP injections, removing mercury amalgams . . . Wow, that's a lot to do. Some of it's got to help."

"That's not quite all. MS is classified as an autoimmune disease. We've found that levels of DHEA, an adrenal hormone, are frequently low in patients with MS and other autoimmune problems. Supplementing to bring DHEA levels back to normal is usually helpful in MS patients."

"I'll get that tested, too."

Since her first visit, I've spoken with Rachel Herndon by telephone once or twice a year. She reports that she's adopted all of the recommendations, and her leg weakness is nearly gone. We both know there's presently no cure for MS, but her symptoms have been well-controlled for the last 5 years.

DR. GABY'S COMMENTARY

A NUMBER OF NATURAL approaches have shown potential in treating MS. Of course, nothing works for all patients, particularly for a condition as complicated and poorly understood as MS. On the other hand, there have been many success stories using natural methods, and some individuals who started treatment early in the course of their disease have remained symptom-free for many years (and possibly permanently).

Dietary Considerations
Role of Allergy

EVIDENCE shows that MS is an autoimmune disease—a condition in which the immune system attacks its own tissues (in this case, the myelin sheath). Of the many different factors that contribute to autoimmune disease, allergy appears to be a relatively common (and frequently overlooked) cause. In a study of 15 patients with MS, symptoms were completely or partially controlled by avoiding allergenic foods, tobacco, or house dust.[1] In another study, 31% of 49 patients improved when they avoided foods to which they were found to be allergic. In those patients, reintroduction of offending foods frequently caused the symptoms to recur.[2]

Reports such as these, although encouraging, have been sporadic, and conventional doctors have ignored the possible connection between allergy and MS. Skeptics argue that, because the symptoms of MS fluctuate spontaneously and unpredictably, it is difficult to prove that any particular treatment actually caused an improvement. However, while it is true that we should view "anecdotal" evidence cautiously, some anecdotes are too convincing to be ignored by open-minded people.

For example, I once saw a young woman with a 9-month history of fairly constant numbness. The diagnosis of MS had been made on the basis of an abnormal MRI. The woman went on an allergy-elimination diet and, within 2 weeks, her numbness was gone. Retesting of foods implicated dairy products as the cause of her symptoms. Over the next 7 years, she remained symptom-free while avoiding milk products. During that time, on several occasions she tried to reintroduce milk into her diet. Each time, the numbness recurred within 24 hours.

Another woman in her late thirties had been diagnosed with MS by three different physicians at Johns Hopkins. Although her MRI was normal, her symptoms of numbness and blurred vision were considered classic for MS. She, too, became symptom-free on an allergy-elimination diet, and eventually identified sulfites (a group of commonly used food additives) as the major cause of her symptoms. Over the next 6 years, she remained well, except for the few occasions when she inadvertently ingested sulfite-containing foods.

The "Yeast Connection"

SOME doctors have suggested that MS may be triggered or aggravated by an allergic reaction to *Candida albicans,* the common yeast germ that often lives in the intestinal tract or vagina.[3] Although this theory has been rejected by most doctors, I believe it deserves a closer look. I have successfully used anti-yeast medication as the primary treatment for 3 patients who had definite or probable MS.

One patient was a male in his thirties who developed classic MS symptoms shortly after receiving a 30-day course of antibiotics for prostatitis. Since we know that certain antibiotics promote the growth of candida in the intestinal tract, I asked this patient to take nystatin, a medicine that kills yeast. After a brief period of time, his MS symptoms disappeared entirely. However, over the next 12 months, every time he tried to stop the nystatin, the symptoms would return within days. He was eventually able to discontinue the medication without experiencing a recurrence.

The Swank Diet

BETWEEN 1949 and 1984, Roy Swank, M.D., prescribed a low-fat diet for 150 patients with MS. Saturated fat was restricted to 20 grams per day or less, and margarine, hydrogenated oil, and shortenings were forbidden. The diet included cod-liver oil (5 grams per day) and vegetable oils high in polyunsaturated fatty acids (10 to 40 grams per day). Long-term follow-up showed that patients who closely adhered to the diet had significantly less neurological deterioration, compared with patients who did not comply. In addition, the death rate was considerably lower in those who followed the diet than in those who did not (31% vs. approximately 80%). The greatest benefit was seen among individuals who had minimal disability at the start of the study. In that group, about 95% of the patients showed little or no disease progression over a 30-year period.[4, 5]

Based on these impressive results, the Swank diet seems like a worthwhile approach for patients with chronic MS. It is important, however, to follow all of Swank's recommendations: i.e., restrict saturated fats, avoid specific fats, and consume cod-liver oil and polyunsaturated vegetable oils. It is likely that more than one component of the Swank diet program is helpful. For example, supplementing with polyunsaturated fat in the form of sunflower oil has been shown to prevent neurological deterioration in patients with MS.[6] Cod-liver oil is known to inhibit autoimmune processes in animals[7] and may, therefore, be helpful for individuals with MS. In addition, evidence shows that consuming a diet low in saturated fats and margarine may enhance the beneficial effects of these oils.

Nutritional Supplements

EVENING PRIMROSE OIL (EPO) has been proposed as a possible treatment for MS. This oil contains gamma-linolenic acid (GLA), a fatty acid that is manufactured in the body of healthy individuals, but which people with MS appear to have difficulty producing. In theory, GLA may help MS patients in 2 ways: by reducing the tendency of the immune system to attack the myelin, and by improving the integrity of myelin itself. In a small study, administering EPO plus the anti-inflammatory drug colchicine produced encouraging results.[8] However, in another report, EPO was ineffective.[9]

Some patients with MS have found that vitamin B_{12} injections improve their energy level and their overall feeling of well-being. In addition, several patients have shown an improvement in neurological function while receiving vitamin B_{12} shots.[10]

Other Treatments

A TIBETAN HERBAL formula known as Padma 28 has been reported to benefit nearly one-half of patients with MS. In a double-blind study, patients given Padma 28 noticed an improvement in general health, an increase in muscular strength, and/or a reduction in bladder dysfunction.[11] For reasons that are not clear, the Food and Drug Administration has prohibited the sale of Padma 28 in the United States. However, a similar product, called Adaptrin, is commercially available in this country.[12]

Adenosine monophosphate (also known as AMP) is a compound that occurs naturally in the body and has been used to treat viral infections and other conditions. In a 1953 study, 16 patients with severe disability resulting from long-standing MS received a series of AMP injections over a period of 6 to 10 months. Marked improvements were noted in the patients' endurance and in bladder dysfunction.[13] This study did not have a control group, so the possibility of placebo effects or spontaneous remissions cannot be ruled out. However, AMP therapy clearly warrants further investigation. As discussed in the chapter on herpes simplex, certain precautions should be followed when administering AMP injections.

Studies have shown that DHEA is helpful for patients with lupus, and some doctors have observed a beneficial effect of DHEA in treating other autoimmune diseases, including MS. Although there is little research on the use of DHEA as a treatment for MS, we consider it reasonable to supplement with small doses of this hormone if laboratory tests indicate a deficiency.

Conclusion

MULTIPLE SCLEROSIS IS a common and frequently serious neurological condition. When the disease is chronic and associated with significant disability, the best one can hope for is partial improvement. However, if treatment is begun early, complete relief of symptoms is sometimes possible. Avoiding allergenic foods and eradicating candida (when appropriate) may produce dramatic results. A fat-modified diet, as described by Swank, may greatly minimize long-term deterioration. Other natural remedies, as described above, are also worth considering.

Summary of Recommendations for Treating Multiple Sclerosis

- Work with food and environmental allergies.

- Swank Diet: Restrict saturated fat, margarine, and partially hydrogenated vegetable oil. Supplement with cod-liver oil, 5 grams (approximately 1 teaspoon) per day, plus sunflower oil, 10 to 40 grams (approximately 2 to 8 teaspoons) per day. Vitamin E, 400 IU per day, to "balance" the extra unsaturated fat.

- Anti-yeast medication, evening primrose oil, vitamin B_{12} injections, adenosine-monophosphate injections, and/or Padma 28 (Adaptrin), in selected cases.

- DHEA, with medical supervision, if levels are low.

Editor's Note: As we go to press, Dr. Wright, Dr. George Gillson and other physicians have been working with a transdermal histamine preparation—an updated version of a 1940s Mayo clinic-originated intravenous histamine treatment, created by Elaine DeLack, R.N. Although, preliminary findings are encouraging with symptom improvement in approximately 70% of individuals observed, further studies are needed. For more information, please contact the Professional Compounding Centers of America at (800) 331-2498 or the International Academy of Compounding Pharmacists at (800) 927-4227.

OSTEOARTHRITIS

OSTEOARTHRITIS (ALSO KNOWN *as degenerative arthritis or degenerative joint disease), is the most common form of arthritis, affecting more than 16 million Americans. This condition becomes more prevalent with advancing age. The joints most often involved are the fingers, knees, hips, and cervical or lumbar spine.*

The cause of osteoarthritis is not known. Although inflammation is present to some extent, it does not appear to be the main cause of joint damage. It is often assumed that osteoarthritis is caused by progressive wear and tear on the joints, resulting in damage to the cartilage. However, although cartilage damage is one of the hallmarks of osteoarthritis, heavy use of the joints does not necessarily cause problems. In fact, many former long-distance runners have perfectly normal hips and knees, while their more sedentary friends become plagued with degenerating joints.

Osteoarthritis differs from the other common form of joint disease, rheumatoid arthritis (see chapter on rheumatoid arthritis), in that it is not primarily caused by inflammation, does not usually lead to severe joint deformity, and does not affect tissues in the body other than the joints.

As with many degenerative diseases, conventional medicine focuses primarily on relieving symptoms, rather than addressing the cause of the problem. For many patients, anti-inflammatory drugs, such as aspirin, ibuprofen (Motrin, Advil), naproxen (Naprosyn), and piroxicam (Feldene) do relieve pain, swelling, and other symptoms, but they do not slow the rate of joint destruction. In fact, there is evidence that taking these drugs may even cause the joints to deteriorate faster.[1] Furthermore, anti-inflammatory drugs can cause bleeding peptic ulcers, and they may occasionally damage the liver or kidneys. Analgesic drugs such as acetaminophen (Tylenol) may relieve pain without risking further damage to the joints. However, repeated use of acetaminophen can also harm the liver.

DR. WRIGHT'S CASE STUDY

Harry Gustafson got up slowly from his waiting-room chair. Leaning on his cane, he walked slowly toward my office. "These knees slow me down a bit, but I'll get there," he remarked. Once seated, he looked at me expectantly.

"What can I do for you?"

"Dunno. My wife Sarah has been in to see you on and off for 2 or 3 years. She said if I don't want to have my knees replaced with plastic parts, I'd better get in here. Well, they aren't getting any better, that's for sure, so here I am."

"How long have your knees been a problem?"

"Going on 10 years, but only this bad for a couple years now."

"You've been to see a doctor?"

"Of course."

"What were you told?"

"It's degeneration, deterioration—a lot of people my age have it. Maybe part of it is my weight—I've always packed a few too many pounds. 'Course I don't think that explains the arthritis in my hands and neck; don't spend a lot of time standing on my head. Osteoarthritis— that's what they call it. Got it in the lower spine too, but definitely the worst is my knees."

"Besides hurting, do your knees stay swollen?"

"A little bit most of the time—sometimes pretty bad. The right's worse than the left, though."

"What sort of treatment were you given?"

"Doctor said there wasn't much but pain pills and aspirins, particularly when it swells. Other than that, nothing to do but surgery when it gets really bad. I took some physical therapy but it didn't help much."

"You were checked for rheumatoid arthritis?"

"Several times. The blood test always came up negative, but the X-rays showed the deterioration, so that's why they told me it was that degenerative type."

I made some notes. "Osteoarthritis, worst in the knees, but also in the hands and spine. Negative rheumatoid arthritis tests. X-rays show deterioration. Treatment—pain pills, aspirin, and wait for knee replacement surgery. That about it?"

"You've got it."

"Other health problems?"

"Not much that I know about. 'Course, I don't have the energy I think I should, but who does at my age? And Sarah says I'm getting more forgetful than I should."

I looked at his medical record. "Let's see, 1923, you'd be . . ."

"Seventy-two in just a few weeks. Figure I have a few good years left, at least. I'd like to do them without major surgery and with better knees, if I can. Right now, doesn't seem likely, though."

"Any family history of diabetes or other significant problems?"

Mr. Gustafson gave me a puzzled look. "Did Sarah tell you?"

"No. I've only asked her about her own blood relatives."

"Huh. Well, my mother got that 'old age' diabetes when she was just over 80, and my older sister had the same at 75, I think. One younger sister's been told she'd better watch it, she's 'borderline'. But how'd you know to ask about diabetes in my family?"

"Over the years, I've noticed some connection between osteoarthritis and 'maturity' (type 2) diabetes. Its certainly not 100% or even close, but it's higher than I'd expect by just random chance."

"OK."

"Other health problems in your family?"

"Yes. Several cases of cancer, and my grandfather on the other side had a heart attack. My kids are OK so far, and no problems with the grandkids except a few allergies."

I took the rest of his health history, then asked him to go to an exam room to check things over. As he'd said, his knees were slightly swollen—the right a bit worse than the left. There was considerable rough, irregular feeling, like a "grating" inside both knees when the kneecap was compressed, and when the knee flexed and extended. As with the swelling, the right was definitely worse than the left.

In addition, Mr. Gustafson had swelling and slight tenderness in several finger joints on both hands. His skin was slightly dry. He appeared to have a bit more gas than usual in the abdomen.

"So, is there anything I can do, Doc? Change my diet? Take any vitamins?"

I looked at my notes again. "Your diet appears fairly good."

"It ought to be. Since Sarah's been coming here, it's been nothing but healthy food—lots of fresh vegetables and fruits, hardly anything processed or canned, whole grains, and a lot more fish and chicken. She reads all the labels, nothing with sugar or chemicals. 'Course I have to admit she's really made a turnaround in her health with that and all the vitamins she's been taking. So she really didn't have a hard time getting me to come here."

"But you're not taking any vitamins yourself?"

"Some vitamin C now and again, but I didn't know if there were any vitamins that would help deteriorating joints. But Sarah asked at the health-food store, and they showed her some things. But since we're both fairly new at the vitamin game, I thought I'd ask you first."

I got out a notepad. "Not much question about the osteoarthritis, so you may as well get started on a few things."

"Hold on. Aren't you going to run some tests or something to find out what I need?"

"Sometimes that's very necessary, and there actually are a few things I think you need checked, but the osteoarthritis isn't one of them. It's obvious. Since there are several supplements which routinely help—sometimes quite a lot—you may as well get started. First is niacinamide. That's a form of vitamin B$_3$. Please obtain the 500-milligram capsules, and use 2 capsules, 3 times a day. Though it's very unlikely, if you have any queasiness or nausea, please stop for a few days, then resume at half the dose."

"What's it supposed to do?"

"The large majority of the time, take the pain and swelling away."

"Take the pain and swelling away? Why haven't I heard about this before?"

I sighed. "Likely the same reason most of us haven't heard about many effective nutrient and other natural therapies. It isn't patentable."

"That means it's not expensive, and no one can make a lot of money on it, right?"

"Right. In this case, excellent-quality niacinamide is available from a number of sources for less than $10 per bottle."

"And it really works?"

"It's been working for the large majority of folks with osteoarthritis in my practice since 1973. Actually, it's been working since the treatment was described by Dr. William Kaufman in 1949."

"1949?"

"That's right. One other thing—you likely won't notice any change for the first 3 weeks. After that it starts being noticeable."

"Three weeks is short enough if it does the job."

"Next, please get some glucosamine sulfate, also 500 milligrams, and take 1 tablet, 3 times a day. Glucosamine is a molecule naturally present in the body that serves as a building block for new joint cartilage. The amount of glucosamine in the body appears to either decrease with age or be used up more rapidly in elderly people. Taking glucosamine as a supplement hasn't been associated with side effects.

"Your skin is definitely a little on the dry side. Considering osteoarthritis and our northwest lack of sunshine, please get some cod-liver oil and take 1 tablespoon daily."

Mr. Gustafson laughed. "My Norwegian grandmother forced that stuff down all of us kids when we were small. Told us 'for your bones, for your teeth'. I hated it!"

"It comes in capsules now."

"No problem. I'll take it. I was just imagining her telling me 'I told you so, Harry!'"

"Lastly, and also to help the osteoarthritis, please get some vitamin E—600 to 800 IU total daily, and selenium, 300 micrograms daily. And to 'back all this up', a good general multiple vitamin-mineral." I finished writing the list and handed it to him.

"That's a lot of stuff there—niacinamide, glucosamine sulfate, cod-liver oil, vitamin E, selenium, and a multiple! But if it all helps . . ." He started to get up slowly to go.

"Very likely it will. But hold on. There is a test or two I'd recommend you get done."

"I thought you said I didn't need any tests for osteoarthritis."

"That's right, you don't. But remember you mentioned low energy and maybe a little forgetful? Those may be 'surface clues' to another problem that over half of us develop by age 65 or so—incomplete digestion of our food and poor assimilation of nutrients. Plainly speaking, the gastrointestinal tract simply gets 'worn out', and doesn't work as well anymore, so even if we eat the very best diet available, we don't derive as much nutrition from food as we did when we were younger. So, of course nothing in the body works as well as it should."

"That's what Sarah's problem was."

"Yes."

"And you think I might have that problem, too—as well as this arthritis?"

"There are enough indications to check for it."

"Let's do it. It sure did Sarah a lot of good."

By the fourth week, Mr. Gustafson reported a definite lessening of his arthritis symptoms, especially in his knees. By 4 months, he was walking around well without his cane, and the pain and swelling were gone. These symptoms have not returned in the 4 years to date. He reported that his wife was warning him against doing too much!

Like his wife, Mr. Gustafson was found to have a partial digestive failure. (The excess abdominal gas found at his examination was a strong clue.) With the help of digestive aids—hydrochloric acid-pepsin capsules, and pancreatic enzymes as well as B-vitamin injections, the nutritional deficiencies caused by this common problem of aging were mostly corrected. By 6 months, he reported that his energy levels were "distinctly improved," and his memory starting to get better.

DR. GABY'S COMMENTARY

THERE ARE SEVERAL safe and effective natural treatments for osteoarthritis. Unlike some anti-inflammatory drugs, natural treatments do not increase the rate of joint destruction. On the contrary, some may actually protect the joints from further damage.

The Role of Food Allergy

IN A SMALL proportion of the patients we see with osteoarthritis, food allergies contribute to their symptoms. With the help of a medically supervised elimination diet, followed by individual food challenges, the offending foods can usually be identified. If these foods are removed from the diet, the arthritis improves, sometimes dramatically.

One of the elimination diets I have used in my practice is presented in appendix A. Some doctors use other tests to identify allergenic foods. The reliability of some of these tests is controversial (see chapter 3 for additional discussion).

The class of foods known as the Nightshades (potato, tomato, eggplant, and bell pepper) also contributes to osteoarthritis in some individuals. The adverse effect of the Nightshade foods is usu-ally not due to an allergic reaction; rather, it is thought to be caused by a toxin called solanine.[2] Some people find that their osteoarthritis improves after they have avoided the Nightshade foods for several months. It should be noted that tobacco is also a member of the Nightshade family.

Nutritional Supplements
Niacinamide

ONE of the oldest and most successful treatments for osteoarthritis is vitamin B_3, in the form of niacinamide. Niacinamide therapy was first described by Dr. William Kaufman in the 1940s, and it has been used successfully by nutrition-oriented practitioners ever since. Kaufman treated 663 arthritic patients, some for as long as 20 years. In most patients, the range of motion of the joints improved, while pain and swelling gradually diminished. Patients usually noticed improvement after 3 to 4 weeks, and the improvement became even more pronounced with continued treatment. However, if patients discontinued niacinamide, their symptoms gradually returned.[3]

Anyone familiar with Kaufman's work realized

that niacinamide therapy showed great promise, because it appeared somehow to control (or even reverse) osteoarthritis, rather than merely relieve its symptoms. Furthermore, when used properly, niacinamide was extremely safe (especially when compared with many of the anti-inflammatory drugs that are in use today). However, except for a small group of doctors, the medical community has ignored this treatment for 50 years.

Until recently, no one even attempted to follow up on Kaufman's research. That changed in 1996, when Wayne Jonas, M.D., and his coworkers published the results of a carefully designed double-blind study. In that study, niacinamide (500 mg, 6 times per day) was found to be significantly more effective than a placebo, as determined by improvements in joint mobility and in the overall severity of arthritis.[4] Hopefully, that report will stimulate new interest in this simple and inexpensive therapy.

Although it is not known how niacinamide works, this vitamin is thought to improve somehow the metabolism of joint cartilage. Effective doses range from 1,000 to 3,000 mg per day. Niacinamide works best when taken in small, frequent doses. For example, 500 mg taken 4 times a day is more effective than 1,000 mg taken twice a day.[5] Kaufman often had his patients take 250 mg, 6 times a day.

Although Kaufman did not observe any significant side effects in his group of more than 600 patients, large doses of niacinamide can, on rare occasions, cause damage to the liver. Nausea and queasinesss are early warning signs of niacinamide-induced liver stress. If these symptoms occur, patients should discontinue treatment for several days and have a blood test for liver enzymes done. If the levels are normal, niacinamide may be resumed at a lower dose. Because of the small risk of liver damage, anyone using therapeutic doses of niacinamide should be monitored by a physician. Individuals taking more than 1,500 mg per day of niacinamide would be well advised to have a blood test for liver enzymes after 3 months of treatment and annually thereafter. If liver-enzyme levels are elevated, then the dose should be reduced. If this precaution is kept in mind, niacinamide is remarkably free of side effects. We have not seen anyone develop significant or permanent liver damage while taking niacinamide. However, if you have liver disease, you should not try this treatment.

Glucosamine Sulfate

ANOTHER effective remedy for osteoarthritis is glucosamine (usually administered in the form of glucosamine sulfate), a compound that occurs naturally in the body. Glucosamine is one of the building blocks of joint cartilage, and it has been shown to prevent the degeneration of joint tissue. Because of these 2 actions, glucosamine seems like an ideal agent for preserving and repairing joints.

In one double-blind study, 20 patients with osteoarthritis of the knee received glucosamine sulfate, 500 mg, 3 times a day, or a placebo for 6 to 8 weeks. Glucosamine sulfate was significantly more effective than the placebo at relieving pain, joint tenderness, and swelling. The results were rated as "excellent" in all 10 patients receiving glucosamine sulfate, whereas all 10 patients receiving the placebo rated the results as "fair" or "poor."[6] A larger double-blind study of 252 patients also found glucosamine sulfate to be effective; however, that study lasted only 4 weeks.[7]

In a separate double-blind study, 40 patients with osteoarthritis of the knee received glucosamine sulfate, 500 mg, 3 times a day, or 1.2 grams per day of ibuprofen (an anti-inflammatory drug) for 8 weeks. Although the rate of improvement (as determined by a reduction in pain) was slower in the glucosamine-sulfate group, the improvement in that group increased as the study progressed. By the eighth week, glucosamine sulfate was significantly more effective than ibuprofen.[8] The slow but progressive improvement obtained with glucosamine sulfate suggests that this compound promotes healing of joints, rather than merely relieving symptoms. That possibility is supported by observations from one study, in which biopsies of osteoarthritic knees taken before and after 30 days of glucosamine-sulfate therapy revealed that degenerating tissue had been replaced by more healthy looking joint cartilage.[9] Evidently, the commonly held belief that osteoarthritis is an irreversible disease is wrong.

No significant side effects were seen in any of the studies that used glucosamine sulfate. Despite the similar names, glucosamine does not contain any glucose, and there is no evidence that it causes problems in diabetics.

Glucosamine/Niacinamide Combination

So far, there have been no studies to determine whether the combination of glucosamine and niacinamide works better than either compound alone. Since it is not known how niacinamide works, one can only speculate on whether niacinamide would add to, or merely duplicate, the effects of glucosamine on joint tissue. We do know from clinical observations and a few scientific studies that the benefits of niacinamide are not limited to the joints. Some of our patients who have taken niacinamide for osteoarthritis have reported that their mood, energy level, and overall well-being also improved. One of my patients, who was in her 60s, returned after 6 weeks of niacinamide therapy and remarked, "I feel like I'm 16 again." Those kinds of improvements do not typically occur with glucosamine. Although additional research is needed, we see no reason at this time why glucosamine and niacinamide cannot be used in combination.

Chondroitin Sulfate

ANOTHER naturally occurring compound that is being used to treat osteoarthritis is chondroitin sulfate. This large and complex molecule is a component of joint cartilage. The body manufactures chondroitin sulfate, using glucosamine as one of its building blocks. In a 3-month, double-blind study, chondroitin sulfate (1,200 mg per day) was significantly more effective than a placebo at relieving the symptoms of osteoarthritis.[10] Moreover, the benefits of chondroitin sulfate became more pronounced with time. In a separate 1-year, double-blind study of patients with osteoarthritis of the knee, supplementing with 800 mg per day of chondroitin sulfate significantly reduced pain, improved overall joint mobility, and appeared to slow the degeneration of joint cartilage.[11] Improvement was evident after 3 months of treatment, and it became more marked after 12 months. Another study also showed that administering chondroitin sulfate may help prevent further joint damage in individuals with osteoarthritis.[12]

Some doctors recommend the combination of glucosamine and chondroitin sulfate to treat osteoarthritis. Others argue that taking chondroitin sulfate is just an expensive way to obtain glucosamine. These doctors believe that chondroitin sulfate is broken down by the digestive enzymes into glucosamine, then reassembled in the joints into chondroitin sulfate. The question of whether orally administered chondroitin sulfate can be absorbed intact is still being debated, although there is some evidence that it can.[13] Also, it is not known whether combination therapy is more effective than glucosamine or chondroitin sulfate alone. It is possible that chondroitin sulfate confers certain benefits that are not obtainable with glucosamine. We usually recommend glucosamine sulfate for our patients, without the addition of chondroitin sulfate. However, we have no objection if someone wants to use the more expensive combination treatment.

Vitamin E and Selenium

VITAMIN E has a mild anti-inflammatory effect, similar to that of aspirin-like drugs. Although vitamin E is not nearly as strong as aspirin and related drugs, it also doesn't produce any of the side effects associated with these drugs. In a study performed in Israel, 29 patients with osteoarthritis were given 600 IU of vitamin E per day for 10 days and a placebo for an additional 10 days. Pain relief was reported by 52% of the patients during vitamin E supplementation, compared with only 4% during the placebo period.[14] Because this study was single-blind (i.e., the researchers, but not the patients, knew which treatment was being given), it is possible that the investigators might have unconsciously influenced the patients' perception of pain. Nevertheless, vitamin E is safe, and it exerts a wide array of beneficial effects in the body. Therefore, we believe that it is reasonable to recommend vitamin E as part of the overall treatment of osteoarthritis.

The trace mineral selenium is often used in combination with vitamin E, because it appears to enhance the effectiveness of the latter. Selenium supplements have been found in some,[15] but not all,[16] studies to relieve the symptoms of rheumatoid arthritis, but it is not known whether selenium is of any value in the treatment of osteoarthritis.

S-adenosylmethionine (SAMe)

THIS compound, which occurs naturally in the human body, has been shown in numerous studies to be effective for osteoarthritis.[17, 18, 19] Used in Europe for more than a decade, SAMe has only recently become available in the United States. Although SAMe itself appears to be quite safe, the purity of many of the products sold in this country has been questioned.[20] Crystalline SAMe degrades rapidly upon exposure to heat and/or moisture, and some of the imported raw material has been said to be partially decomposed upon arrival. Therefore, it may be preferable to use the pharmaceutical-grade finished product that is imported in tablet form from Europe, rather than other preparations that are currently being sold in the United States. Although we do not have any clinical experience with SAMe, the published research demonstrating its effectiveness has been impressive. However, this compound is quite expensive, particularly the tablets that are im-ported from Europe (this product has been chemically stabilized so it does not decompose rapidly).

Conclusion

OVERALL, THE NATURAL approach to osteoarthritis is successful at least 75% of the time and is remarkably free of side effects. Natural medicine can relieve symptoms at least as effectively as conventional drugs. In addition, unlike drug therapy, the natural approach may prevent the progression of the disease, and in some patients may even reverse it.

Summary of Recommendations for Treating Osteoarthritis

PRIMARY RECOMMENDATIONS:

- Diet: Work with food allergies. Consider a several-month trial of avoiding Nightshades (potato, tomato, eggplant, bell pepper, tobacco).

- Niacinamide, up to 3,000 mg per day, taken in 3 to 6 divided doses. Because of a small risk of liver toxicity, niacinamide therapy must be monitored by a physician.

- Glucosamine sulfate, 500 mg, 3 times a day. May use in combination with chondroitin sulfate, 800 to 1,200 mg per day.

OTHER RECOMMENDATIONS:

- Vitamin E, 400 to 800 IU per day.

- Selenium, 100 to 200 mcg per day.

- Vitamin C, 500 to 1,000 mg, 2 times a day (to strengthen connective tissue).

- Multiple vitamin/mineral (adjust doses of other nutrients according to the amounts in the multiple).

- S-adenosylmethionine (SAMe), 400 to 600 mg per day, in selected cases, with medical super vision.

OSTEOPOROSIS

OSTEOPOROSIS IS DEFINED as thin or porous bones. It is a major epidemic, affecting as many as 30% of postmenopausal women and about 5% of men in the United States. More than 1.2 million fractures (primarily of the hip, spine, or wrist) occur each year as a direct result of osteoporosis. Conventional therapy, which consists mainly of calcium supplements, estrogen, and exercise, does not reverse or even fully prevent osteoporosis; it merely slows down the rate at which bone loss occurs. In addition, estrogenic drugs such as Premarin are not without risk, as underscored by recent studies showing higher rates of breast and ovarian cancer in estrogen users. Newer treatments such as calcitonin and alendronate (Fosamax) have shown some benefit, but the long-term safety of these drugs has not been demonstrated.

DR. WRIGHT'S CASE STUDY

Mary Hallgren looked happy. As she sat down, she handed me some papers—the reports from her recent bone-density test. "Three percent overall improvement in just one year!" she said. "And at my age, too, after getting worse on every previous test! Don't say you can't teach an old lady like me new tricks!"

I opened her record and pretended to search. "And you're looking awfully good for a 99-year-old."

"You know darn well I'm only 63," she said. "But I expect you to help me make it to 99 or past there." She thought for a moment. "You know, my golf score has improved this year, too."

"Good. Before I go over a new test development with you, . . . let's review everything you're doing already. Obviously, you must be doing things right or your bone density wouldn't have improved like that, but still . . ."

"That's what I'm here for—to stay on track. I brought my list with me so we can go through it together. Here's a copy."

"Thank you. Let's see . . ." I read through her general diet plan. "Good. I see you've really increased the proportions of vegetables and fruits, and cut back the animal protein and grains."

"You know, I was so surprised when you told me I was overdoing those grain products! 'Specially since I was using whole grains—wheat, rye, rice, and oats. I thought they were really good for me and Jack, and that we could eat as much as we wanted—as long as we watched our weight, of course. I remember what you said: excessive intake of grains—even whole grains— and animal protein leads our bodies to lose calcium, even if we're taking a big calcium supplement, whereas vegetables and fruits help our bodies retain calcium. So you can see I've made sure more than half our diet is vegetables and fruits. And no milk or dairy in our house anyway. Every once in a while I cheat when we're out, though." She smiled a sly smile.

"You mean you're not absolutely perfect?" I asked. "I have that problem, too. Well, come as close to it as you can."

"You know, it still amazes my friends that I have osteoporosis, and I don't drink any milk or eat dairy."

"Amaze them some more with that 3% increase in bone density," I said. "Cow's milk is for . . ."

"Little cows. I know, I know. You've mentioned that a few dozen times, at least."

"As I said, 'I'm not perfect', but I'm glad I got the point across."

I looked back at her list. "Good. You're using 4 to 6, 10-grain betaine hydrochloride capsules with every meal, depending on size. Digestive enzymes after meals."

"You know, it seems every woman I've met at this clinic who's being treated for osteoporosis is taking those same digestive aids. Isn't anyone's stomach or digestion normal anymore?"

"Women with osteoporosis almost always have significant underproduction of hydrochloric acid and pepsin. I can remember only 2 patients in the last 10 years with osteoporosis and perfectly normal stomach and digestive function."

"Sort of makes sense. I've read that many minerals, not just calcium, aren't separated out from the food as well if the digestion isn't functioning well. So there wouldn't be as much calcium and other minerals available to keep the bones in good repair."

"That's so. And even supplementing with hydrochloric acid and pepsin and other digestive enzymes doesn't do as well as a fully functional, normal digestive system. But it's better than letting it go. You're still taking your B_{12} and folate injections?"

She made a face. "Oh yes, about once a week. I get tired more easily if I don't. You know, I was reading recently about homo—what's it called?"

"Homocysteine?"

"That's it, homocysteine. The newspaper said blood levels of homocysteine go up after menopause, and it causes bone loss and atherosclerosis. It also said that folate, vitamin B_6, and vitamin B_{12} bring homocysteine levels back down again."

"Glad it made the newspapers," I grumbled. "That's only been known for a few decades now. The homocysteine story originated with a professor at Harvard—Dr. Kilmer McCully—in the late 1960s! I suppose that's progress, though. It took us only 2 or 3 generations of doctors to learn to wash our hands. Now, let's check your calcium numbers."

I added up her calcium. "Let's see—600 milligrams from the 'bone-building formula', slightly over 1,000 milligrams from hydroxyapatite and other sources, and a total close to 1,700 milligrams daily. And a total of about 500 milligrams of magnesium. Looks like enough."

"I guess so. My bones are getting better. And I'm so glad all those other bone-building nutrients come in one formula—to 'back up' the calcium. Magnesium, manganese, zinc, copper, silicon, boron, strontium, vitamin K, vitamin D—I can't remember them all. I can't imagine having to find all of those nutrients individually, but I've read they're all necessary for strong, healthy bones."

"That's right. The details are all in Dr. Gaby's book *Preventing and Reversing Osteoporosis.*"

"I got that one as soon as you told me. It's a terrific book!"

"Now, let's review your hormone program."

"I'm taking them all—the triple-estrogen, progesterone, testosterone, and DHEA."

"Let's see—you're using 2.5 milligrams of the triple-estrogen."

"In a cycle, like you said. It sure feels better in my head than that Premarin I took years ago. Don't know how to explain it, it just feels right."

"It should. Triple-estrogen contains the same estrogen molecules—in approximately the same proportions—as those found in women's bodies from the onset of menstruation until menopause. Just doesn't make sense to put a horse's estrogen—which has a different molecular structure—into a human, just because her own estrogen has dropped off."

"Makes sense if you're a drug company, I guess."

"Now about progesterone . . ."

"I decided to continue using the progesterone cream that I'd found just before I came in here. It helps with vaginal dryness, too. I might as well put it there as in my stomach. But I asked your nurse to write me a prescription so I'd get a standard strength and no chemical preservatives."

"And the DHEA and testosterone?"

"I was a little nervous about that testosterone until you explained there's a normal level produced by women's ovaries, as well as estrogens and progesterone. And testosterone is a major bone and muscle builder! So the nurse and I did several of those testosterone and DHEA tests until we got just the right dosage for me. I'm really glad the price has come way down on those tests lately, even though the 24-hour urine collection is more of a nuisance.

"Also, I've been reading up on DHEA a lot lately. Looks like it not only helps regain bone like you said, but it can improve my immune system, cut my risk of cancer, and maybe help me make it to 99."

"That's right. I'm glad you got that, too." I scanned through her list once more. "Looks like everything. Now tell me what you're doing for exercise."

"Never did like exercise just for the sake of exercise," she said. "So I started a major re-landscaping project at my place. I'm doing almost all of it myself, and it'll take me another 2 or 3 years to finish. When the weather's just too bad, I tackle all the heavy housekeeping that I don't usually do like washing walls and so on. Jack says he's never seen anything like it. I've got him exercising right along with me. The house looks terrific, and he's had to take me golfing more often, just to get away from the house and yard."

I looked up from her paperwork. "Was that part of the heavy housework plan?"

She smiled slyly again. "Don't tell Jack."

"I'll leave that to you." I closed her folder. "Before you go, there's a new test I'd like to tell you about. It provides a way of keeping track of your bone health in between those bone-density tests, which are done only once every year or 2, since bone density changes very slowly. This new test allows us to measure bone loss as often as we want, with much less expense, and no radiation at all."

"Why haven't I done this one before?"

"Just released, literally days ago. It's called NTx, and is done with a urine specimen. It measures a very specific type of collagen that comes only from bone."

"So the more there is in the urine, the more bone is being lost?"

"Exactly. So we can tell if a program is working to stop bone loss."

"Doesn't tell you if bone is being rebuilt?"

"No, we still need a test for that which would show changes more rapidly than the bone-density test. However, it's a very reasonable inference that if a first test shows considerable bone loss, and later tests show a decline to a minimum—hopefully no more than a young woman loses—and you're doing everything else right . . ."

"That I might regain bone." She looked puzzled. "But I already have. Will this test do me any good anymore?"

I smiled at her. "Remember you told me you weren't absolutely perfect about your program at all times? Well . . ."

She flashed her sly smile back. "So doing this test every so often might motivate me just a little more toward perfection?"

"I hope so."

She got up to go. "You can keep that test report," she said. "I've got my own. Framed! See you next year!"

DR. GABY'S COMMENTARY

NEW APPROACHES ARE needed if we are to have a greater impact on the osteoporosis epidemic. Fortunately, research into natural alternatives has given us new ideas and new hope. Osteoporosis no longer looks like an irreversible disease, an inevitable consequence of aging. It now appears that bone loss is not only preventable, but reversible, as well. We have seen a number of patients who showed increases in bone mineral density (indicating an improvement in their osteoporosis) after undertaking a natural approach.

As with other chronic illnesses, a comprehensive treatment plan is likely to work better than any single therapy alone. In the case of osteoporosis, important factors include a good diet, regular exercise, nutritional supplements, hormone therapy when appropriate, and avoiding certain environmental toxins.

Dietary Considerations

AN OSTEOPOROSIS-PREVENTION diet should be low in refined sugar, caffeine, and alcohol, each of which has been shown to promote the loss of calcium from bones. Excessive intake of animal protein may also cause the body to lose calcium. Although it is not clear exactly how much animal protein is "too much," I advise some of my osteoporosis patients to limit their total intake of meat, chicken, fish, and eggs to 4 helpings per week. On the other hand, protein deficiency may also result in bone loss,[1] so moderation is important where protein intake is concerned.

Milk is frequently promoted as being a bone-building food because of its high-calcium content. However, in a 12-year study of 77,761 women, those who drank more than 14 glasses of milk per week had 45% more hip fractures, compared with women who consumed 1 glass per week or less.[2] Moreover, in certain areas of the world where dairy products are not consumed, osteoporosis is uncommon. Although these studies do not prove that drinking milk worsens bone health, they also do not support the notion that consuming more dairy products will help solve the osteoporosis epidemic. Considering the other potential problems associated with ingesting dairy products (see chapter 1), we often encourage our patients to obtain their calcium from other sources, such as dark green vegetables (except spinach), whole grains, beans, and calcium supplements.

Soybeans contain two isoflavones, genistein and daidzein, that appear to have beneficial effects on bone. Administering either of these compounds[3] or a soy-based diet[4] to rats partially prevented the loss of bone resulting from surgical removal of the ovaries. Preliminary studies in humans also suggest that ingesting soy products may help prevent osteoporosis.[5]

Nutritional Supplements

THE IMPORTANCE OF calcium for healthy bones is well known. Numerous double-blind studies have shown that supplementing with calcium slows the rate of bone loss in postmenopausal women. Most doctors recommend a total daily calcium intake (from diet and supplements) of 1,200 to 1,500 mg. Major dietary sources of calcium include dairy products, sardines and salmon (canned with bones), green leafy vegetables, beans and nuts. However, as the typical American diet provides only about 400 to 800 mg of calcium per day, it appears that many individuals could benefit from taking a calcium supplement.

Calcium supplements are available in many different forms. Calcium carbonate is often used, because it is inexpensive and contains a larger amount of calcium per tablet, compared with other forms of calcium. For example, 1 gram of calcium carbonate provides about 400 mg of calcium, whereas 1 gram of calcium citrate provides only about 210 mg of calcium. However, if stomach-acid production is low (see chapter 2), a common problem among individuals with osteoporosis, the absorption of calcium carbonate is poor, while the absorption of calcium citrate is normal. A nutritionally oriented doctor can help you determine which type of calcium supplement might be best for you.

While calcium is important, it is not the only nutrient needed to maintain healthy bones, and it may not even be the most important one. A number of other vitamins and minerals, including vitamin K, magnesium, manganese, boron, strontium, silicon, zinc, copper, folic acid, vitamin B_6, and vitamin C, play a role in osteoporosis prevention. Many of these nutrients are in short supply in the American diet, as a result of food processing, modern farming methods, and unwise food choices. A growing body of research suggests that each of these nutrients must be present in adequate amounts if bone loss is to be prevented effectively.

Vitamin K

VITAMIN K is required to manufacture osteocalcin, a unique protein found in bone that attracts calcium to bone tissue. Without adequate vitamin K, normal bone mineralization is impaired. Vitamin K deficiency is common in individuals with osteoporosis,[6] and supplementing with vitamin K has been shown to reduce calcium loss from the body.[7] In a study of 72,327 women, low intake of vitamin K was associated with an increased risk of hip fracture.[8] The best dietary sources of vitamin K are green vegetables.

Magnesium

IN a small study from Israel, 16 of 19 women with osteoporosis had laboratory evidence of magnesium deficiency. In each of these women, bone biopsies revealed abnormal bone mineral crystals. On the other hand, the 3 osteoporotic women with normal magnesium levels each had normal crystal formation.[9] This study suggests that magnesium deficiency is common in women with osteoporosis and may result in abnormal mineralization of bone, possibly rendering bones more susceptible to fracture. In another study, 32 postmenopausal women took 250 to 750 mg of magnesium per day for 2 years. Bone mineral density increased by 1 to 8% in nearly 75% of cases.[10] These results with magnesium therapy are remarkable, because women typically lose bone at a rate of 3 to 8% per year around the time of menopause.

Manganese

MODERN farming techniques and food processing have reduced the quantity of the trace mineral manganese in the American diet. Manganese deficiency produces osteoporosis in animals, and blood manganese levels are often below normal in women with osteoporosis. In the 1970s, NBA basketball star Bill Walton had repeatedly been suffering fractures, one of which was refusing to heal. A medical evaluation showed that he had osteoporosis, a surprising finding in a young male athlete. Blood tests revealed undetectable levels of manganese, as well as deficiencies of a few other minerals. After receiving a supplement containing these minerals, he recovered rapidly, and he had no further problems during his basketball career.[11]

Folic Acid

FOLIC acid prevents the buildup of a compound call homocysteine, which is thought to be one of the triggering factors for osteoporosis. Folic-acid requirements seem to increase around the time of menopause (the same time that bone loss accelerates), and supplementation may become necessary at that time.[12]

Boron

EVIDENCE shows that boron may enhance the production of compounds that are related to bone health, including estrogen, testosterone, DHEA, and vitamin D. In a study of postmenopausal women who were fed a boron-deficient diet, supplementing with boron increased blood levels of estrogen and reduced calcium losses.[13] While the capacity of boron to increase estrogen levels might raise concerns about possible cancer risks, there is no evidence that populations with a high intake of boron (such as the French) have an increased incidence of hormone-related cancers. Boron is found in fruits, vegetables, and nuts.

Hormone Therapy

THE OVARY MANUFACTURES 4 hormone: estrogen, progesterone, dehydroepiandrosterone (DHEA), and testosterone. At the time of menopause, a deficiency of any of these hormones can occur. Evidence suggests that each of the 4 ovarian hormones plays a role in osteoporosis prevention, and that combination therapy may be more effective—as well as safer—than taking estrogen alone.

Estrogen

CONVENTIONAL estrogen-replacement therapy (ERT) reduces the incidence of fractures by 50%, but may increase the risk of gallbladder disease, blood clots, and some cancers. Some natural-medicine doctors have been taking a different approach to ERT—using a combination of the 3 estrogens that occur naturally in the human body, rather than using Premarin (horse estrogens) or pure estradiol (one of the 3 estrogens). The rationale for using this approach is explained in chapter 4. The most commonly prescribed "natural estrogen" formula, known as "triple-estrogen," was developed in the early 1980s by Dr. Wright. It contains 80% estriol, 10% estrone, and 10% estradiol. Triple-estrogen is generally effective against hot flashes and other menopausal symptoms, and it appears to cause fewer side effectsthan Premarin. However, there have been no studies on the long-term safety of triple-estrogen or on

whether it can prevent osteoporosis. Triple-estrogen is available by prescription through compounding pharmacists.

Progesterone

PROGESTINS (progesterone-like compounds, such as Provera) are frequently prescribed along with estrogen to prevent the uterine-cancer-promoting effect of estrogen. However, progestins are not the same as the natural progesterone manufactured by the ovary. Natural progesterone is not only much safer than progestins, but possibly more effective against osteoporosis. John Lee, M.D., a pioneer in natural-progesterone therapy, reported that administering progesterone as a skin cream almost invariably increased bone density and prevented fractures in women with osteoporosis.[14] Lee also recommended dietary modifications, various nutritional supplements, and an exercise program, so the benefits he found were probably not entirely due to progesterone. In addition, because there was no control group in Lee's study, the results are difficult to evaluate. A double-blind study published just as this book went to press has failed to demonstrate a bone-building effect of progesterone.[15] Therefore, the effectiveness of this hormone against osteoporosis is now in doubt. However, some practitioners of natural medicine have observed that taking both progesterone and a "bone building" nutritional supplement has a greater effect on bone density than taking either treatment by itself.

It must be pointed out that the amount of natural progesterone found in some over-the-counter skin creams is not enough to prevent the uterine-cancer-promoting effect of Premarin. Therefore, it could be dangerous to switch on your own from a progestin to natural progesterone, while continuing your estrogen preparation. On the other hand, a larger dose of natural progesterone (available by prescription) can be used as a safer alternative to progestins. A physician trained in natural medicine can help you decide whether a natural-hormone regimen is appropriate for you.

Testosterone and DHEA

ALTHOUGH testosterone and DHEA are considered androgens ("male hormones"), they are both produced by the ovaries. Both of these hormones are considered "bone builders," in that they stimulate the formation of new bone. DHEA levels (measured as DHEA-sulfate) are frequently low in postmenopausal women, whereas testosterone deficiency is common only in women whose ovaries have been surgically removed.

When androgen deficiency is identified, supplementing with the appropriate hormone(s) will sometimes relieve menopausal hot flashes, fatigue, and depression as well as improving libido and immune-system function. According to some studies, supplementation will also delay the aging process and help prevent cancer. The potential to improve bone density is an added benefit of these hormones.

One recent study shows that supplementing with DHEA does increase bone mineral density in postmenopausal women.[16] However, the amount of DHEA used in that study (300 to 500 mg per day) was much larger than what would be considered normal "replacement therapy." While there have been no studies showing that "physiologic" doses (such as 5 to 25 mg per day for women) will increase bone density, we have seen such a benefit in a few of our patients.

In males, testosterone levels tend to decline with advancing age, and this decline appears to be a risk factor for the development of bone loss. In one study, supplementing testosterone-deficient men with testosterone for 18 months resulted in a significant 5% increase in bone mineral density (measured at the lumbar spine).[17] Other studies have also shown a beneficial effect of testosterone on bone.[18]

Because of the potential for testosterone to cause side effects, it should be prescribed by a physician who is experienced in its use.

Ipriflavone

A SEMI-SYNTHETIC flavonoid known as ipriflavone has recently been found to be helpful in the treatment of osteoporosis. Ipriflavone is metabolized in the body into daidzein, one of the osteoporosis-preventing compounds found in soy. Numerous studies have shown that supplementing with ipriflavone (200 mg, 3 times per day) can prevent bone loss in postmenopausal women.[19, 20, 21] Because ipriflavone appears to be quite safe, it may be a viable alternative to some of the drugs currently being used to treat osteoporosis.

Ipriflavone inhibits an enzyme (cytochrome P450) that breaks down certain drugs. Therefore, this compound could potentially interact with other medications. For example, treatment with ipriflavone has been shown to increase blood levels of the asthma drug theophylline.[22] For this reason, the use of ipriflavone should be supervised by a doctor.

Effect of Pollution

TOXIC METALS, SUCH as aluminum, lead, cadmium, and tin, are widely distributed in the environment. Animal studies have shown that each of these metals can cause osteoporosis. It is possible that the increased incidence of osteoporosis over the past 40 years is due in part to the proliferation of toxins in our environment.

Some simple steps can be taken to reduce your exposure to toxic metals. Drinking bottled water eliminates one of the major sources of aluminum and lead—the municipal water supply. Many municipalities add aluminum salts to the reservoirs as a means of reducing particulate matter in the water. In addition, a study by the U.S. Environmental Protection Agency revealed excessive concentrations of lead in the water supply of 130 cities, including Boston, New York, Philadelphia, Washington, Seattle, San Francisco, and Phoenix.[23] To reduce your aluminum exposure further, do not use aluminum cookware or drink beverages stored in aluminum cans (which leach aluminum into the beverage). Additionally, wrap your food in something other than aluminum foil. If you avoid foods packaged in tin cans, you will greatly reduce your exposure to tin. If you must use such foods, do not let the food sit in the can after it has been opened, because exposure to air increases the rate at which the tin migrates into the food.

Conclusion

MOST DOCTORS BELIEVE osteoporosis cannot be prevented; that the best we can hope for is to slow down the inevitable loss of bone that occurs with age. However, if one follows a comprehensive approach as outlined above, osteoporosis appears to be both preventable and reversible. A more detailed discussion of the natural approach to osteoporosis can be found in my 1994 book, *Preventing and Reversing Osteoporosis* (Prima Publishing, Rocklin, CA).

Summary of Recommendations for Treating Osteoporosis

DIET AND LIFESTYLE:

- Avoid refined sugar and caffeine.
- Avoid excessive intake of alcohol and animal protein.
- Use soy products.
- Do not smoke cigarettes.
- Exercise 3 to 5 times per week, particularly weight-bearing exercise such as walking or jogging.
- Reduce exposure to toxic metals.

SUPPLEMENTS:

- Calcium, 600 to 1,200 mg per day.
- Magnesium, 200 to 600 mg per day.
- Manganese, 5 to 20 mg per day.
- Vitamin K, 100 to 500 mcg per day.
- Silicon, 1 to 2 mg per day.
- Boron, 1 to 3 mg per day.
- Strontium, 0.5 to 3 mg per day.
- Vitamin D, 200 to 800 IU per day.
- Multiple vitamin/mineral that provides zinc, copper, folic acid, and vitamin B_6. Adjust doses of other nutrients as needed.
- Ipriflavone, 200 mg, 3 times per day, in selected cases.

HORMONE THERAPY:

- Estrogen, progesterone, DHEA, and/or testosterone, in selected cases.

ULCERATION OF THE *stomach or duodenum—commonly known as peptic ulcer—is a major problem in industrialized nations, affecting 10 to 15% of men and 4 to 15% of women at least once in their lives. It is estimated that more than 8 million work-days are lost each year in the United States due to peptic ulcer, and more than 80,000 ulcer patients are chronically disabled.*

Conventional treatment for peptic ulcer includes avoiding caffeine, alcohol, and cigarettes, decreasing stress levels, and taking medication. Taking drugs that reduce stomach-acid secretion usually relieves pain and aids in healing, but the drugs do not prevent recurrences. In fact, when individuals discontinue the use of acid-blocking drugs such as Tagamet, Zantac, or Pepcid, they may experience a "rebound" effect, making it more likely that the ulcer will come back. In addition, because stomach acid is needed for the absorption of many nutrients, long-term use of these drugs can lead to malnutrition.

While antacids may also relieve symptoms, the presence of aluminum in many antacids is cause for concern. The long-held scientific belief that the body does not absorb aluminum has turned out to be incorrect. Carefully performed studies have revealed that ingesting aluminum-containing antacids increases the level of aluminum in both brain and bone tissue,[1] and could therefore promote the development of Alzheimer's disease and osteoporosis, respectively.[2]

*New research has shown that some individuals with peptic ulcer have a bacterial infection (*Helicobacter pylori*) in their stomach or duodenal lining. This organism can be eradicated by a combination of bismuth (Pepto-Bismol) and antibiotics, and such treatment can promote ulcer healing and prevent recurrences. H. pylori can be identified by a standard blood test, which determines who is likely to benefit from the bismuth/antibiotic treatment.*

DR. WRIGHT'S CASE STUDY

Peter Shaughnessy came in clutching his stomach. "I know it's important not to eat before a check-up and blood tests," he said. "But I don't know if I can last. This ulcer hurts when there's nothing in my stomach."

"We can always reschedule any tests that require fasting," I said. "Or cover things as rapidly as we can, now."

"Let's do that. It's settling down—but it comes and goes. It's tough to get time away from the job, anyway. So what do we do?"

"Tell me about the ulcer. How long has it been a problem, what sort of tests have been done, and what sort of treatment have you had?"

"It goes back years, at least 20. I'm in stocks, bonds, and commodities, it's an occupational hazard. My wife keeps telling me to quit, and get another job. But I'm pretty good at what I do, and would need to start from zero anywhere else. So I just put up with it most of the time, and these days just see doctors when it gets really bad."

I looked at his record. "So this must have started when you were . . ."

"Twenty-four—2 years out of college, and 2 years into the brokerage. I had X-rays taken, and they told me it was a peptic ulcer. The guys at work told me, 'welcome to the club.'"

"What treatment did you use?"

"I've used practically everything they have over the years. At that time it was bland diet and antacids. I should have bought stock in an antacid company back then, I've certainly been keeping them in business. As soon as those acid-blocking drugs were available, they put me on those. I've had 'em all—Tagamet, Zantac, Prilosec—I can't remember which ones I used at which time."

"Those drugs cause malnutrition better than anything else I know, besides simply not eating," I remarked.

"That's what my wife says, too. She reads your stuff, and she reads health magazines. She's why I'm here. She says over 20 years of on-and-off ulcer trouble is way too much, and if I won't quit the job, then I have to come here."

"Only married a few years?"

"Five. How did you know?"

"It's a pattern I've heard before. I assume you've had X-rays more than once?"

"Oh yes, several times over the years. Also, that 'scope thing, gastroscope twice, and a whole raft of blood tests. They never find anything besides the peptic ulcer. Sometimes they haven't found that, but the symptoms are so typical they give me the treatment anyway."

"Have you been tested for helicobacter?"

"You mean that bacterial infection thing that's supposed to be the cause of a lot of peptic ulcers?"

"That's the one."

"The last couple of times I was checked—a few months back and about 4 years ago. Both times they couldn't find it. The last time, they tried me on that Pepto-Bismol and antibiotic treatment anyway, but it didn't seem to help. So they're back to recommending I take those acid-blocker drugs every day like I did for years before I met my wife. Once she pointed it out to me, I had to admit that they really did drain my energy."

"Has she got you off caffeine yet?"

He groaned. "Yes! A broker without coffee! Not only that, she's slowly worked me off sugar, and she manages to limit my alcohol to 1 or 2 drinks on weekends or special occasions. She's got a way of doing that."

"Smart woman. Sugar, caffeine, and alcohol all contribute to peptic ulcer."

"I have to admit I've been better since we've been married and she's been watching things."

"You're not a smoker?"

"That's one occupational vice I never took up."

"Good thing. Tobacco smoking really contributes to peptic ulcer, too."

"I was better—not cured—but definitely better for quite awhile there. But a few months ago, it really started to come back. That's when she started her campaign for me to quit the job or come over here. She figures that all those years of poor diet, antacids, and acid-blocking drugs have left me depleted in all kinds of nutrients. She said I should get over here and find out which ones. She even told me that, based on her reading, my stomach might be low—rather than high—on hydrochloric acid and pepsin."

"After 20 years of chronic peptic ulcer, she might be right. But we can't even begin to address that issue until the ulcer is very well healed. Another thing: as far as you're aware, have you ever had any food allergies or other allergies?"

"Not as far as I know."

"Anyone in your family have allergies?"

"My grandmother, but that's all I know about."

We finished his health history and went to the exam room for his check-up. Aside from signs of chronic fatigue and tenderness over the expected area of the stomach, things appeared physically normal.

"So what do I do now?"

"There are a few tests that would be useful. Your wife's right—we should check for minerals, vitamins, and amino acids because of all those years you took those acid-blocking drugs. As I mentioned before, I've observed they're a major cause of malnutrition. We also should check for intestinal microflora—normal and abnormal bacteria and so on. They're important to the health of the intestinal tract and in fact the whole body. Unfortunately, both acid-blocking drugs and antibiotics can really make a mess of them.

"So far, these tests are mostly to look for the consequences of the ulcer and the treatments you've tried—some of which may impair healing now. Also, even though you have no history of it, please get screened for food allergy. It's possible for allergy to be a direct cause of peptic ulcer, and we don't want to overlook a possible cause."

"Do I need more X-rays or scope exams?"

"No, you've had enough of those."

"Anything I can start on?" He put his hand over his stomach again. "I think I need something soon."

"Well, you could start on some licorice."

"Did you say licorice? You're not serious!"

"In fact, I am. Research has shown that licorice is just as effective as acid-blocking drugs in helping peptic ulcers to heal, and even more effective at preventing relapse. But to be on the safe side, please get a particular type, deglycyrrhizinated licorice. For a very few people, the glycyrrhizin naturally present in licorice can raise the blood pressure, and lower the body's potassium level."

"Are you sure? All these years I've been paying $80 to $100 or more per bottle of acid-blocking drugs, and I could have been eating licorice? You sure there isn't a mistake somewhere?"

I smiled. "I could tell you volumes about mistakes in health care—using costly, toxic, patented medicines or even surgery, when safe, inexpensive diet adjustment, nutrients, and other natural treatments would do as well or better. But we'd better stick with your problem. There's no mistake. Dozens of people have told me how much licorice has helped their peptic ulcers. Please chew and swallow two of the deglycyrrhizinated-licorice tablets at least 3 to 4 times daily, in between meals."

"They really work?"

"They really work. But the licorice isn't all. I'll write the list for you. First, zinc—30 milligrams, twice daily, in the form of zinc picolinate or zinc citrate. Take this one with food—a few folks say it irritates an empty stomach. Zinc is well known to help ulcers heal anywhere they occur. Make sure to take 4 milligrams of copper from copper sebacate at a different time of day, to make sure that no problems arise from zinc/copper imbalance."

"What kind of problems?"

"If they happen at all, they take months, but if copper levels are too low, extra zinc can raise total cholesterol, lower HDL-cholesterol, and even in rare instances cause heart-rhythm disturbances. Unless you know for sure that your copper levels are OK, it's wisest to use a bit of copper as 'insurance' when taking extra zinc.

"Next, vitamin A. Vitamin A promotes healing of all the cells that line the gastrointestinal tract. Until you're better, 50,000 IU daily. Make sure it's vitamin A, not beta-carotene.

"Also, please use 1 gram of glutamine, twice daily for now. Glutamine is the principal energy source for the cells lining the upper part of the intestinal tract. Years ago, Professor Shive demonstrated that glutamine helps heal peptic ulcers.

"Also, add in vitamin C, 1 gram twice daily. Extra vitamin C is another nutrient important to healing. Make sure to find a 'buffered' type, which has less chance of irritating your stomach. Lastly, a high-strength multiple vitamin-mineral with at least 50 milligrams of vitamin B_6."

Mr. Shaughnessy took the list. "That's a lot of

stuff, but my wife said it would be if I was to heal this thing once and for all. I assume there'll be other recommendations as my tests come in."

"Especially after all those years on acid-blocking drugs. Even though your wife did her best with helping you change your diet, it's not a surprise that the ulcer has had a hard time healing. . . . And speaking of that, please check with the nurse for 2 or 3 shots of vitamin B_{12} and folate over the next 2 to 3 weeks. Absorption of these nutrients is specifically impaired by acid-blocking drugs, and is often poor in a malfunctioning stomach, which you likely have. And these two vitamins are key—along with zinc—in helping the formation of new cells by stimulating DNA production."

Mr. Shaughnessy got up to go. "Sounds like I'm going to be the healthiest stock and bond broker I know! Well, I'm going home to tell my wife that I'm going to do all this to the letter, and hang on to my job. Maybe I'll feel so good I can work twice as hard—as long as I get home from the office on time, of course!"

In 3 months, Mr. Shaughnessy's peptic-ulcer pain was entirely gone. By his own description, he'd become "a licorice junkie" as he'd found it immediately helpful for his ulcer. Six years later, his peptic ulcer has not returned.

DR. GABY'S COMMENTARY

DESPITE THE MEDICAL advances in the treatment of peptic ulcer, millions of Americans continue to suffer from this problem. Fortunately, there are a number of safe natural treatments that show great promise.

Dietary Considerations
The Role of Food Allergy

As with many other chronic illnesses, food allergy appears to be a significant factor in some individuals with peptic ulcer. We have seen a number of patients whose ulcers did not heal properly and whose pain did not subside until they stopped eating foods to which they were allergic. One doctor has pointed out that the tissue changes that are characteristic of peptic ulcer closely resemble those resulting from the Arthus reaction, a type of allergic reaction.[3]

In a study of 12 individuals with both peptic ulcer and respiratory allergies, all 12 were able to control their ulcer symptoms and prevent recurrences by avoiding allergenic foods.[4]

Herbal Supplements
Licorice Extract

PERHAPS the most effective natural remedy for peptic ulcer is an extract of licorice. Herbalists have long known about the ulcer-healing properties of licorice. However, the use of licorice for this purpose was limited by concerns about potential side effects. Licorice contains a compound called glycyrrhizin, which has properties similar to those of cortisone. In large doses, glycyrrhizin can cause high blood pressure, potassium deficiency, and heart problems.

Fortunately, scientists discovered a way to remove about 97% of the glycyrrhizin from licorice without destroying its anti-ulcer effects. This licorice extract, known as deglycyrrhizinated licorice (DGL), has been shown to be quite effective as a treatment for both gastric[5] and duodenal[6] ulcer. In fact, this herbal extract works as well as the acid-blocking drugs Tagamet and Zantac,[7] while causing considerably fewer side effects. Moreover, DGL is a lot less expensive than prescription anti-ulcer drugs. DGL works by improving the health of the mucus-secreting "goblet cells" that line the stomach and duodenum and protect these tissues from damage. In contrast to most conventional treatments, DGL does not shut off or neutralize stomach acid and therefore does not promote malnutrition. In addition, because DGL works in a completely different way than acid-blockers, when necessary, these treatments can be combined to produce an effect greater than either one alone can achieve. DGL is also helpful for individuals who experience gastric upset from anti-inflammatory drugs.

DGL is available in 380-mg chewable tablets. For the treatment of peptic ulcer, we usually recommend chewing 2 tablets, 3 times a day, 20 minutes before meals. For maintenance, or to prevent side effects of anti-inflammatory drugs, 1 tablet 2 or 3 times a day, is usually sufficient. Chewing the tablets, rather than swallowing them whole, appears to enhance the effectiveness of the treatment, possibly by increasing the amount of DGL that comes in contact with stomach and duodenal tissue.

Nutritional Supplements
Glutamine

GLUTAMINE is an amino acid that is found naturally in the body and in food. Glutamine helps improve the integrity of gastrointestinal tissues. In one study, supplementing with glutamine reduced the incidence of stomach ulcers in rats treated with aspirin.[8] In a double-blind study published in 1957, 7 patients with peptic ulcer received 1.6 grams of glutamine per day, while 14 others were given a placebo. After 4 weeks, the ulcer had healed in all 7 patients receiving glutamine, compared to healing in only half of those given the placebo.[9] Unfortunately, this small, preliminary study has never been repeated, so glutamine is not a well-documented treatment for peptic ulcer. Nevertheless, since this amino acid is nontoxic and inexpensive, we usually recommend it as part of a comprehensive ulcer-healing program.

Zinc

SINCE it helps promote tissue healing, zinc may be helpful as a treatment for peptic ulcer. In animals subjected to various stresses or toxic substances, the development of peptic ulcers was inhibited by supplementing with zinc.[10, 11] In a double-blind study, 15 individuals with stomach ulcers were given either zinc or a placebo for 3 weeks. The ulcers healed about 3 times as fast in the zinc group as in the placebo group.[12] A few milligrams of copper should be used in conjunction with zinc, since copper has ulcer-healing properties of its own,[13] and zinc supplements increase the need for copper.

Vitamin A

VITAMIN A is known to promote the health of epithelial tissues, which include the cells that line the stomach and duodenum. When ulcers were induced in rats by subjecting them to stress, treatment with vitamin A significantly reduced the size of the ulcers.[14] Similar results have been found in humans. Stomach ulcers are a common occurrence following severe physical trauma, such as major burns or serious injuries. Vitamin A levels usually decline in response to severe stress, and this decline may play a role in the increased susceptibility of trauma victims to gastric ulceration. In one study, 52 trauma patients were divided into 2 groups, one of which received intramuscular injections of vitamin A. Ulcers developed in 18% of the patients treated with vitamin A, compared with 63% of those not given the vitamin.[15]

Other Nutrients

OTHER studies have shown that blood levels of vitamins C, E, and B$_6$ are often low in individuals with a peptic ulcer. Each of these nutrients helps promote tissue healing and each is therefore recommended as part of a comprehensive ulcer-healing program. We generally prefer buffered vitamin C, such as calcium ascorbate or sodium ascorbate, since ascorbic acid is mildly acidic and may cause irritation in ulcer patients.

Peptic Ulcer and Helicobacter: A "New" Natural Treatment?

HELICOBACTER PYLORI was first identified as a cause of peptic ulcers by Dr. Barry Marshall of Australia. Despite initial skepticism by the medical community, infection with *H. pylori* is now considered to be a major factor in ulcer disease. Conventional treatment of *H. pylori*-associated peptic ulcer includes an "acid-blocker" (such as Zantac, Pepcid, or Prevacid) and antibiotics (such as metronidazole plus tetracycline, or amoxicillin). While this treatment can eradicate helicobacter, it often causes undesirable effects, and it may result in significant disruption of normal intestinal flora.

Mastic gum is a resinous extract from the tree *Pistacia lentiscus,* that has recently been found to kill *H. pylori* in the test tube.[16] In a double-blind study, 20 patients with duodenal ulcers took 1 gram of mastic powder once a day before breakfast for 2 weeks, while another 18 patients received a placebo (lactose). Endoscopic examination showed ulcer healing in 70% of those taking mastic, compared with only 22% of those taking the placebo.[17] In another study, 6 individuals with gastric ulcers took 1 gram of mastic powder twice a day for 4 weeks. Complete relief of symptoms occurred in all patients after an average of 1 week, and the ulcers healed in 5 of the 6 patients after 4 weeks.[18]

Mastic has no significant side effects. The Ministry of Agriculture (United Kingdom) has stated that mastic is safe for use as a flavoring in foods, chewing gum, and "breath sweeteners." It is also traditionally used in dentistry. Mastic became available in the United States in 1999, and Dr. Wright has just started to use it for patients. Preliminary reports of its effectiveness are encouraging.

Vitamin C has also been shown to be effective against *H. pylori*. In one study, supplementing with vitamin C (5 grams per day in divided doses) eradicated *H. pylori* infection in 30% of 27 patients with chronic gastritis.[19] Additional research is needed to determine whether a higher dose of vitamin C would produce a greater success rate; however, this preliminary study suggests that high-dose vitamin C might be an effective treatment for peptic ulcer that is caused by *H. pylori*. Of course, buffered vitamin C would probably be better tolerated than ascorbic acid by patients with active peptic ulcers.

Conclusion

ALTHOUGH ADVANCES HAVE been made in the conventional treatment of peptic ulcer, natural alternatives are still the safest—and often the most effective—treatments available. A combination of dietary modification, stress reduction, and appropriate nutritional and herbal supplements will often eliminate the need for potentially dangerous drugs and surgery.

Summary of Recommendations for Treating Peptic Ulcer

- Diet and Lifestyle: Avoid refined sugar, caffeine, alcohol, and tobacco. Participate in a stress-reduction or relaxation program. Work with food allergies in selected cases.

- Deglycyrrhizinated licorice (DGL): Chew 2 tablets, 380 mg each, 3 to 4 times per day, 20 minutes before meals. Reduce dose as improvement occurs.

- Glutamine, 500 to 1,000 mg, 2 to 3 times a day.

- Zinc (picolinate or citrate), 30 mg, 1 to 2 times per day. Balance with copper, 2 to 4 mg per day.

- Vitamin C (buffered), 500 to 1,000 mg, 2 to 3 times per day.

- Vitamin E, 400 IU per day.

- Vitamin A, 10,000 to 25,000 IU per day, or as recommended by a doctor.

- High-potency B-complex vitamin.

- High-potency multiple vitamin/mineral (adjust doses of other nutrients as needed).

- For possible eradication of *Helicobacter pylori,* mastic or high-dose vitamin C, as prescribed by a doctor.

PREGNANCY *(preventing and treating toxemia)*

🌿 TOXEMIA OF PREGNANCY *(also known as preeclampsia or, in its more severe form, eclampsia) occurs in some women during the late stages of pregnancy. The condition is characterized by high blood pressure, edema (fluid retention), and protein in the urine. If not adequately controlled, preeclampsia can progress to epileptic seizures and threaten the health and life of both mother and child.*

The conventional approach to severe toxemia is to hospitalize the patient and treat her with intravenous infusions of large doses of magnesium. While that treatment is helpful, it is not without risk.

DR. WRIGHT'S CASE STUDY

Alice Higgenbotham arrived with her grand-daughter. "I know it's short notice and you haven't seen Cindy before, but your nurse said it was OK. It's really urgent. She's 7½ months pregnant, and they want to give her diuretics because her blood pressure's starting to go up, and her ankles are swelling. They're calling it preeclampsia, which is the same thing as early toxemia, isn't it? I've read both your books. In one of them, you helped that Barbara Morton, so I got Cindy tickets. She lives in Pittsburgh." She paused for breath.

"That's a long way to come," I said. "Barbara Morton—that book was published in 1979!"

"The doctors in Pittsburgh still haven't read it," Alice declared. "At least not the ones Cindy was seeing. So I convinced her and her mother to start her on vitamin B₆ and magnesium . . ."

"And when that did more good than anything else, I agreed with Gram to come out here," Cindy said.

"Glad you're here. What's happened with the vitamin B₆ and magnesium so far?"

"Well, I only took 50 milligrams of the B₆ a day, because my doctor said it might not be safe. I took 200 milligrams of magnesium. But I lost 4½ pounds in one week, and I can see my ankle bones a little better."

"That's a start. Did Grandma tell you about eating more protein?"

"Yeah, and I've been trying. But Sam—that's my husband—he's been off work, and we couldn't afford much, and Mom can't help . . ."

"Which is another reason Cindy's going to stay with me until this is entirely straightened out," Alice said. "Now, can you give Cindy those IVs you wrote about—the ones with magnesium and vitamin B₆?"

"Very shortly," I said "But I need a little health history first, and we need to check Cindy's blood pressure, weight, and have a urinalysis done."

"My doctor in Pittsburgh says there's protein in my urine," Cindy reported.

Cindy was 23. Her blood pressure was 160/105, she was 5' 5", and she weighed 181. Her urinalysis showed "2+" protein. "You have more than just a little problem," I said to Cindy. "But it's very likely you can reverse it entirely. We're going to put some amino acids in your IV, along with the magnesium and vitamin B6. Please stop by a natural-food store on your way home and get a bottle of predigested protein. Make sure to use 10 grams twice daily for now, along with eating extra protein. Raise the vitamin B6 to 200 milligrams twice daily, and the magnesium to 300 milligrams twice daily. These can all be reduced as you do better." I wrote this all on a note and gave it to her. "Oh, and make sure to get a good prenatal vitamin/mineral if you don't have one already."

Cindy looked even more tired the next day. "I couldn't believe how many times I was up to the bathroom," she said. "And the nurse said I've lost 6 pounds, and my blood pressure's dropped 10 points already!"

"What did I tell you, Cindy?" Alice said. "Just like that Barbara Morton!" She turned to me. "You didn't give Barbara Morton another IV, but Cindy's a little worse. Could you give her one more?"

I laughed. "What a memory. If we all had grandmothers like you, we wouldn't need as many doctors!"

"Might be better off, too," Alice grumbled.

"But you're right. I had planned one more IV—a little less this time. That should do it, as long as Cindy sticks to her program."

"I will," Cindy said. "Gram's already making me lists of foods for when I get home. I'm going to start eating more eggs. Gram says they're cheap protein and really complete nourishment."

"Of course—everything is in there that is needed to grow a baby chicken if the egg was fertilized, so it ought to be good for growing a baby. And this whole eggs-and-cholesterol thing is way overrated," Alice said.

Cindy lost 4 more pounds after her second (and last) IV. By the time Alice let her go home

3 weeks later, her blood pressure was 132/80, her weight 162, she had no more edema fluid, and the protein was gone from her urine. We subsequently received a picture of Cindy with her baby, and a note saying she'd had no further toxemia problem at all.

A Discussion on Preventing Toxemia

THOSE OF US familiar with the history of medicine will not be surprised to learn that, even today, young mothers are still getting ill and sometimes dying from an entirely preventable disease—toxemia of pregnancy. Also termed eclampsia (the convulsive and sometimes fatal stage) and pre-eclampsia (all stages prior to convulsions), this sometimes-fatal problem has been known to be a disease of malnutrition since the work of Strauss and Burke at Harvard in the 1930s and 1940s.

From 1971 through 1974, a team from the National Institutes of Health (NIH) studied the records of Dr. Tom Brewer at public-health clinics in Contra Costa County, California. The NIH researchers compared those records with records of women from the same clinics who were not under Dr. Brewer's care. Using standard medical care of the time, with the added dimension of nutrition edu-cation, Dr. Brewer virtually eliminated toxemia among his patients, and drastically cut the incidence of low-birth-weight infants. Yet to this day, the team from NIH has not published its findings!

During 25 years in practice, I've observed that Dr. Tom Brewer (and his few predecessors) are correct about the prevention and reversal of toxemia or preeclampsia. The consumption of high-quality protein and supplements (especially vitamin B6 and magnesium) reverses to normal the early to middle stages of this potentially life-threatening disease. Even in later, more serious stages, administering amino acids or human albumin, vitamin B6, and magnesium intravenously will eliminate the problem. There's just no excuse for allowing death from toxemia to claim the lives of more mothers.

Following is an interview with Dr. Tom Brewer. We challenge the NIH to release their decades-old study of his work!

The Work of Dr. Tom Brewer

FROM 1963 through 1976, Dr. Tom Brewer conducted a prenatal-care and nutrition-education project in Contra Costa County, California. His public prenatal clinic served low-income, high-risk women with a program that incorporated nutrition education into routine prenatal care. The incidence of low-birth-weight babies born to women in Dr. Brewer's care over those 12 years was 2.8%, as compared with 13.7% among women seeing other obstetricians in the same county's low-income clinics. During the same time, he demonstrated the effectiveness of good nutrition in preventing toxemia of late pregnancy.

In 1966, Dr. Brewer first published *Metabolic Toxemia of Late Pregnancy: A Disease of Malnutrition,* and he updated the book in 1982. He has also co-authored *What Every Woman Should Know: the Truth About Diet and Drugs in Pregnancy* (1985 revised edition, Penguin Books, New York) and *The Brewer Medical Diet for Normal and High-Risk Pregnancy* (Simon and Schuster, New York, 1983). From 1962 onward, he published 40 scientific papers concerning toxemia and other complications of pregnancy in such journals as *The American Journal of Obstetrics and Gynecology, The Journal of Obstetrics and Gynaecology of the British Commonwealth,* and *Australia-New Zealand Journal of Obstetrics and Gynaecology.*

In 1969, he founded the "Nutrition Action Group," which he still chairs. From 1972 to 1982, he was President of the Society for the Protection of the Unborn through Nutrition (SPUN), headquartered in Chicago, an organization that works to prevent toxemia and other complications of pregnancy through good nutrition.

An Interview with Dr. Tom Brewer

Q: *Figures recently released by the World Health Organization and others state that approximately 75,000 women worldwide die each year of toxemia of pregnancy. For decades, you've taught that toxemia is an entirely preventable disease—a disease of malnutrition. Following your lead and a few other clues, I've helped women eliminate early to moderate cases of toxemia (technically "preeclampsia"). Why isn't your work taken more seriously?*

A: The major criticism of my work is that I wouldn't do "controlled studies." I contend that any such study is unethical—who wants to be assigned to the "poor-diet control group" and risk harming herself or her child?

Q: *When did you first become interested in the problem of toxemia of pregnancy?*

A: Almost 50 years ago. I was a medical student at Tulane University, on obstetrics in my third year. My instructor was James Henry Ferguson, M.D., who had been to the Mississippi countryside studying maternal deaths, particularly among poor black and white mothers. Ferguson told us students the classic picture of toxemia: high blood pressure, edema, protein in the urine, progressing to headaches, spots in front of the eyes, dizziness, nausea, vomiting, and in the end a lethal situation of coma or convulsions or both, heart failure, kidney and liver damage, and death. Toxemia was more common among the poor, teenagers, black women, unmarried women, older women with many children, women with diabetes, women with high blood pressure prior to pregnancy, lupus, and so on. There were a whole gamut of things associated with toxemia—it had been and still is studied to death. Yet then and even now the official line is "nobody knows what causes toxemia."

Ironically, our instructor Ferguson had studied in Chicago with William Dieckmann, the author of a textbook *Toxemias of Pregnancy.* Dieckmann is the only American author I know who cited the work of Pinnard, a French professor at the Hospital of LaMaternité in Paris who discovered in 1893 that milk could totally prevent seizures in toxemia. The "régime latté absolut," he called it. So there's been evidence toxemia is a nutritional problem for over 100 years now. But I'm digressing.

Q: *You were telling us you were a third year medical student . . .*

A: Yes. I went out to the toxemia wards. In those days, the black and the white patients were on opposite sides of the hospital. Even the blood banks were segregated into "black blood" and "white blood."

Q: *Excuse me, you said toxemia wards? There were whole wards with toxemic women?*

A: Yes.

Q: *How many women in each one?*

A: About 20. As a student, my job was to take and record blood pressures, collect urine specimens, run tests in the lab. I took medical histories. Do you remember doing that in school? They ran to 20 or 30 pages—and one of the sections was for diet. Someone would tell me, "I had fatback and cornbread and clay dirt and sago starch and sorghum," and so on. I'd ask, "did you drink milk, eat any eggs, what about meat?" They mostly said no. After taking histories, including diet from several hundred women with toxemia and then some who didn't have toxemia, it occurred to me that toxemia must be a disease of malnutrition.

I then began to tell my fellow students, the interns, occasionally a resident, "These women here, they're malnourished. That's why they're sick. They're seriously malnourished." They usually told me, "They can't be." When I found out the serum proteins in these women were very low, I thought that confirmed it, but the medical literature from all around the world said it was because protein was being lost in the urine. But I found out that isn't true—the protein loss into the urine doesn't

start until the toxemia has well-progressed all over the body.

Q: *Didn't Professor Maurice Strauss of Harvard publish in the 1930s about low serum albumin in women with toxemia?*

A: Exactly. He influenced my thinking. And a fellow Harvard faculty member, Bertha S. Burke worked it out very clearly that women who ate over 60 grams of protein a day simply didn't get toxemia. That was in the 1930s and 1940s. But one of the most important influences on my thinking was my experience in the war in the Pacific, where I observed directly that people could get malnourished enough to get sick from it.

But nobody wanted to listen to me. I was just a student, and besides at that time I was making a racial issue of it, as there were many more malnourished blacks than whites. It didn't help at all that I was a lower-middle-class white antisegregationist Texan in Louisiana in the late 1940s and early 1950s. But I'm digressing again.

They were using a potent diuretic made with mercury, Mercuhydrin.

Q: *Which works by actually damaging the kidneys?*

A: Yes. We were actually ordered to give mercury diuretics to these pregnant women. Later, I worked in the outpatient clinics, and we would have as many as 300 women, occasionally 350 a day.

Q: *All with preeclampsia?*

A: Every one. And all that we did in those clinics was check the blood pressure, give the mercurial diuretic, weigh them, and give drastic warnings about not gaining weight or eating salt or they might swell up with water and have seizures and die. That's where I first encountered what I called iatrogenic starvation. They were putting women I knew to be malnourished onto starvation diets. I complained and said, "These women simply need more and better food, not starvation and all these drugs." That didn't make me any more popular with the professors in charge—remember, I was still a medical student.

After I graduated from medical school, I started an internship at Charity Hospital, but it was all the same. I couldn't do anything about it. I got discouraged and dropped out, worked as a carpenter's helper, and delivered milk for a couple of years. I went back to another internship in Houston in 1953.

Q: *We're happy you didn't quit medicine entirely.*

A: I thought about it. After I finished the internship, I was a general-practice resident for a year. This was in Independence, Louisiana, which was a very, very poor rural area. About 25% of the women delivered there had one stage or another of toxemia. At Charity Hospital in New Orleans it had been 19%. Again I took dietary histories and got the same stories—fatback, cornbread, sorghum, grits, soda pop, and maybe an apple a week or so. No good quality sources of protein. None of this was formal research, though. But after the residency, a partner and I took over a practice in Fulton, Missouri, and we saw only one woman of the first hundred we delivered with toxemia. Only 1%! It was easy to predict—she was very poor, lived in a shack on an easement by the Missouri River, and was malnourished.

While I was in Fulton, drug company "detail men" were calling me all the time. They were promoting the latest diuretics for toxemia. It drove me crazy. By early 1958, I just had to do research on toxemia, so I went to Miami where my former instructor James Henry Ferguson was now professor. He was the only one who would listen to me. He couldn't get me any money for research, so I became an Ob/Gyn resident in his department, because he would let me do research "on the side." I didn't really want to be an Ob/Gyn specialist, but it was the only way. I finally got a paper published in the *American Journal of Obstetrics and Gynecology* about the limitations of diuretics and the meaning of low serum albumin in toxemia.

Q: *That was in 1962?*

A: Yes. By 1963, I had done another study where I gave intravenous human albumin to a few toxemic women with massive edema. These were women with already-low serum albumin—the lowest was 1.2 grams per hundred grams of blood. It was just dramatic. Women who were in shock came right out of it, their edemas lessened, their blood pressures lowered, and they felt much better. It seemed almost miraculous, but it was just simple physiology. Every gram of albumin given intravenously could draw 50 cc of edema fluid back out of the tissues into the bloodstream where it belongs.

Q: *Starling's Law.*

A: You're onto this, aren't you? Starling, *Journal of Physiology*, 1895, Volume 19, pages 312–336. His paper on "Absorption by Blood Vessels." That was Maurice Strauss' take-off point.

Q: *How many women did you give intravenous human albumin?*

A: I personally gave it to 13, and all 13 had marked diuresis, loss of edema fluid.

Q: *That would support your theory. What happened?*

A: No one would accept the results.

Q: *So you kept working on it?*

A: During my entire residency in Ob/Gyn, from 1958 through 1962. Then I went to the University of California, San Francisco, as an NIH Fellow Instructor in the Ob/Gyn department. But when I started a program of trying to teach the women at the Outpatient Clinic to eat right, to gain any weight they wanted as long as it came from a good diet, the other Ob/Gyn instructors and professors wouldn't support me. You'd have thought I was the worst food faddist in the world. I got so frustrated all over again. Somebody else would see one of my patients and lecture her about not gaining weight and put her on a low-salt low-calorie diet and give her amphetamines to promote weight loss. Honest to God, they were giving amphetamines to pregnant mothers! I nearly went mad and told myself, "I can't stay here another year. I have to go somewhere and do this on my own!"

So the next year I went across the Bay to the Contra Costa County Health Services, and I started my program in Richmond. I talked to every woman who came in there about good nutrition on her first visit. I told them this was the most important part of prenatal care. Just as importantly, I eliminated all the stuff about low calories, low salt, diuretics, and so on. I just stopped all that.

Q: *What were the results?*
A: After I had been there a few years, the NIH agreed to come in with a sophisticated team and go over the records. They compared records from patients in my program at Richmond to records from Richmond patients prior to my program. They found a 10-fold reduction in what they called "pregnancy-induced hypertension" in first pregnancies.

Q: *Did they publish that anywhere?*
A: No.

Q: *Why not?*
A: I don't know; it's political, I guess.

Q: *How long were you with Contra Costa County Health Services?*
A: Twelve and a half years.

Q: *Were any other statistics collected during that time?*
A: NIH actually carried out an extensive study. They hired 7 clerks. They brought a big trailer office, set it up on the hospital grounds, and supposedly abstracted every record of every woman delivering a baby there for a 5-year period. They coded them as to whether they were from the Richmond Clinic with Brewer or not Brewer, the Martinez Clinic with Brewer or not Brewer, and the Pittsburgh Clinic with or without Brewer. I thought, "What wonderful statistics we're going to have." They checked every serum protein, every urinalysis was recorded, every blood pressure was coded on cards and tape—and they came out with nothing at all.

Q: *Where is all this data?*
A: Supposedly the NIH still has it. They gave me a copy of the computer tape. I sent it to 5 different computer experts, and they couldn't decipher it. I finally gave up. I'm not a computer person.

Q: *They studied 5 years worth of records?*
A: Yes. Several women clerks were working 5 days a week, 8 hours a day from 1971 through sometime in 1974. I kept asking, when is something going to show? I know personally there were no cases of toxemia in my patients. I had people visit to see if I was doing anything wrong from the University of California-Davis, University of California-Berkeley, Planned Parenthood, March of Dimes, and so on. No one could find anything the matter, but none of them publicly acknowledged my work. By the way, have you heard of the 1958 Vanderbilt Study?

Q: *No.*
A: It was done by Darby, one of the so-called leading nutritionists at Vanderbilt, and someone from the Ob/Gyn department. They concluded from a study of reasonably well-fed middle class white women that nutrition had nothing to do with toxemia, or for that matter with low birth weight or infant mortality. It was believed by all the academics. I was up against that, and to some degree, we still are.

Q: *It would seem so. Since you left the Contra Costa County Health Services, what have you been doing?*

A: I've been involved with 'SPUN' (Society for the Protection of the Unborn through Nutrition), writing, lecturing, doing telephone consultations, and promoting my book *Metabolic Toxemia of Late Pregnancy: A Disease of Malnutrition.*

Q: *Where can we obtain your book?*
A: Frequently you can get it through your local health food store, or directly from NTC Contemporary Publishing Group, (800) 323-4900.

DR. GABY'S COMMENTARY

Nutritional Factors

A NUMBER OF years ago, Dr. Tom Brewer found that women who consumed ample amounts of milk, cheese, lean meat, liver, fish, chicken, soybeans, fruits, vegetables, and whole grains during pregnancy could substantially reduce their risk of developing toxemia.[1] While the benefits of Brewer's diet have been attributed to its high protein content, other nutrients may have exerted a protective effect, as well. Dr. Wright's patient (Cindy) was given amino acids (the building blocks of protein) intravenously, as well as a predigested protein supplement, in order to help correct a presumed protein deficiency. Although giving amino-acid and protein supplements has not been studied as a treatment for preeclampsia, it seems like a good way to improve protein status rapidly.

Obtaining adequate amounts of magnesium and calcium is important for preventing preeclampsia. In one study, high-risk women who received a magnesium supplement had a lower-than-expected incidence of preeclampsia.[2] A review of 14 studies on calcium and preeclampsia was published in the *Journal of the American Medical Association* and concluded that supplementing with calcium—in doses ranging from 375 to 2,000 mg per day—reduced the incidence of preeclampsia by an average of 62%.[3] Some studies have failed to find a beneficial effect of calcium supplementation; however, the women in those studies were, in general, already consuming substantial amounts of calcium in their diet.

Research on the effect of vitamin B_6 has been conflicting. In one study, 820 pregnant women were given a daily multivitamin containing 10 mg of vitamin B_6 or the same formula without vitamin B_6. The incidence of preeclampsia was significantly lower by 61% in the women who received vitamin B_6, compared with the incidence in women who did not receive the vitamin.[4] However, in another study, supplementing with vitamin B_6 was associated with an increase (though not statistically significant) in the incidence of toxemia.[5]

Dr. Evan Shute, an early proponent of vitamin E therapy, reported more than 50 years ago that supplementing with vitamin E could reduce the incidence of toxemia.[6] Other studies suggest that high-fiber foods[7] and foods that contain flavonoids[8] (such as fruits and vegetables) may have a protective effect.

Intravenous Therapy

FOLLOWING UP ON the work of Dr. John Ellis,[9] Dr. Wright has found that the dose of intravenous magnesium can be greatly reduced if vitamin B_6 is also included in the infusion. One of Dr. Wright's typical injections contains 1 gram of magnesium sulfate and 300 mg of vitamin B_6. Of the half dozen or more preeclamptic patients who have received this treatment, all improved rapidly and dramatically. In contrast, conventional protocols require the injection of 20 grams or more of magnesium sulfate over a 24-hour period. Such a large dose of magnesium can potentially cause heart-rhythm disturbances or depressed breathing.

Furthermore, while magnesium therapy does prevent seizures, it is not particularly effective against fluid retention. The addition of vitamin B_6, on the other hand, results in a marked loss of edema fluid, while allowing for a much lower (and safer) dose of magnesium.

Of course, if a woman consumes a nutritious diet (supplemented with moderate amounts of vitamin B_6, magnesium, calcium, and other nutrients) throughout her pregnancy, she will probably not need to be "rescued" late in the pregnancy with intravenous injections.

Summary of Recommendations for Preventing Toxemia of Pregnancy

- Diet: Consume ample amounts of high-protein foods, whole grains, fruits, vegetables, and legumes. Avoid nutrient-depleted foods such as sugar and white flour.

- Calcium, 1,200 to 1,500 mg per day; magnesium, 400 to 600 mg per day (total, from diet and supplements).

- High-potency multiple vitamin/mineral that contains 10 to 20 mg of vitamin B_6. Adjust doses of calcium and magnesium as needed.

PREMENSTRUAL SYNDROME

> ❧ PREMENSTRUAL SYNDROME (PMS) *is a symptom complex that affects a large proportion of women in the United States. It is estimated that between 70 and 90% of women of childbearing age suffer from PMS and that, in 20 to 40% of these women, symptoms are severe.*
>
> *PMS usually begins several days to 1 week before menstruation, although some women have symptoms for 2 full weeks prior to each period. Symptoms often become more severe as menstruation approaches and stop abruptly as soon as the period begins. The most common symptoms are depression, anxiety, irritability, clumsiness, cravings for sweet or salty foods, headaches, weight gain, fluid retention, breast pain and swelling, abdominal bloating, and flare-ups of acne on the face or shoulders.*

DR. WRIGHT'S CASE STUDY

Kathy Dantley seemed nervous. "I have this like, well, terrible PMS," she started. "I promised Dave here to do something about it, 'cause he's been terribly, terrifically understanding—at least mostly. And we just got married last year and all. But these 'witch weeks'—that's what we call my PMS—are getting worse, and you know, lasting longer, so my grandmother and mother said I should come here, because I was here when I was much younger, and you told my mother totally what was wrong, so here I am!" She stopped to catch her breath.

I'd looked at Kathy's record, and noted she'd last been in 10 years before about a skin problem. "You're 24 now? How long have you had premenstrual symptoms?"

"Ever since I've known her, and that's about 4 years," Dave interjected. "But her 'witch weeks'

definitely seem worse since we've been married. Maybe we're just together more."

"My mother says I've had PMS at least for sure since I was 17. It started about a year or so after I got my driver's license and was away from home more. I noticed it totally got worse when I went away to college. Some of my roommates didn't notice it, but one girl moved out. She said she just couldn't handle my mood changes every month. After awhile I quit dating right before my periods 'cause I, you know, scared off most of the dudes—until I met Dave here." She paused and smiled at Dave.

"I have 3 older sisters, and they all have PMS," Dave shrugged. "I thought it was normal, but it is sort of hard to live with sometimes, and Kathy's mother and grandmother told me it isn't normal at all. Since it's getting worse and lasting longer, we've all encouraged Kathy to come in and see you."

"I made sure to make this appointment in the

first part of my cycle when I'm more steady, so I wouldn't get, you know, all upset about Dave saying stuff about me or you asking questions. When I'm being witchy and all like that, I can't always tell I'm being that way, and I get angry and upset and everything."

"You have a quick temper at that time of the month?"

"Lightning," Dave said.

"What other symptoms do you have?"

"You know, I get all depressed for no reason. I totally swell up—like 6 or 7 pounds—and my face breaks all out. Sometimes I can't sleep and other times I sleep way too much. I get mass foggy . . ."

"Mass foggy?"

"She means she can't think or concentrate as well," Dave interpreted.

"He's so patient with me," Kathy said. "And the really, totally worst part is getting angry for no good reason. I spend like hours apologizing later."

"All this happens every month? For how many days?"

"Never until after I ovulate. I can tell when that happens—so could my mother and grandma—it runs in the family. We all get this little pain. Of course Grandma doesn't any more but she did, you know."

"And how long do these symptoms go on?"

"Usually 12 days," Dave said. "I can almost tell the day Kathy's period starts because the symptoms just quit. That's why I don't really blame her—it's obviously related to her hormones or chemistry or something like that." He smiled at his wife and took her hand.

"Please tell me something about what you eat, Kathy."

Kathy looked embarrassed again. "Mother told me you'd ask, and she's always telling me I'd do better if I quit eating junk and ate like she raised me—you know—totally whole grains and lots of vegetables, and no sugar or pop, and taking mass vitamins. She says that's why my PMS started about a year after I got my driver's license—

because, you know, I'd go out and get mass stuff I never got at home that all my friends ate—like candy and pizza and everything like that. When I got to college, it was totally worse, and I started doing more beer and like party stuff."

"So what do you eat now?"

"Well, we're totally in a hurry to get to work, so I don't usually eat breakfast, but I do drink a couple of cups of coffee because it, you know, wakes me up."

"She's definitely better with it than without it," Dave murmured.

"And after I get to work, there's always doughnuts and stuff, so the first, like, real food is at lunch when we usually all go out to a fast-food or sometimes a Chinese restaurant or whatever."

"Can you give me some examples of what you eat at lunch?"

"Usually I go to, you know, the fast-food salad bar 'cause I'm starting to remember to do like I really should; but PMS time I get mass sugar cravings, and I like a lot of grease, like, you know, burgers and fries; but at the Chinese I do better—maybe egg or pork fried rice and bean sprouts and Chinese vegetables. And usually I have a Coke or Pepsi or like that."

"And in the evening?"

"Since we've been married we've both done a better job. We take turns cooking—not like every day—but we trade off. Dave does a lot of meat and potatoes and salads and like that, and I do pasta and chicken more."

"Do you eat fish?"

Kathy wrinkled her nose. "Not really. Fish usually smells totally gross."

"What about nuts or seeds?"

"I like peanuts," Dave offered, "But otherwise we don't usually have them around much."

"What snacks do you eat?"

"Mostly ice cream, or apples or other fruit, or pop. Sometimes cookies. Like I said, I get mass sugar cravings at PMS time, so the sugary stuff and pop totally goes up," Kathy reported.

"Do you take vitamins?"

"Just vitamin C when I'm feeling like I'm getting a cold or something. I really totally hated the mass vitamins Mom made me take when I was a kid, and I totally stopped when I left home. I guess I was being rebellious; but dude if it makes this PMS stop I'm all over it. Grandma goes, 'Take vitamin B$_6$'. Mom goes 'vitamin E'. And I go, 'I'll just wait until I got it all together over here'. I just don't want to put us through this anymore."

"Have you ever had allergies, or are there any in your family?"

"You mean like hay fever or asthma?"

"Yes."

"Not that I know about. Do allergies cause PMS?"

"For some people. I've worked with many women who improved a lot by avoiding foods like milk and dairy or wheat, and many other foods. Quite a few women are allergic to their own hormones, especially progesterone."

Kathy stared. "Allergic to their own hormones? How can that happen? That would be totally awful—you couldn't get away from it. It'd like follow you around worse than a shadow."

I laughed. "Fortunately, it's almost always possible to desensitize people to their hormones when they're sensitive to them. It doesn't sound as if you have that problem, but it's easy to check and shouldn't be overlooked."

"OK."

I looked through the forms Kathy had been sent to fill in when she made her appointment. "It looks like you forgot to take your temperature."

"I'm sorry. We're mass rushed in the morning, and I asked Mom what that was for and she said maybe thyroid testing but I know you can check that on blood tests or something, can't you?"

"We can, and we will, but blood test aren't the final word. Sometimes we learn a lot from observing the body temperature every day. Dr. Broda Barnes, a pioneering endocrinologist, showed us that decades ago. He even wrote a book about it called *Hypothyroidism: The Unsus-*pected Illness, which is still available in most health-food stores. If you can, please take your temperature every morning according to the instructions printed on the back of this temperature record. Unfortu-nately, I can't tell whether it's important for you until you do it."

"If it helps, I'm all over it, for sure! I just wanted to wait until I talked to you, and now that I know for sure it could possibly be related to my PMS I'll make sure and do it." She took the blank temperature chart and put it in her purse. "Besides that, what do I do?"

"We should do a check-up, but likely I'll recommend what we've talked about: allergy/sensitivity tests for both foods and hormones, thyroid testing, diet-change recommendations, and some vitamin and mineral supplements. But let's do your check-up first."

Aside from dry skin, slightly flaky on her legs, Kathy's check-up was normal. "But dry skin almost always means insufficient essential fatty acids in the diet," I told her. "And that contributes to PMS. I'll be sure to put those on a supplement list. In the diet, essential fatty acids are found in fish, raw nuts and seeds, and salad oils. Try to eat more of those if you can. Also, dry skin could be an indicator of a weak thyroid.

"But before we get to supplements, about the rest of your diet . . ."

"I think I know what you're going to say. After all, my mother's been coming here for years. She brought me here 10 years ago, and she totally doesn't have any sugar or caffeine in the house; she uses only like whole grains and mass vegetables and soy and stuff like that."

"It's very possible you'll have withdrawal symptoms," I said. "But withdrawal only lasts for a few days, and if you continue to want it you can try coffee later—once the symptoms are gone—to see how much difference it makes. And you're right, please eliminate all the refined sugar and white flour, and load up on vegetables. Lots more vitamins and minerals there.

"Now about supplements. Your mother is right about vitamin B$_6$. It particularly helps against hormone-related fluid retention and acne, and usually depression, too. To start, please use 100 milligrams, 3 times a day,

"Next, magnesium. It works with vitamin B$_6$, and also helps on its own to calm the nerves. Again, to start, use 200 milligrams, 3 times a day. For essential fatty acids, in addition to diet changes, please use flaxseed oil, 1 tablespoon or 9,000 milligrams daily. And grandma was right about the vitamin E—you should take 400 IU daily. In addition to the individual supplements, remember the multiple vitamin-mineral. Go to your local health-food store for a high-potency type—usually it'll be in several capsules or tablets daily—not just 1 or 2."

"Awesome. If I can do this whole list of supplements and make all these diet changes, I should be major better, shouldn't I?"

"Nothing's guaranteed, Kathy, but there's a good chance it'll make a difference. Check back in a few months and let me know. And please don't forget the allergy/sensitivity tests, and the thyroid tests (both blood tests) and taking your temperature as the form says."

Seven months later, Kathy and Dave returned, this time for a problem of Dave's. Kathy

informed me she was, "like, totally mass better."

Although Kathy turned out to be not particularly allergic or sensitive to her own hormones (or anything else), for a minority of women with PMS this is a major problem. Hormone (particularly progesterone) sensitivity was first clinically documented by physician-members of the American Academy of Environmental Medicine, using special skin-testing techniques called "dilution-titration" and "provocative neutralization." Using these techniques, I observed women literally having their symptoms "turned on and off" by a technician using precisely varying (and incredibly minute) quantities of progesterone. While using these incredibly minute dilutions of progesterone in "desensitization drops," I was even more impressed by husbands who simply refused to leave my office without obtaining a "refill" of these drops for their wives! (Fortunately, only 1 or 2 refills are usually necessary to complete the desensitization.)

It's not known at all how an individual can become sensitive to an internally-produced molecule, but it's very likely that such sensitivity is not an "allergy" as defined by current medical science.

DR. GABY'S COMMENTARY

ALTHOUGH CONSIDERABLE RESEARCH has been done on the subject, no one can say for sure what causes PMS. Some evidence suggests that hormonal imbalances are at the root of the problem, primarily an excess of estrogen and/or a deficiency of progesterone. (As we discussed in chapter 4, progesterone is a hormone produced by the ovaries that opposes the effects of estrogen.) Other research suggests that deficiencies of some of the brain's chemical messengers, such as serotonin or dopamine, are involved in PMS. Whatever the cause, a number of natural remedies have been found to be helpful.

Dietary Considerations
Diet and Lifestyle

WE have found that women who avoid refined sugar, caffeine, alcohol, and excessive salt intake experience greater relief from PMS symptoms than women who do not change their diet. In fact, some women hardly improve at all until they make some dietary adjustments. For many women, refined sugar is the greatest dietary contributor to PMS. Other women find that avoiding dairy products also helps. Perhaps these individuals are sensitive to the estrogenic chemicals from the environment that concentrate in milk, or perhaps they are just allergic to dairy products. Additionally, a study of 295 college women revealed that caffeine consumption was strongly related to the presence and severity of PMS.[1]

In addition to dietary changes, aerobic exercise is also valuable for women with PMS. In one study, women who participated in an exercise program, such as running 1.5 miles per day, 5 days a week, had a significant improvement in their premenstrual symptoms.[2]

Nutritional Supplements
Vitamin B6

VITAMIN B6 exerts a number of effects in the body that might be expected to relieve symptoms of PMS.[3] First, vitamin B6 may increase the concentrations of serotonin, dopamine, and progesterone, compounds which are thought to be low in women with PMS. This vitamin also reduces some of the adverse effects of estrogen. Consequently, vitamin B6 seems like an ideal nutrient for the treatment of PMS. In one double-blind study, 25 women with moderate to severe PMS received vitamin B6 for 3 months and a placebo for another 3 months. Eighty-four percent of the women reported greater improvement during treatment with vitamin B6 than during treatment with the placebo.[4] These findings were confirmed in another study of 70 women with various premenstrual symptoms. Of those who complained of depression, 60% were cured or markedly improved by vitamin B6 therapy. For other premenstrual symptoms, the proportion of women who responded to vitamin B6 were as follows: swelling and bloatedness, 60%; irritability, 56%; headaches, 81%; lethargy, 52%; lack of coordination, 27%; and breast tenderness, 52%.[5] Another study found that premenstrual acne flare-ups were improved in about three-quarters of women who took vitamin B6 supplements.[6]

Most women respond to 50 to 100 mg of vitamin B6 per day, although, for some women, taking larger amounts during the week prior to menstru-ation is helpful. Larger doses of vitamin B6 are occasionally necessary to obtain satisfactory results. However, excessive amounts of this vitamin can cause damage to the nervous system, resulting in loss of sensation in the hands and lower legs. Any-one taking more than 200 mg of vitamin B6 per day for prolonged periods of time should be monitored by a health-care practitioner who is knowledgeable about nutrition. Vitamin B6 may also cause mild irritability or sensitivity to noise, possibly by inducing a deficiency of magnesium. Taking vitamin B6 appears to increase the body's need for mag-nesium, and supplementing with magnesium usually prevents these vitamin B6-related side effects.

Magnesium

IN a study of 105 women with PMS, 45% were found to be deficient in magnesium (as determined by low levels of magnesium in their red blood cells).[7] Some of the symptoms of magnesium deficiency, such as apathy, personality changes, muscle spasm, anxiety, and depression, are the same as those reported by women with PMS. In a double-blind study, 32 women with PMS received either magnesium or a placebo for 2 months. The treatments were given daily from day 15 of the menstrual cycle until the onset of menstruation. Magnesium was significantly more effective than the placebo in relieving premenstrual mood changes.[8] In another double-blind study, magnesium supplementation (200 mg per day) alleviated symptoms of premenstrual fluid retention, such as weight gain, swelling of the extremities, breast tenderness, and abdominal bloating.[9]

Calcium

IN a recent double-blind study, 497 women with moderate to severe PMS were randomly assigned to receive 1,200 mg of calcium per day or a placebo for 3 menstrual cycles. Premenstrual symptoms were reduced to a significantly greater extent in the calcium group than in the placebo group

(48% reduction vs. 38% reduction).[10] Although these results with calcium were not dramatic, calcium supplementation appears to be a useful addition to the overall treatment of PMS.

Vitamin E

A DOUBLE-blind study of 75 women with fibrocystic breast disease provided an opportunity to determine the effect of vitamin E on the symptoms of PMS. In that study, the women were randomly assigned to receive vitamin E (150 to 600 IU per day) or a placebo for 2 months. Compared with the placebo, vitamin E significantly relieved the symptoms of PMS.[11] Whether vitamin E relieves PMS in women without fibrocystic breast disease is not known.

Essential Fatty Acids (EFAs)

WOMEN with PMS have been shown to have abnormalities of essential-fatty-acid (EFA) metabolism. Supplementing with a specific fatty acid called gamma-linolenic acid (GLA), which is found in evening primrose oil (EPO), is sometimes helpful for conditions such as PMS that are associated with abnormal EFA metabolism. In one study, 17 women with PMS received 8 capsules of EPO per day during the last 14 days of their menstrual cycle, for 5 consecutive months. After 1 cycle, the women experienced significant improvements in premenstrual symptoms, and these improvements became more pronounced over the following 4 cycles.[12] However, in another study, evening primrose oil was no more effective than a placebo.[13]

While EPO may be helpful for PMS, it is also quite expensive. A less costly source of GLA is borage oil. If the active ingredient in EPO is GLA, then borage oil should work just as well as EPO, although the former has not been tested as a treatment for PMS. Flaxseed oil is also commonly recommended as a source of EFAs. Additional research is needed to determine which EFA supplement is best for women with PMS.

Hormone Therapy
Thyroid Hormone

Some of the symptoms of hypothyroidism (underactive thyroid gland) are the same as those of PMS. In a study of 54 women with PMS, 94% had laboratory evidence of subtle hypothyroidism. Thirty-four of these women were treated with thyroid hormone, and all 34 experienced complete relief from PMS.[14] However, in another study of 14 women with PMS, no thyroid abnormalities were found.[15]

Progesterone Therapy

TREATMENT with the naturally occurring ovarian hormone progesterone has been reported to relieve the symptoms of PMS.[16] In our experience, women who fail to improve with the treatments described above will often respond to natural-progesterone therapy. Progesterone can be given in the form of a skin cream or as a vaginal or rectal suppository. Although several research studies have failed to confirm the effectiveness of progesterone, the results in our clinics are so obvious in many cases, that we are convinced the negative research was in some way flawed. Possible explanations for these conflicting observations are that the doses of progesterone used in the "negative" studies were too low, or that the failure to restrict dietary sugar may have somehow prevented progesterone from doing its job properly.

It should be noted that natural progesterone is not the same as progestins (such as medroxyprogesterone acetate: Provera). Progestins, which are often prescribed by conventional doctors along with estrogen therapy, have some of the same actions as progesterone, but they also exert anti-progesterone effects. In addition, progestins cause considerably more side effects than natural progesterone. For these reasons, we do not recommend progestins for the treatment of PMS.

Some women appear to be "allergic" to their body's own progesterone. These women improve after receiving treatments that "desensitize" them to this hormone. Although it is difficult to understand how someone could be allergic to her own hormones, the treatment is safe and it appears to work.[17]

A Comprehensive Approach

WE HAVE DESCRIBED a number of different treatments that help alleviate PMS. We find that the most effective approach is a comprehensive one that includes dietary modifications, exercise, and nutritional supplements. In specific instances, thyroid hormone, progesterone supplementation, or progesterone desensitization is necessary. At least 80% of women who follow the natural approach tell us that their PMS improves, and many women report dramatic and long-lasting relief from a problem that had plagued them for years.

Summary of Recommendations for Treating Premenstrual Syndrome

PRIMARY RECOMMENDATIONS:

- DIET AND LIFESTYLE
  ➤ Avoid refined sugar and other refined carbohydrates, caffeine, and alcohol. Reduce or eliminate intake of dairy products, in selected cases.

  ➤ Participate in an aerobic-exercise program, equivalent to jogging 1.5 miles per day, 3 to 5 days a week.

- SUPPLEMENTS
  ➤ Vitamin B$_6$, 50 to 200 mg per day; larger doses are sometimes used, with medical supervision. Dosages greater than 200 mg per day for prolonged periods of time can cause nerve damage and must be monitored by a doctor.

  ➤ Magnesium, 200 to 600 mg per day (divided doses for intakes at the higher end of the range). Reduce the dose if diarrhea occurs.

  ➤ Vitamin E, 400 to 800 IU per day.

  ➤ Calcium, 600 to 1,000 mg per day, especially when intake of dairy products is being restricted.

OTHER RECOMMENDATIONS:

- Essential fatty acids—options include:
  ➤ Evening primrose oil or borage oil, providing a daily dose of approximately 200 to 400 mg of gamma-linolenic acid (GLA), or

  ➤ Flaxseed oil, 1 to 3 teaspoons per day.

- High-potency multiple vitamin/mineral (adjust doses of other nutrients as needed).
  ➤ Thyroid hormone, in selected cases.

  ➤ Progesterone therapy, in selected cases.

  ➤ Progesterone "desensitization," in selected cases.

PSORIASIS

PSORIASIS IS A *common, hereditary skin disorder that affects more than 1 in 100 individuals. The lesions of psoriasis may develop on the scalp, limbs, or other parts of the body. They typically appear as red, slightly raised areas with a thick, silvery overlying scale. One of the hallmarks of psoriasis is the tendency of new lesions to appear at healing sites of trauma, such as burns or scrapes. Psoriasis may cause itching or pain of varying intensity, although some individuals do not suffer anything more than the "heartbreak" of a cosmetic problem.*

The skin lesions result from overproduction of a protein called keratin. An excessive inflammatory response in the skin also plays a role in the development of psoriasis, and some treatments are aimed at reducing inflammation.

Conventional therapy includes topical application of steroids or other medications, ultraviolet-light therapy, or (in severe cases) internal administration of powerful drugs such as methotrexate. None of these treatments cures psoriasis, but the condition can often be kept under control. Unfortunately, psoriasis tends to recur shortly after treatment is discontinued. Furthermore, most conventional therapies are not without risks and side effects.

DR. WRIGHT'S CASE STUDY

"There must be something better for this psoriasis," Woodrow Dooley said. "I've used steroid creams and ointments, various 'tar' preparations, things I've ordered from catalogs, and even a big dose of prednisone once when it got really bad. But nothing ever takes it away completely or even keeps it down very far. That treatment with psoralen and light helps. I've had it twice, but it's a little expensive, and when I quit, the psoriasis comes right back."

"Sounds like a bad case."

"No kidding! Why else would I have long sleeves and trousers on an 87° day in Seattle, not to mention no current girlfriend. The only woman who can stand me is my mother!"

"It's really that bad?"

"You're right, I'm exaggerating a little . . . but I just don't feel very social or confident when it's this bad, so I don't try very hard."

"Let's go through your health history and then take a look."

Woodrow Dooley was 28 years old. Except for the psoriasis and a teenage acne problem treated with long-term antibiotics, he'd been relatively healthy. The first signs of psoriasis had come on when he attended the university.

Unfortunately, it had progressed rapidly, reaching nearly to all parts of his body in just over a year. Several relatives had lesser degrees of psoriasis, and others had allergies. Otherwise, his older relatives had lived into their 80s and 90s.

As he'd said, the psoriasis was nearly everywhere. It was worst on his legs, covering the front surface between his knees and ankles almost entirely with silvery-yellow scales over angry red skin. About half the surface of his calves was also covered. Both surfaces of his upper legs had numerous psoriatic patches of varying sizes, with a large cluster at the base of the spine. His arms showed a pattern similar to his legs: worst between wrists and elbows, less but still a lot up to his shoulders. There were many patches on his trunk, both front and back, several small ones in his scalp. The only areas free of psoriasis were his hands, face, and feet.

"And this is how I look when I've been slathering the latest steroid on myself," he said. "Now, don't get me wrong, but if you were a young woman would you want to date me?"

"Sure—after I learned what a good person you are—kind, thoughtful, always living up to his word, and hard-working. There are fewer of those around than perfect physical specimens, you know."

"You sound like my mother."

"So, listen to your mother, already. Also, listen to how you can get this better. Notice I didn't say 'cured' right off. Psoriasis is a tough problem, and you've got a tough case. Sometimes the best we can do is persuade it to go down a lot, but not completely go away."

"So what do I do? Any tests I should have run?"

"Before we get to tests, let's go over some dietary basics."

"Wait. Mom says, 'Woody, you've got to quit drinking, cut out the sugar and caffeine, eliminate the food chemicals, and stay out of those fast-food hamburger places'. So, should I listen? How much of that is just basic good-health stuff like a lot of moms say, and how much is really relevant to psoriasis?"

"What's wrong with basic good health stuff? Your mom's right on all counts about that. But if you want to narrow it down, there is some correlation between alcohol intake and psoriasis. And for some people, cutting back on protein and saturated fat makes a difference. By the way, the first thing on your 'mom said' list was quit drinking. Have you had a problem there?"

"Well, I did go a little overboard at the university, but not since then."

"As part of your overall program, I recommend you stop entirely and wait until your psoriasis is a lot better before you try it again, to see what happens. Also, for now, cut down on the protein and fat and go for a lot more vegetables and fruits. That's often directly relevant to psoriasis, too."

"OK. And as long as I'm doing that, I'll do the rest for Mom, too."

"Good. Can't hurt. Now, about tests. First, please turn in a stool specimen at the lab. Remember all those antibiotics you took when you had acne? Chances are they disrupted the 'friendly bacteria' internally. There's no absolute proof but strong suspicion that abnormal bowel microorganisms contribute to psoriasis. And it might just be coincidence that your psoriasis started shortly after you'd taken all the antibiotics and did more drinking—but maybe it's not a coincidence, either.

"Secondly, have a gastric analysis done. I've observed a strong correlation between weak stomach acid-pepsin function and psoriasis. It appears the worse the psoriasis, the worse the stomach function in most cases."

"How could that affect it?"

"Don't know exactly, but psoriasis usually improves with supplemental hydrochloric acid and pepsin if the test shows a need. Hydrochloric acid and pepsin are very necessary for appropriate digestion, and they affect which microorganisms grow in the mid- and lower bowel."

"Like a pH effect?"

"Exactly. You a chemist?"

"Nope, but I remember a little from the university."

"If your stomach function is low, I'll ask you to try fairly heavy—but safe—quantities of vitamin B_{12} and folic acid by injection. Some folks report that it helps a lot, some say it doesn't. That's reflected in conflicting research articles, too, but it's harmless and worth a try."

"Next, screening for food allergy and sensitivity. Do you have a family history of allergy?"

"I don't know of any personally."

"You may not have any, but sometimes there are surprises."

"I'll get the tests done, but isn't there anything I can start right away that might help?"

"If you'd just won the lottery, I'd suggest 1,25-dihydroxyvitamin D cream. There's some very promising research going on. But with as much surface as you have to cover, right now it'd be way too expensive. But don't be discouraged, there are several other things to try that have helped others. To start, cod-liver oil as well as a fish-oil concentrate that contains a fatty acid called EPA. Please use 1 tablespoon of cod-liver oil and 3 grams of 'MaxEPA' twice daily. Take 400 IU of vitamin E and a high-lipase digestive enzyme each time you take these supplements, to help ensure that the whole thing gets into your system as well as possible.

"Next, a tricky one, with some possible adverse effects to watch out for. Some people find that a derivative of a natural metabolite called fumarate can lessen or even eliminate psoriasis. It's both swallowed and rubbed on. But the oral quantities occasionally cause low-blood-sugar reactions, and some people get flushes—like a hot flash—with no warning. And, though I've never seen it happen, liver and kidney problems have been reported, and regular blood tests are advised."

"What's 'occasionally'?"

"The folks I've worked with, 5% or less."

"You know what . . . even though that stuff's a natural metabolite, it still sounds a little tricky. Does the rub-on fumarate cause those symptoms, too?"

"No one using just the rub-on version has reported any of those problems. But it doesn't work quite as well as using the capsules."

"For now, I'll use the rub-on, and wait and see how I do."

"Sounds reasonable. For now, use the cod-liver oil, MaxEPA, vitamin E, high-lipase digestive enzyme, and topical fumarate. Make sure to have your tests done. As you said, we'll see how you do."

Like many others with moderately severe psoriasis, Mr. Dooley's gastric analysis was quite abnormal. He was advised to take hydrochloric acid-pepsin capsules with each meal, along with self-injections of vitamin B_{12} and folate. Due to the degree of his psoriasis, he was asked to start these injections every day, tapering the dose down as he progressed. He was found to have many food sensitivities he wasn't aware of, and re-arranged his diet to avoid them while desensitizing. He also quit alcohol, and put into effect his mother's "general good-health recommendations." In addition to supplements recommended, he took a multiple vitamin/mineral and extra vitamin C.

During the first month after starting his program, progress was slow. He noted mostly a significant decrease in the "angry, red" appearance of the involved skin areas. By the end of the second month, the involved areas started to recede, and by the end of 11 months, there were very few areas of psoriasis left, even though he hadn't used topical steroids for several months. At that visit, he introduced us to his new girlfriend.

DR. GABY'S COMMENTARY

Nutritional therapy is not universally successful in treating psoriasis. However, it does provide additional options, which are quite helpful for many patients. In our experience, about 50% of psoriasis patients respond to nutritional therapy, and for some patients, the problem resolves completely. One of the advantages of the nutritional approach is that it is relatively free of adverse side effects.

Dietary Considerations

SOME INDIVIDUALS WITH psoriasis appear to be particularly sensitive to refined sugar and alcohol. Eliminating these items from the diet will occasionally result in substantial improvement. Evidence also shows that food allergy plays a role in psoriasis. In one study, 11 of 16 patients with severe psoriasis showed "remarkable improvement" on a diet free of gluten (wheat, oats, barley, and rye). Intestinal biopsies performed on the patients who improved showed evidence of celiac disease (moderate or severe atrophy of the lining of the jejunum), an intestinal disorder caused by gluten intolerance.[1] Other investigators have also found an association between gluten intolerance and psoriasis.[2]

I typically advise patients with psoriasis to follow an allergy-elimination diet, followed by individual food tests. While gluten grains are a factor for some patients, other foods may be involved, as well. One of the elimination diets I have used in my practice is presented in appendix A. Some doctors use other tests for allergy and sensitivity, as well as desensitization techniques. The reliability and effectiveness of some of these methods is controversial (see chapter 3 for additional discussion).

Nutritional Supplements
Essential Fatty Acids

RESEARCH has shown that fish oil can produce some improvement in individuals with psoriasis. In a double-blind study, 28 individuals with chronic psoriasis received 10 grams of a fish-oil concentrate per day or a placebo for 8 weeks. There was a significant lessening of itching, redness, and scaling in the fish-oil group, but not in the placebo group.[3] Additional research has confirmed these findings; however, some investigators have failed to observe any benefit from fish oil.

Another oil that shows promise in the treatment of psoriasis is flaxseed oil. Although no studies have been done, we have found that taking 1 to 3 tablespoons of flaxseed oil per day provides substantial benefit for some patients. Fish oil and flaxseed oil probably work by reducing inflammation and promoting tissue repair. Unsaturated oils should always be balanced with a vitamin E supplement to prevent the formation of dangerous free radicals.

Vitamin D

SINCE vitamin D is known to inhibit excessive cellular proliferation, it has been investigated as a possible treatment for psoriasis. The vitamin D present in food and that formed by sunlight exposure actually has little or no biological activity. In order to become effective, it must first be converted by the liver and kidney into one of its active byproducts (1alpha-hydroxyvitamin D or 1,25-dihydroxyvitamin D). These are the forms of vitamin D that have been used in clinical studies of patients suffering from psoriasis. In some reports, the vitamin was applied to the skin, and in others it was taken orally. The results obtained with this treatment have been consistently positive, and in some cases have been dramatic.[4, 5, 6]

Activated forms of vitamin D are very powerful, and they can cause potentially dangerous elevations of serum calcium. Consequently, these products are available only by prescription. However, when used appropriately and monitored adequately, this treatment is unlikely to cause any problems. Some conventional dermatologists are now using vitamin D therapy for psoriasis.

Folic Acid

THE use of folic acid as a treatment for psoriasis was first described by cardiologist Kurt Oster. Dr. Oster had found that large doses of folic acid, when taken in combination with vitamin C, can inhibit xanthine oxidase, an enzyme involved in the production of uric acid. Allopurinol, a drug that inhibits xanthine oxidase, had previously been shown to be an effective treatment for psoriasis.

Oster therefore postulated that the folic acid-vitamin C combination would also be helpful. In his study, 7 patients with long-standing psoriasis were given 20 mg of folic acid, 4 times per day, in combination with an unspecified amount of vitamin C. Marked improvements were seen in these patients after 3 to 6 months of treatment. However, of 3 other patients who had previously received methotrexate (a drug that interferes with folic acid) for their psoriasis, 2 became decidedly worse after taking folic acid.[7] Dr. Wright and I have tried Oster's regimen with a few patients. As with other nutritional treatments for psoriasis, it appears to help some patients but not others.

Vitamin B$_{12}$

IN one study, 34 patients with chronic psoriasis that had failed to respond to treatment were given daily intramuscular injections of vitamin B$_{12}$ for 10 days, followed by injections 1 to 2 times per week. The lesions disappeared in 32% of the patients and improved in an additional 62%.[8] However, other investigators failed to find any beneficial effect of vitamin B$_{12}$.

These conflicting results may be explainable by one doctor's observation that it takes at least 30 injections before results are seen, and that the improvement is often delayed for up to 6 weeks after the treatment is stopped.[9] The doctors who failed to observe benefits may not have continued the treatment for a long enough period of time.

Other Treatments
Fumaric Acid

IN the 1980s, doctors reported that derivatives (esters) of fumaric acid, a compound that occurs naturally in the body, can relieve some cases of psoriasis. Apparently, fumaric acid is formed in the skin of healthy people during exposure to sunlight. Individuals with psoriasis have difficulty manufacturing fumaric acid, and that deficiency is thought to contribute somehow to the development of the skin lesions. Controlled trials have confirmed the effectiveness of fumaric-acid esters.[10, 11] However, this treatment can cause a number of side effects, including low blood sugar and (on rare occasions) kidney damage. Fumaric-acid esters should be used only under medical supervision.

A Yeast Connection?

ACCORDING to one theory, psoriasis is caused by an excessive inflammatory reaction to certain microorganisms, particularly *Candida albicans* (the common yeast germ) or other fungi. There are a few case reports in the medical literature in which psoriasis responded well to orally administered antifungal drugs, such as nystatin or ketoconazole (Nizoral). The relationship between yeast infections and psoriasis may explain why eating sugar often makes psoriasis worse (sugar tends to promote the growth of yeast).

Thyroid Hormone

ONE DOCTOR HAS used large doses of thyroid hormone (thyroxine) to treat psoriasis. Patients generally tolerated the treatment well, although it was necessary to administer a beta-blocker (propranolol) to prevent the patients from developing a rapid pulse. Both the skin lesions and the arthritis that is sometimes associated with psoriasis improved greatly with this treatment.[12] Thyroxine is available only by prescription. Large doses should be given with caution, and patients must be monitored closely.

Conclusion

PSORIASIS REMAINS A confusing disorder, and the results of treatment are unpredictable and sometimes disappointing. Nevertheless, many individuals respond well to the natural treatments described here, and in some cases the results are dramatic.

Summary of Recommendations for Treating Psoriasis

- Diet: Avoid refined sugar and alcohol. Work with food allergies.

- Essential fatty acids: cod-liver oil, fish-oil concentrate, or flaxseed oil; dosage varies according to the severity of the condition.
  (NOTE: *Because of its vitamin A and vitamin D content, cod-liver oil in doses greater than 1 tablespoon per day should be monitored by a physician.*)

- Folic acid and vitamin B$_{12}$, in selected cases.

- "Activated" vitamin D (by prescription), topically or orally, in selected cases.

- Other treatments that have been used with some success include antifungal medication, fumaric-acid esters, and thyroid hormone. These treatments should be monitored by a physician.

RECURRENT INFECTIONS

> 🌿 RECURRENT INFECTIONS ARE *among the most common medical problems. Infections can be caused by bacteria, viruses, or fungi. They can affect many different areas of the body, including the respiratory and urinary tracts, skin, intestines, gums, and sexual organs.*
>
> *Our capacity to withstand the assault of disease-causing microorganisms is related in part to the strength of our immune system and to the integrity of our tissues (which function as a physical barrier against microbes). These, in turn, are influenced by dietary and nutritional factors. It may therefore be possible to reduce the recurrence rate of infections by modifying the diet and using appropriate nutritional supplements. A growing body of published research supports our clinical observation that natural medicine can be of great benefit for most people who "get sick all the time."*

DR. WRIGHT'S CASE STUDY

"Every year for the last 6 or 7 years, I've gotten at least half a dozen colds, the flu once or twice, and bronchitis at least once," Jenny Wallgren said. "I've taken so many antibiotics, I'm on a first-name basis with all my pharmacists. One of them even asked me out! In between infections, I feel pretty good, but there must be something the matter with my immune system or I wouldn't be getting sick so much. Elmer . . . he's the pharmacist who asked me out . . . referred me to an infectious-disease specialist last year. She ran a bunch of tests, and said she couldn't find anything the matter with my immune system." She dug into her purse, emerging with several sheets of paper she handed to me. "Keep them, they're copies."

"Let's see. You have a normal white-blood-cell count, normal immune-cell profile and immune globulins, and normal protein electrophoresis. These certainly look OK."

"Well, supposedly my immune system is OK, but since I saw her last year I've had my usual 'hard flu' and half a dozen colds. So I've been reading about this natural-medicine thing in magazines, and thought I'd give it a try. It sure can't do any worse than having to take antibiotics, antihistamines, and stuff like that all the time."

"If you don't get sick, you might not see Elmer as much."

"Well . . . that's OK, we're seeing each other even when I'm not sick."

"Sounds good. So what have you done so far?"

"I've started taking some vitamin C—a couple of grams a day, and lots more when I get sick. It hasn't reduced the number of colds I'm getting much, but I think I'm getting better quicker."

"That's a good summary of what many studies have shown about vitamin C. Are you doing anything else?"

"Elmer said probably a multiple vitamin and mineral would be a good idea, but he also said I should probably see a doctor who knew something about all this, and I agree, so here I am."

"You said between infections you feel well? No other health problems?"

"None that I know about."

"Good. Let's review a few other areas." We covered her prior health history, her family history, and other parts of her life as related to her health. We got to a diet history.

"I probably could be eating a little better," Jenny admitted. "But I'm single, working one job full time and another part time to try to save some money. I'm just busy all the time. But I really do try. The last two years, I've made sure to have something for breakfast every day. I was skipping that for several years."

"What do you eat in the morning?"

"One of those instant oatmeal things."

"With cow's milk and sugar?"

"Yes."

"And lunch?"

"What I call 'good fast food'. I always go to one of those places with a salad bar as well as tacos, chicken, or burgers. I always get the salad first and whatever else second. And I always ask for whole wheat instead of white bread for sandwiches."

"And dinner?"

"Pretty much the same thing, except when I go to my parents to visit or out to eat with someone. And at least twice a week, I order a pizza with lots of vegetables."

"What do you eat for snacks?"

"Not much. I'm busy, and watching my weight besides. Maybe I have a cookie or candy bar once a week or so, but mostly it's apples, oranges, and bananas."

"Drink any coffee, tea, soft drinks, water, or alcohol?"

"Not much alcohol except if I'm out for an evening and not working the next morning. I drink several glasses of water every day. I've read it's good for me, and helps me control my weight, I think. I drink coffee only when I need to stay awake. Mostly I drink tea, and I probably average one cola or other soft drink a day."

"Where does the water come from?"

"City water, I guess."

"You're doing a little better than average for a busy single working woman," I said. "But there are at least 2 areas in your diet you could change right away that would help your immune function, and 1 area to investigate."

"But I thought there was nothing the matter with my immune system."

"You're correct. There's nothing wrong with those particular tests. They show numbers of immune cells, amount of immune globulins, and so forth. But they don't say what those cells are actually *doing*. For example, have you read or heard what sugar does to the ability of white blood cells to literally 'eat' and kill bacteria?"

"No."

"In the 1970s, research demonstrated that ingesting sugar could significantly interfere with the ability of white cells to kill bacteria for 4 to 5 hours before they recovered. But if one had, say, sugar with oatmeal at breakfast, a soft drink for lunch, and something else with sugar in the evening, then the white cells could be significantly impaired all day."

"Just from eating sugar?"

"That's right. It's one of many reasons that so many of us get colds so often."

"Good grief. Well, I'll just get rid of the sugar, though it might be a little tough. Mom's been doing it recently, and she says there's sugar in everything."

"Initially, it involves a lot of label reading and asking questions when you're out to eat . . . but it pays off, and after awhile it's easy. Like learning to ride a bicycle."

"OK, I'll try it—no sugar. What's the second area?"

"The water you're drinking."

"What? I thought water is good for me!"

"Water, yes. It's all the other stuff in the water that's not so good for your immune system—specifically the fluoride and chlorine in city water. Even National Cancer Institute scientists have published articles showing an increase in cancer risk from chlorinated water. If cancers are increased, the immune system must be weakened. And there are many studies showing that fluoride at the levels found in our drinking water—and in our tissues if we drink that water—interferes with both the mobility of our white blood cells and their ability to engulf and kill germs."

"So what do I substitute for water?"

"Please keep drinking lots of water—it is good for you. But make sure it's water without chlorine, fluoride, and other chemical additives. Usually that means bottled water when you're out, and distilled water (which is cheaper) or bottled water at home, too."

"What about the good minerals in the water."

"You can obtain more beneficial minerals in 1 or 2 multiple vitamin/mineral capsules per week than you can from drinking city water every day."

"Bottled water is more expensive."

"Probably not as expensive as all those antibiotics and doctors you've seen."

"Good point. So, no sugar and no fluoridated or chlorinated water. What else?"

"We need to screen you for allergies and sensitivities."

"As far as I know, I'm not allergic."

"You might not be, but a basic principle of natural, nutritional medicine is to always check for allergies and sensitivities whenever there are recurrent infections. When we find allergies and sensitivities—and we almost always do in cases of recurrent infection—and eliminate or desensitize them, recurrent infection nearly always decreases."

"OK. Now what about my vitamin C and any other supplements?"

"Please continue the vitamin C, at least 1,000 milligrams, twice daily. You can take twice that much if it doesn't give you gas or loose bowels. Next, make sure your vitamin A intake is approximately 40,000 IU daily—that's vitamin A itself, not beta-carotene. We'll reduce the dose of vitamin A as you improve. However, while you are taking this amount of vitamin A, it's important that you do not become pregnant, as there is some evidence that taking more than 10,000 IU of vitamin A per day can increase the risk of certain birth defects."

"Oh, you don't have to worry about that."

"Also, zinc—the citrate or picolinate form is best—50 to 60 milligrams daily. Make sure to 'offset' the zinc with 2 to 3 milligrams of copper daily. And please continue a multiple vitamin and mineral to 'back up' the individual nutrients." I wrote a specific recommendation for each item.

"There are a wide variety of botanical remedies that boost the immune system. I'd suggest you start with just two inexpensive ones—goldenseal and garlic. Goldenseal has both immune-stimulating and direct bacteria-inhibiting actions. Garlic also stimulates the immune system, and has anti-viral, anti-bacterial, and anti-fungal activity. Please use 500 milligrams of a standardized goldenseal preparation twice daily, and 2 of the pure garlic-oil capsules daily."

"Except when I'm going to see Elmer, of course."

"Maybe he won't mind a little garlic breath if you don't get sick much anymore."

Tests showed she had food sensitivities she hadn't known about. She eliminated some foods, and desensitized the rest. As recommended, she eliminated the sugar, fluoride, and chlorine, and took the vitamins, minerals, and two botanicals mentioned above. She was pleasantly surprised that over the next 4 years, she averaged less than 1 cold per year, and no flu or bronchitis at all.

Recurrent infections can be annoying and cause individuals to miss a great deal of work and/or school. Conventional medicine offers little help for individuals who are prone to infections. But natural treatments—including diet and supplements—can help strengthen the immune system and reduce the number of infections.

Dietary Considerations

Effect of Sugar

Eating refined sugar has been shown to have an adverse effect on the immune system. In one study, healthy young adults drank 24 ounces of a cola beverage (containing about 66 grams of sucrose). Within 45 minutes, the ability of their white blood cells to engulf bacteria dropped by about 50%.[1] Similar effects were produced by ingesting 100 grams of glucose, fructose, honey, or even orange juice.[2] This decline in immune function was greatest about 2 hours after consumption of the sugar, and it persisted for at least 5 hours. In another study, the ability of rats to manufacture antibodies (one of the key components of the immune system) was reduced by 50% when the diet contained as little as 10% sucrose.[3]

For these and other reasons, we advise patients with recurrent infections to discontinue all refined sugar (including fruit juices in more severe cases). Some people find that making this single dietary change greatly reduces the number of infections they experience. Cutting out refined sugar is especially important for people with recurrent yeast infections,[4] because sugar is the fuel that allows yeast organisms to thrive and multiply.

Food Allergy

For many individuals with recurrent infections, food allergy is a major underlying factor. One way

in which allergy may predispose people to infection is by causing inflammation and irritation of various tissues. For example, inflamed and irritated bronchial passages are more susceptible to invasion by bacteria than are healthy bronchi. Likewise, chronic vaginitis that results from allergy appears to be an enabling factor for vaginal yeast infections.

I typically advise patients with recurrent infections to undergo a supervised elimination diet, followed by individual food challenges. Many of these patients have other symptoms suggestive of allergy, such as nasal congestion, headaches, joint pains, fatigue, abdominal complaints, or fluid retention. These symptoms usually disappear or improve greatly on the elimination diet, and recur when allergenic foods are reintroduced. When the symptom-provoking foods are eliminated from the diet, the incidence of infections often declines dramatically.

One of the elimination diets I have used in my practice is presented in appendix A. Some doctors use other tests for allergy and sensitivity, as well as desensitization techniques. The reliability and effectiveness of some of these methods is controversial (see chapter 3 for additional discussion).

With careful attention to allergy, many types of infections improve—from recurrent colds and bronchitis to yeast infections and herpes simplex outbreaks. While there is not much published research in this area, the clinical results are usually fairly obvious. One study did show a clear relationship between food allergy and infection. Of a group of children with recurrent middle-ear infections, 78% were found to have food allergies. Excluding the offending foods from the diet led to significant improvement in 87% of the children, and subsequent challenges with suspected foods caused a flare-up in 94% of those who had improved.[5]

Nutritional Supplements

MANY DIFFERENT NUTRIENTS support the functioning of the immune system and/or the integrity of the tissues. Nutrients that are recommended by nutrition-oriented doctors to prevent infections include vitamin A, vitamin C, zinc, selenium, and essential fatty acids.

Vitamin A has been known for more than 50 years as the "anti-infection" vitamin. When animals are fed a vitamin A-deficient diet, they frequently die of respiratory or urinary-tract infections or develop otitis media (middle-ear infection). In developing countries, where vitamin A deficiency is common, supplementing with this vitamin reduced childhood mortality (usually from infection) by as much as 35%.[6] In a study done in Australia, 147 pre-school children with frequent respiratory illnesses were randomly assigned to receive 1,500 IU of vitamin A per day (equivalent to the Recommended Dietary Allowance) or a placebo for 11 months. Children receiving vitamin A had a significant 19% reduction in respiratory symptoms, compared with those receiving the placebo.[7]

The effects of vitamin C include enhancement of immune function, direct killing of some bacteria, promotion of tissue integrity, and reduction of allergic inflammation in various tissues. Each of these actions would be expected to reduce the incidence of infections. Supplementing with vitamin C has been shown to decrease both the incidence and severity of the common cold,[8] although this vitamin appears to be more effective as a treatment than as a preventative measure.[9] Some doctors have observed that large doses of vitamin C can help prevent or treat infections in patients with AIDS.[10]

Zinc also functions as an immune stimulant and increases tissue integrity. Zinc supplements have been shown to be effective in cases of recurrent furuncles (boils—caused by a staphylococcal infection)[11] and to reduce the incidence of opportunistic infections (infections that occur only when the immune system is weak) in HIV-infected patients.[12] In a double-blind study of preschool children living in New Delhi, India, supplementing with 10 mg of zinc per day reduced the incidence of respiratory infections by 45%.[13] Although zinc intake in developing countries is often lower than in the United States, it is noteworthy that the average American diet contains less than two-thirds of the Recommended Dietary Allowance for this mineral.[14]

Many other nutrients, including vitamin B6, vitamin E, iron, copper, and selenium, also play a role in enhancing immune function and preventing infection. Consequently, we recommend a broad-spectrum approach to nutritional supplementation, rather than merely picking a few of our favorite nutrients. The importance of a comprehensive approach is illustrated by a double-blind study in which a very low-dose (but relatively complete) vitamin-and-mineral supplement reduced the incidence of infections in elderly people by more than 50%.[15]

Role of Thyroid Hormone

THE THYROID GLAND plays an important role in immune function. For example, white blood cells from hypothyroid individuals have an impaired capacity to kill bacteria. This defect can be corrected by treatment with thyroid hormone.[16]

In our opinion, some patients with recurrent infections have subtle hypothyroidism that is overlooked by conventional doctors, because standard blood tests for thyroid function do not always give an accurate picture of what is going on at the cellular level (see chapter 4). Other symptoms that suggest suboptimal thyroid function include fatigue, depression, cold extremities, dry skin, constipation, thinning hair (women), and menstrual irregularities. When individuals are treated for "clinical" (as distinguished from laboratory-diagnosed) hypothyroidism, their symptoms disappear or improve, and their resistance against infection often increases considerably.

Environmental Factors

IT SEEMS THAT the incidence of chronic and recurrent infections has been steadily increasing during the past several decades. Diseases that were unknown as recently as the 1970s (particularly AIDS and chronic fatigue syndrome due to the Epstein Barr virus) have now become epidemics. Other opportunistic infections (such as herpes simplex and candidiasis) have also become much more common. During the past 20 years, we have also heard stories of ocean seals dying of strange herpes infections and giant turtles in Florida contracting AIDS-like diseases.

One might speculate that the thousands of toxic chemicals that we are releasing into the environment are taking a toll on the immune systems of exposed animals. It is also reasonable to assume that humans are being affected by these same poisons. When researchers study the effects of various chemicals on the immune system, they almost always test one substance at a time. However, preliminary evidence shows that administering a combination of chemicals—each at a dose that by itself produces no observable toxicity—can have a pronounced adverse effect on the immune system. Although there is no firm scientific proof that we are poisoning our immune systems, prudence dictates that we do our best to minimize our exposure to potentially toxic chemicals.

The increased incidence of opportunistic infections might also be related to the vaccinations that most of us have been given. When we stimulate our immune systems to mount a powerful defense against a few specific infectious agents, how do we know that we have not diminished our capacity to respond to other organisms? That question has sparked a great deal of controversy, and it should certainly be a topic of future research.

Conclusion

FOR MILLIONS OF individuals, recurrent infections are a persistent problem for which conventional medicine has little to offer. Fortunately, a natural-medicine program that includes dietary modifications, nutritional supplements and, in some cases, thyroid hormone, will often reduce the frequency and severity of infections or eliminate them completely.

Summary of Recommendations for Recurrent Infections

- Diet: Eliminate refined sugar, processed foods, and food additives. Emphasize whole foods. Restrict alcohol intake. Work with food allergies.

- High-potency multiple vitamin/mineral.

- Vitamin C, 500 to 1,000 mg, 2 to 3 times per day.

- Additional quantities of other nutrients, including vitamin A, vitamin B_6, vitamin E, zinc, iron, copper, and selenium may be helpful. However, these nutrients should be prescribed and monitored by a nutritionally oriented physician.

- Thyroid hormone in selected cases.

RHEUMATOID ARTHRITIS

RHEUMATOID ARTHRITIS (RA) *is a chronic disease of unknown cause, usually manifesting as inflammation of multiple joints. The severity of the disease varies from person to person, ranging from minor pain and discomfort to severe pain and inflammation, with joint damage and deformity. RA can also attack other parts of the body, resulting in heart disease, anemia, nerve damage, lung disease, and general debility. RA is considered an autoimmune disease, since the immune system goes awry and attacks the body's own tissues. RA differs from the other common form of joint disease, osteoarthritis, in that there is a greater amount of inflammation and joint deformity with RA. In addition, unlike RA, osteoarthritis does not affect tissues other than the joints.*

Conventional therapy includes drugs such as aspirin, ibuprofen, or other "nonsteroidal anti-inflammatory drugs" (NSAIDs). In more severe cases, doctors may prescribe cortisone-like drugs such as prednisone. Other so-called "anti-rheumatic drugs," such as gold or methotrexate are sometimes recommended in the hope of arresting the progress of the disease. Unfortunately, all of these anti-rheumatic drugs are relatively toxic, and we have only limited evidence that they improve the long-term prognosis of patients with the disease. Recently, a new class of drugs known as COX-2 inhibitors has been introduced. Although these drugs are being promoted as a safer alternative to NSAIDs, reports of adverse effects are already beginning to appear.

DR. WRIGHT'S CASE STUDY

"I know there aren't any cures for rheumatoid arthritis," Teresa Clancy said. "And I don't expect that some of my joints will ever look normal again." She held up her hands. "But I would like to prevent any further deformities, and get rid of as much swelling and inflammation as I can without using that prednisone again, and with as little aspirin as possible. My neighbor Emily has rheumatoid arthritis, too. She started with your clinic 3 years ago, and she doesn't even take aspirin, except when she messes up on her diet. I

kept waiting for her to flare up again, because my rheumatologist keeps saying that diet, vitamins, and herbs have nothing to do with rheumatoid arthritis. But it's obvious to me that they make a lot of difference for her—so here I am."

"What are you doing now?"

"For my arthritis, you mean? Right now, about 12 aspirin a day. Some days more, some days less."

"How's your stomach?"

"About like you'd expect with all that aspirin. Some heartburn and some indigestion."

"Any other medications?"

"No other drugs," she smiled slyly. "But I

have been taking some of the things you told Emily about—the ones that seemed harmless anyway, especially those ginger capsules. I swear they've taken down some of the swelling in my fingers and knees, and you know what, they make my stomach feel better, too. Is that possible?"

"Ginger is one of the best herbal remedies for stomach problems of all kinds. And you're right, it helps rheumatoid arthritis, too. But before we talk about any more specific remedies, let's go over your diet. Have you made any changes there?"

"Well . . ." She looked at her feet. "That's part of why it took me 3 years to get here. Emily says I'm one of the worst junk-food junkies she's ever seen. My husband says there's no point spending the money to come in here if I'm not ready to make a big diet change." She took a deep breath, "So I'm ready."

"You're sure?"

"Yes. And Emily says she'll help."

"Before we even get to individual food allergies and sensitivities, which play a big part in aggravating rheumatoid arthritis . . ."

"I know. Emily can't have any milk or dairy or her joints let her know. No pork or tomatoes, either. I'm just hoping I'm not allergic to all my favorites."

"Before we test you for your individual sensitivities, there are some dietary rules for good health that apply to all of us. One basic rule is to eat whole, unprocessed foods, with no added sugar—no so-called 'soft drinks.'"

"That'll be a big one to get over for me."

"Also, no added chemicals, such as artificial flavorings, colorings, or preservatives. Only whole grains—if you're not allergic or sensitive to them. No artificial sweeteners, only small amounts of alcohol . . ."

"I don't drink the stuff anyway."

"No caffeine, no nicotine . . ."

"I'm OK there, too."

"When you put all this together with strict allergy and sensitivity avoidance—at least until some desensitization is done—it can be very difficult. Make sure to see our nutritionist here at the clinic as soon as your testing is done, as well as talking to Emily."

"Oh, I'll make sure to do that. Emily told me how important it is to get my diet right from the start. In fact, she said she wouldn't help me unless I did that first."

"Also, please have your digestion checked, especially your stomach's production of acid. A malfunctioning stomach is a common problem for people who have rheumatoid arthritis."

"Is that the test with the radio capsule and the string that Emily told me about?"

"Yes. If your stomach and other digestive organs are working well, then a whole-food, no-allergy diet, and all the supplements are much more likely to help you along."

"That makes sense. But I thought it was just the aspirin bothering my stomach."

"Could be, but more often than not, people with rheumatoid arthritis have very poor stomach function regardless of taking aspirin or other drugs."

"OK. I'll do it."

"I'll make you a list of supplemental items that can help lessen the symptoms of rheumatoid arthritis, but you probably won't be able to use them all right away. Chances are that testing will show you're sensitive to some of them."

"Emily's told me about that, too. She says to begin with, you didn't want her to take anything without screening it first. Now that she's much better, she just tries things one at a time, and she can tell if they bother her. Why couldn't she do that from the start?"

"She could, and you could too, if no testing were available. But doing it that way is much more tedious and time-consuming. Also, many people with rheumatoid arthritis have so many sensitivities and allergies that telling one from another at the beginning can be nearly impossible."

"So, what's on the list?"

"Just as a reminder—a good diet, individualized for you, is most important. And that'll very likely go along with digestive aids. Without those, the supplements won't work nearly as well."

"I got it! I promised my husband before I ever came here I'd do it all!"

"To start—and remember to get all these items screened—cod-liver oil, 1 tablespoonful, twice daily, or the equivalent in capsules. Research studies show that the omega-3 fatty acids found in cod-liver oil are effective against rheumatoid arthritis. The vitamin D in cod-liver oil is important for your bones. To make sure that 2 tablespoonfuls of cod-liver oil don't contain too much vitamin D, we'll monitor your serum calcium—but don't worry, in 20 years or more I've seen no problem. Also, whenever we take extra oils, it's necessary to use extra vitamin E. Please take 400 IU daily." I wrote these down for her.

"Next, niacinamide. Years ago, Dr. William Kaufman conducted an extensive clinical study of the effect of niacinamide on both osteoarthritis and rheumatoid arthritis. He observed that niacinamide helped reduce swelling, and in some cases it actually helped to partially remobilize rheumatoid joints that had been immobile for years."

"Wow." She lifted her hands again. "I wonder if these two fingers can be less crooked again."

"It'll take months to find out. Please take niacinamide, 500 milligrams, 3 times daily. It's unlikely, but if you notice any nausea or queasiness, stop the niacinamide and let us know. We'll do a blood test periodically to monitor your liver enzymes, because there is a very small chance that taking niacinamide can put stress on the liver."

"Alright."

"Next are copper, zinc, and boron. Copper is a major help in reducing inflammation. Many people who are taking aspirin, ibuprofen, and other anti-inflammatories of that type find they need much less if they take copper, too. Please use copper (sebacate), 4 milligrams daily for now—we'll need to monitor this one a little more closely. Next, zinc. Get zinc picolinate or zinc citrate, and use 30 milligrams of elemental zinc, 3 times daily for now. Again this one will need monitoring. Then there's boron . . ."

"Boron? Is that the stuff they were putting

in the gasoline awhile ago?"

"Boron is an element. There are some very intriguing studies showing an inverse correlation between boron in the soil and the incidence of all types of arthritis. Less boron, more arthritis, and vice versa. Unfortunately, there's not a great deal of study of boron and rheumatoid arthritis, but occasionally it really does well, especially in children with rheumatoid arthritis. Please use 3 milligrams, 3 times daily."

"What about my ginger capsules?"

"We won't leave those out. How much have you been using?"

"Well, I noticed the more I took, the better my joints did, and my stomach, too. I couldn't find anywhere that large quantities of ginger were dangerous, and obviously I didn't react—so I'm taking 9 grams a day; 3 grams, 3 times daily." She finished in a rush, and looked at me sideways. "Is that OK?"

"I'm glad you looked it up before taking a lot. Not all herbs are safe in large quantities. Fortunately, ginger is. Especially since it's helping, keep it up." I added it to her list. "Other herbs have been found helpful for some people with rheumatoid arthritis, too. Yucca, 'Devil's claw', and cayenne pepper—that one's often used as a 'rub-in'. Also, bromelain is a helpful anti-inflammatory. These are all possible tools."

"Should I use any of them?"

"Stick with the ginger for now, since it's working. If you don't do as well as we'd like with the first list, or if you're sensitive to too many of them, the others are available to try."

"Anything else?"

"That should do for now."

"Whole-food diet, no allergies or sensitivities, cod-liver oil and vitamin E, niacinamide, copper, zinc, boron, and ginger. I won't have time to do anything else."

"Not until you're organized, anyway. Remember to be checked for sensitivities first—you may not be able to use some of these items until after you're desensitized to them. And there's one more test, too."

"Another test? What's that?"

"For DHEA, an adrenal hormone. It's an important regulator of the immune system, and it is often useful in autoimmune diseases. It's also often lower than normal in people with a variety of autoimmune diseases, including rheumatoid arthritis."

It took Mrs. Clancy 2 months to get her tests done and her diet and supplement program entirely organized. Her progress was a little slower than usual, but after a year she was off the daily aspirin entirely, and the pain and swelling in her joints were almost completely gone. She even had a little more mobility in her worst joints. After another year, she reported that, "just like Emily, my joints tell me when I mess up," and that her husband couldn't believe how well she was sticking to her program. As she told me, "They're the only joints I have." Five years later, she continues to do well.

DR. GABY'S COMMENTARY

NATURAL MEDICINE HAS a number of promising treatments to offer people who are suffering from RA. While these treatments do not work every time, they are remarkably safe and sometimes produce dramatic results.

Dietary Considerations
The Food-Allergy Connection

FOOD allergy has been reported to play a role in a number of inflammatory and autoimmune conditions, including RA. In one study, 22 patients with RA followed an allergy-elimination diet. Twenty (91%) of the patients noticed an improvement in their arthritis, and 19 reported that specific foods repeatedly caused their symptoms to worsen. The average time on the elimination diet before improvement occurred was 10 days, while the longest time was 18 days. Patients reacted to an average of 2.5 foods, the most common of which were grains, milk, nuts, beef, and egg.[1]

Highly allergic or chemically sensitive individuals may also develop arthritic reactions to pesticides or to other food-derived chemicals. Consequently, consuming organically grown foods may be helpful for some individuals with RA.[2] The important role that food allergy plays in RA has been confirmed in a blinded, placebo-controlled study, which demonstrated that the improvements associated with dietary changes cannot be explained merely by a placebo effect.[3]

In my practice, I have found that avoiding allergenic foods is most often successful for younger female patients (ages 25 to 40) with less severe cases of RA. In fact, of the 15 or so patients I have seen over the years who fit that description, just about everyone improved dramatically with diet changes alone. Older patients and those with more aggressive arthritis also frequently responded, but the improvement was usually only partial, and some did not improve at all.

One of the elimination diets I have used in my practice is presented in appendix A. Some doctors use other tests for allergy and sensitivity, as well as desensitization techniques. The reliability and effectiveness of some of these methods is controversial (see chapter 3 for additional discussion).

Nutritional Supplements
Zinc and Copper

ZINC is known to exert a mild anti-inflammatory effect and may, therefore, be of value in treating individuals with RA. In a double-blind study, 24 patients with moderately severe RA received either zinc (sulfate), 50 mg, 3 times a day, or a placebo for 12 weeks. Compared with placebo treatment, zinc significantly reduced joint swelling and morning stiffness, and significantly improved the patients' overall condition.[4] In another study of patients with more severe RA, zinc therapy was ineffective.[5] Thus, the therapeutic effect of zinc may depend on the severity of the disease.

Copper is also known to have anti-inflammatory activity. Indeed, folk wisdom teaches that wearing a copper bracelet can relieve arthritic symptoms. Although most conventional doctors consider that claim to be nonsense, research confirms that the copper bracelet does have an effect. In a double-blind study of patients with RA, those who wore a copper bracelet fared significantly better than did those who wore an identically colored placebo bracelet.[6] Surprisingly, the weight of the bracelet decreased by 13 mg after patients wore it for 1 month. The results of this study suggest that copper can be absorbed through the skin into the body, where it exerts an anti-inflammatory effect.

We frequently prescribe 30 to 90 mg of zinc and 2 to 4 mg of copper per day for patients with RA. Both of these supplements can cause nausea, particularly if they are taken on an empty stomach. Since taking zinc alone can cause copper deficiency, we do not recommend using zinc by itself.

Copper may be an even more effective anti-arthritic agent when it is chelated (a type of chemical binding) with an established arthritis medication. For example, the copper chelate of aspirin, known as copper aspirinate, is both more effective and less toxic than aspirin itself. Whereas most of the anti-inflammatory drugs can cause peptic ulcers, the copper chelates of these same drugs have actually promoted ulcer healing in animal studies.[7] Copper aspirinate can be obtained by prescription through a compounding pharmacist. It seems to work very well for some arthritis patients, whereas other patients either do not respond or experience excessive nausea.

Selenium

THE trace mineral selenium is also known to have anti-inflammatory effects. Serum selenium levels were significantly lower in a group of 87 patients with RA than in healthy individuals. The reduction in serum selenium was greatest among patients with the most severe disease.[8] In a double-blind trial, 15 women with RA received either 200 mcg of selenium per day (from selenium-rich yeast) or a placebo for 3 months. Pain and joint inflammation were reduced in 6 of 8 women treated with selenium, but there was no significant change in the placebo group.[9] Selenium was ineffective in another study,[10] possibly because the patients in that study had more severe arthritis.

Although vitamin E has not been tested as a treatment for RA, we usually recommend it along with selenium, since these 2 nutrients work together in the body.

Essential Fatty Acids

RA has also been shown to respond to supplementation with several different oils. In a double-blind study, 37 patients with active RA received either 1.4 grams of gamma-linolenic acid (GLA; from borage oil) per day or a placebo (cottonseed oil) for 24 weeks. Treatment with GLA resulted in a statistically significant and clinically important reduction in disease activity, compared with no change or a deterioration in those receiving the placebo. GLA reduced the number of tender joints by 36%, the tender-joint score by 45%, and the swollen-joint score by 41%. No serious side effects occurred, although a few patients reported minor intestinal discomfort from borage oil.[11]

In another double-blind study, 16 patients with RA received 12 capsules of fish oil per day or a placebo for 12 weeks, then the other treatment for an additional 12 weeks. Fish oil was significantly more effective than the placebo in reducing joint swelling and morning stiffness.[12] Supplementing with black-currant-seed oil has also been shown to relieve the symptoms of RA.[13]

It should be noted that different oils exert different effects in the body. Borage oil, evening primrose oil, and black-currant-seed oil contain GLA (one of the so-called "omega-6" fatty acids), whereas fish oil contains eicosapentaenoic acid

(EPA) and docosahexaenoic acid (DHA), both of which are omega-3 fatty acids.

Additional research is needed before we will know what dosages and combinations of oils are best for individuals with RA. Some individuals may respond best to omega-3 fatty acids, others to omega-6, and still others to a combination. When in doubt, measuring essential-fatty-acid concentrations in the blood may provide some guidance.

Niacinamide

DR. William Kaufman's pioneering work from the 1940s with niacinamide was discussed in the chapter on osteoarthritis. Although most of his patients had osteoarthritis, those with RA appeared to improve, as well. Kaufman's original observations on osteoarthritis[14] were confirmed several years ago in a double-blind study.[15] However, no one has attempted to replicate his findings in people with RA. Considering the relative safety of niacinamide (when used properly), additional research is warranted.

Herbal Supplements
Ginger Root

GINGER HAS BEEN used for thousands of years in Ayurvedic medicine and other systems of traditional medicine as an anti-inflammatory agent. In one study, 6 patients with RA consumed 5 grams of fresh ginger or 0.5 to 1 gram of powdered ginger daily. After 3 months, every patient reported pain relief, better joint mobility, and less swelling and morning stiffness, even though they had stopped taking their anti-inflammatory medications. No side effects were reported.[16] Ginger appears to inhibit the inflammation-promoting enzyme cyclooxygenase, and in that respect acts similarly to (but is safer than) aspirin, ibuprofen, and related drugs.

Conclusion

RHEUMATOID ARTHRITIS CAN be a severe and debilitating disease. The safety and effectiveness of conventional treatment leave a lot to be desired. Patients with RA frequently respond to the natural approach, which includes working with food allergies and supplementing with zinc, copper, selenium, vitamin E, fatty acids, niacinamide, and ginger.

Summary of Recommendations for Treating Rheumatoid Arthritis

(NOTE: Treatment should be medically supervised)

PRIMARY RECOMMENDATIONS:

- Work with food allergies.

- Zinc (picolinate or citrate), 30 mg, 1 to 3 times per day. Balance with copper, 2 to 4 mg per day.

- Essential fatty acids (choose one of the following):

  ➤ Borage oil, providing 750 to 1,500 mg of gamma-linolenic acid per day.

  ➤ Fish-oil concentrate, 5 to 10 grams per day; or cod-liver oil, 1 to 2 tablespoons per day. (Note: Because of their vitamin A and D content, doses of cod-liver oil greater than 1 tablespoon per day should be supervised by a doctor.) Black-currant-seed oil, 5 to 10 grams per day.

- Vitamin E, 400 IU per day, to balance essential fatty acids or to support selenium.

OTHER RECOMMENDATIONS:

- Fresh ginger root (5 grams per day) or ginger-root powder (0.5 to 1.0 gram per day), or as directed by a physician.

- Niacinamide, 500 mg, 3 times per day. Reduce dose if nausea occurs. Monitor blood test for liver enzymes periodically.

- Selenium, 200 mcg per day.

SHINGLES *(herpes zoster)*

HERPES ZOSTER *(also known as shingles) is caused by the same virus that causes chicken pox (Varicella zoster). The condition occurs in partially immune individuals (i.e., those who have previously had chicken pox). The skin lesions of herpes zoster are similar in appearance to those of herpes simplex, and they can be quite painful. These lesions usually heal within 7 to 10 days, although in some individuals they persist for 2 to 4 weeks. In more than half of individuals over the age of 50 (and less commonly in younger people), pain may persist for many months or even years at the site of the previous infection. Known as post-herpetic or post-zoster neuralgia, this chronic pain is often frustrating for both patient and doctor.*

Herpes zoster is common in people with cancer, AIDS, and other diseases that are associated with impaired immune function. However, more subtle immune-system deficiencies may also increase the risk of developing zoster. For that reason, a comprehensive prevention-and-treatment plan should include measures that enhance immune function. These include avoiding refined sugar, eliminating allergenic foods from the diet, getting adequate amounts of sleep and exercise, and keeping stress at tolerable levels.

Conventional therapy consists mainly of anti-viral drugs, which are helpful to some extent. However, these drugs are rather expensive, and they can cause side effects.

DR. WRIGHT'S CASE STUDY

Grace French was obviously in considerable pain. She walked slowly, holding her left arm away from her side. Her daughter supported her right side. She made her way into the examination room and sat down. It was obvious she'd been crying.

"It's this shingles," she said. "I don't want to take any drugs. I'm just against it, but I can't stand the pain. Linda called in and your nurse said there were some vitamin shots that might help. So we got here as soon as we could."

Her blouse wasn't tucked in, and she lifted the left side. She had a series of angry-looking small, clumped red blisters roughly in a line from near her spine around to the front of her ribs.

"Have you put anything on it?" I asked.

"Not today. I wanted you to see it."

"We'll do the injection first. And while you're getting that done, I'll also write down the formula for a 'nutrient goo' that should help considerably, also."

"What kind of injection?"

"Today, tomorrow, and maybe the next day an IV given here at the clinic. As soon as the pain has diminished enough, you can continue with a modified version intramuscularly at home. Linda can do the shots for you."

"What's in the IV?"

"Several things—vitamin B$_{12}$, B-complex with an emphasis on vitamin B$_1$, vitamin C, adenosine monophosphate, lithium, selenium, and glycyrrhizin."

"All natural?"

"Yes."

"Well, give me the shot first, and explain what it's all about afterwards. I'm in too much pain to listen now."

Approximately 2 hours later she was back. She appeared to be in considerably less pain. "Don't know if it was the shot or the 'nutrient goo' that's under this bandage, or what, but I surely am feeling better. In fact, the pain is better than half-gone already. Now, tell me what all this stuff is," she said.

"You know what vitamin B$_{12}$, B-complex, and vitamin C are," I started, "and you know lithium and selenium are minerals . . ."

"Yes. But I thought lithium was for manic-depressive people. I sure was feeling depressed, but that's not the same."

"Every mineral or vitamin has dozens—even hundreds—of uses and purposes. Lithium has been found to inhibit reproduction of some viruses, including the herpes viruses. Can't say it's directly responsible for pain relief this quickly, but it's making a start on stopping this outbreak, anyway. Selenium inhibits herpes virus reproduction in a slightly different way."

"You mentioned 2 other things I don't remember in that IV, too."

"Yes, adenosine monophosphate and glycyrrhizin. Glycyrrhizin is a portion of licorice that also inhibits viruses. Adenosine monophosphate is actually a natural metabolite found in our bodies. Years ago, a researcher found that injections of adenosine monophosphate helped many shingles sufferers relieve their pain."

"And this 'nutrient goo?'"

"It's a combination of aloe vera, vitamin E, zinc oxide, lithium cream, glycyrrhizin, and vitamin B$_{12}$, all rubbed in with DMSO. DMSO is dimethylsulfoxide—a wood-pulp extract that helps transport all of these compounds through the skin."

"I thought I detected a familiar odor. But that's OK if it helps that awful pain."

"It does, and it helps it heal more rapidly too. It also reduces the chance of 'post-herpetic neuralgia.'"

"That doesn't sound good at all. What is it?"

"Post-herpetic neuralgia is pain that persists even when all visible signs of the shingles—the herpes zoster—are gone."

"I definitely don't want that."

"Please come back tomorrow for another IV. From the looks of things, that might be the last one you'll need. After that, we'll ask your daughter to give you intramuscular injections of vitamin B$_{12}$, B-complex, and adenosine monophosphate at home. Of course, you should continue to use the 'nutrient goo', and there are some supplements you should take until this is completely gone."

"What're those?"

"Vitamin C, 4 grams, 3 times a day. Also, L-lysine, 2 grams, 3 times daily in between meals. Selenium, 250 micrograms twice daily, and a very temporary prescription for lithium."

"And I can eat lots of licorice for that glycyr . . . whatever, right?"

"Glycyrrhizin. Sure, licorice is fine unless you have high blood pressure." I checked her record. "You don't, but even if you did, it'd need to be very high for a few days of licorice to bother it. However, please limit the licorice to a maximum of 1 week, as prolonged use of large amounts can cause high blood pressure, potassium deficiency, or other problems. Make sure to get the kind with no artificial colors or sugar."

"Always did like licorice." She got up. "Let's go, Linda."

She reported later that the "shingles" pain was completely gone within 3 days, and her skin was back to normal within 3 weeks. Most important, Grace French did not develop post-herpetic neuralgia, the chronic painful condition that more than 50 percent of elderly individuals develop after a bout of shingles.

DR. GABY'S COMMENTARY

THE TWO MAIN goals in the treatment of herpes zoster are to accelerate healing of the lesions and to prevent the development of post-herpetic neuralgia. Although there are only a few studies on the use of natural remedies to treat herpes zoster, some of the research related to other viral diseases (see the chapter on herpes simplex) may be applicable to the treatment of herpes zoster. Dr. Wright's use of vitamin C,[1] zinc,[2] licorice extract,[3] and selenium[4] is based on their reported anti-viral effects.

Nutritional Supplements
Vitamin E

IN one study, 13 patients with chronic post-zoster neuralgia were given vitamin E orally (400 to 1,600 IU per day), and applied the vitamin to the skin at the area of discomfort. Nine of the 13 patients experienced complete or almost complete relief of pain and the others had slight or moderate relief. Two of the patients who were cured had had painful neuralgia for 13 and 19 years, respectively.[5] To obtain the maximum benefit from vitamin E therapy, it is important to avoid ingesting inorganic iron at the same time—either as medication, in vitamin tablets, or in the form of cereal or white bread fortified with iron. Inorganic iron combines with and inactivates vitamin E.

Vitamin B₁₂

IN one study, intramuscular injections of vitamin B_{12} appeared to accelerate the healing of acute herpes zoster.[6] Vitamin B_{12} has also been reported to relieve various types of neuritis and neuralgia. Some doctors give B_{12} injections to patients with zoster, in the hope of preventing post-herpetic neuralgia.

Other Treatments
Adenosine Monophosphate

ADENOSINE monophosphate (AMP) is a compound that occurs naturally in the body. It is known to have activity against herpes viruses and to enhance immune function. In 1 study, 130 patients with herpes zoster received a series of AMP injections, beginning early in the course of their illness. The treatment regimen was similar to that used for herpes simplex. Their lesions healed unusually rapidly, and none of the patients developed post-herpetic neuralgia over a 2-year follow-up period.[7] No significant side effects were seen. The beneficial effect of AMP against herpes zoster was later confirmed in a double-blind study.[8]

Because AMP appears to prevent the development of post-herpetic neuralgia, it would seem like a good idea to give patients a series of injections as soon as possible after the onset of acute herpes zoster. AMP would be particularly helpful for people over age 50, who are at greatest risk of developing neuralgia.

Intramuscular injections of AMP occasionally cause temporary chest pain. Although this pain is not related to the heart, it can be alarming. Chest pain can usually be prevented by giving half of the full dose, waiting 20 minutes, then giving the other half. Dr. Wright has observed that AMP works better when given intravenously rather than by the intramuscular route. However, if administered too rapidly, intravenous AMP can cause life-threatening heart-rhythm disturbances. For that reason, intravenous AMP should be given very slowly (over at least 30 minutes) and only by a physician knowledgeable in its use. I have been satisfied with the results using intramuscular AMP, and I have not given it intravenously.

Capsaicin

APPLYING a cream containing capsaicin (an extract of chili pepper) can relieve the pain of post-herpetic neuralgia.[9] This product is sold over the counter under the name Zostrix. Capsaicin cream produces a burning sensation with each application during the first few days, but the pain does subside, and relief is often seen shortly thereafter. Care should be taken to keep capsaicin away from the eyes.

Summary of Recommendations for Treating Herpes Zoster (Shingles)

- Injections of adenosine monophosphate, vitamin B_{12}, vitamin C, and possibly other antiviral agents, in selected cases.

- Vitamin C, 3 to 10 grams per day orally for acute treatment.

- Vitamin E, 400 to 1,600 IU per day, for prevention and/or treatment of post-herpetic neuralgia.

- Capsaicin cream (supervised by a doctor) for treatment of post-herpetic neuralgia.

- Various other antiviral agents (including zinc, selenium, licorice extracts, and lithium) have been used either orally or topically by some doctors of natural medicine; however, there is little research on their effectiveness for herpes zoster.

ULCERATIVE COLITIS

ULCERATIVE COLITIS IS *a disease in which the colon becomes inflamed, resulting in abdominal pain and bloody diarrhea. In its milder forms, ulcerative colitis is merely a nuisance, or it may produce no symptoms at all. However, in some patients, the diarrhea and bleeding can be severe enough to cause dehydration and anemia. Inflammatory bowel disease (a term which includes ulcerative colitis and Crohn's disease) is a common medical problem, affecting millions of Americans. Individuals with ulcerative colitis often develop complications, including nutritional deficiencies, arthritis, skin and eye disorders, liver disease, kidney stones, and colon cancer.*

Although the cause of ulcerative colitis is not known, it is considered to be an autoimmune disease—one in which the body's immune system attacks its own tissues. Various abnormalities of immune-system function have been identified in individuals with this condition. Standard treatment consists primarily of cortisone-like drugs and other anti-inflammatory medications and in some cases antibiotics. If the condition becomes severe or debilitating, surgical removal of some or all of the colon may be necessary. Although conventional therapy relieves the symptoms in many cases, it is often ineffective. Furthermore, there are many risks and complications involved with the standard drug-and-surgery approach.

DR. WRIGHT'S CASE STUDY

"I want to get rid of this ulcerative colitis," Jim Olson declared. "I'm told it's chronic, and there's nothing to do except take medications indefinitely and hope for the best. Right now, the bleeding's back again. So I can hardly go anywhere or do anything without making sure there's a bathroom handy. I've had to start the prednisone again." He handed me two prescription bottles.

"Prednisone, sulfasalazine," I read. "Fairly standard. How long have you had colitis?"

"Eight years since they told me that's what it was. But I've always had a tendency to bowel trouble—loose stools, gas—that sort of thing. My mother tells me I had a lot of stomach aches as a child."

"Any idea why it worsened 8 years ago?"

"I was under a lot of stress at work, and started having a lot of bleeding. I'd had a little bit of blood on and off for years, but never thought much of it. That time, it was really a lot, so I went to the doctor and they did X-rays and that scope thing and told me it was ulcerative colitis and that the stress caused it. They put me on these medications, and it gradually slowed down. Since then it's never been completely gone, and it gets bad regularly. I've noticed stress can make it worse, but not always. Sometimes it's really bad when I'm not stressed at all. So, I'm sure that's not the whole answer."

"After the X-rays and scope thing, where did they tell you the problem was?"

"Mostly in the lower colon, maybe a little bit further up."

"You're how old now?"

"I'm 37. I was 29 the first time it really got bad."

"Besides bleeding and diarrhea, do you notice mucus?"

"Usually. Sometimes that happens by itself, too, without any other symptoms."

"Do you get heartburn or indigestion?"

"Not much heartburn, unless I eat too much. I had a lot more of that when I was younger. I do get a lot of indigestion, but they tell me that's just part of the colitis."

"Any other symptoms?"

"Nothing major. I'm more tired than I think I should be, but if it weren't for this colitis thing I'd be doing pretty well."

"Anyone else in your family have colitis?"

"I'm told my grandfather did. My mother's pretty healthy—she gets migraines though. My father's had hay fever and sinus most of his life, and so do both my brothers." He thought for a moment. "There's diabetes and cancer in the family, too—grandparents and aunts and uncles. That's all I can think of."

"No children?"

"Not yet. Only been married 2 years."

"What sort of things do you eat?"

He smiled. "That's been changing some since we got married. Now I'm eating breakfast instead of just a cup of coffee. Usually oatmeal or no-sugar cornflakes with milk and a glass of juice. Lunch has stayed mostly the same. Because of my job, I'm always in a hurry, so it's fast food or Chinese or Mexican take-out."

"And dinners?"

"Definitely an improvement the last 2 years. Not near as many pizzas and sandwiches, more green stuff. We have chicken, beef, pasta, and the usual run of things, but Barbara's been on a program to eliminate the sugar and junky snacks, eat whole grains, and so on. Doing it slow so I don't complain too much. She's even got me taking a one-a-day type vitamin."

"Sounds good. Has it helped the colitis?"

"Seemed to, at first. But it started getting bad again 6 months or so back, and Barb's been persuading me to come over here ever since. One of her friends did, and got a lot better, and they've been reading health magazines ever since."

After completing Mr. Olson's health history, we went to the exam room. Aside from slight abdominal tenderness and a bit more gas than average, his exam was generally normal.

"Now what? Take some more vitamins or something?"

"That's part of the program, but first the basics. Please have food allergy and sensitivity screening done. I'll be recommending you eliminate for at least several months the foods that test positive. And you may as well eliminate all milk and dairy products starting now."

Mr. Olson looked surprised. "Allergies? My father and brother have allergies, but I never had any, that I know of, anyway."

"Everyone I've ever worked with who has ulcerative colitis is allergic to foods. Milk and dairy are nearly always a problem, that's why I recommended stopping them now. Even if that weren't the case, it's basic in natural, nutritional medicine to screen people for allergies if other family members have them. You have allergy on both sides of your family. There's usually allergic involvement with sinus problems and nearly always with migraine headaches, too."

"Really? I'll tell my mom."

"After you've been screened for allergy, please bring your wife in for a visit with our nutritionist. Usually a fairly big diet change is required for at least several months."

He looked hopeful. "Not permanent?"

"I do recommend permanently eliminating the milk and dairy products, and your wife has you started on a few other changes which should be permanent—no sugar, white flour, food chemicals, hydrogenated vegetable oils—that sort of 'dietary housecleaning'. But most allergies and sensitivities to good, wholesome food can be desensitized, so the foods can be re-introduced later on without causing bowel problems again.

"Next, please have your stomach tested for normal acid and pepsin production."

"What's my stomach have to do with it? It's my colon that's the problem—or so they tell me."

"We check everyone with ulcerative colitis for stomach function, and the large majority are abnormal—some severely so. Remember you told me you get some indigestion? That's likely due to weak stomach function. If your food isn't completely digested, it's more irritating to the colon, which isn't really a digestive organ."

"Makes sense. What else?"

"Vitamins and minerals next. Please have these tests done." I handed him a lab request slip. "Some of these vitamins and minerals are quite standard for helping to heal an ulcerated colon. After you have them screened for sensitivity, you might as well start right away while you're waiting for other test results."

"Screened for sensitivity—to vitamins? I didn't know it was possible to be sensitive to vitamins or minerals."

I laughed. "Unfortunately, it's possible to be allergic or sensitive to nearly anything. As long as you're having allergy screening anyway, it's best to be careful." I started to write a list. "First, please use zinc (as zinc picolinate), 30 milligrams, 3 times daily. Zinc promotes healing of ulcers anywhere in or on the body—colon, peptic ulcer, leg ulcers—it's a general healing promoter and accelerator. Next, vitamin A. Start with 150,000 IU daily . . ."

"Isn't that an awful lot of vitamin A?"

"Not when you've got bleeding ulcerative colitis. Vitamin A stimulates healing and normalization of the cells lining the colon and the rest of the gastrointestinal tract. In addition, prednisone interferes with normal healing and impairs normal immune function, and vitamin A helps to reverse those effects. As you improve, we'll cut the vitamin A back, as it might be too much once things are more normal."

"OK."

"Whenever we use extra vitamin A, it's wisest to add vitamin E. It keeps the A from breaking down too rapidly, and it helps on its own. Please use 400 IU daily. Vitamin C promotes healing, too, but with a diarrhea problem, use only 1,000 milligrams of a buffered type daily. Try to find one with some flavonoid content." I wrote this all down.

"That's a lot of stuff."

"That's what it takes—but we're almost done for today. Just two more things. Keep using a multiple vitamin-mineral—a good high potency one. And last, enemas with sodium butyrate."

Mr. Olson groaned. "Enemas? I've had to use those cortisone enemas twice, a few years back when the colitis got so bad they were going to hospitalize me. The enemas worked, but it isn't that bad right now. Can't I try this other stuff first?"

"Remember you want to get rid of the colitis. Butyrate is one of our more important tools. Butyrate is a naturally-occurring fatty acid, and it's the principal source of energy for the cells that line the colon. If we give them a lot of their major energy source, they get stronger and healthier in a lot less time."

"Can't I just swallow it?"

"Sure, but it doesn't work very well. You said the problem's mostly in the lower colon. Why not put the butyrate right where the problem is—right on those sick colon cells—so they can soak up the energy before the rest of your intestine gets at it?"

"OK, OK. It makes sense when you explain it that way. If this will cure the problem, I'll do it."

"The overall program has a very good chance of doing just that. You'll need all the supplements, very likely help for your stomach, and careful allergy work to get the job done. Especially careful about allergies and sensitivities, as they likely triggered the problem, and you've probably had them most or all of your life. Remember what your mother said about your childhood stomach aches? And you mentioned you've always had a tendency to excess gas and loose bowels."

He looked thoughtful. "Allergies, huh? Wish I'd known."

"One more thing . . ."

"Thought you said that was all."

"Nothing more to swallow today, just a blood test. It's for DHEA—an adrenal hormone that's often helpful with more severe allergies and in autoimmune conditions. Actually, ulcerative colitis is one of a 'family' of autoimmune problems, so please check to see if your DHEA levels are low. If they are, using supplemental DHEA can be another major help in eliminating the problem."

Jim Olson was found to be sensitive to a total of 37 foods, which his wife said politely "makes for some interesting meal planning." His stomach test disclosed very low acid production. He reported that supplementing with hydrochloric acid and pepsin capsules with meals not only eliminated his indigestion, but made a significant reduction in his diarrhea and gas. He was able to use all the recommended supplements, along with

30 milligrams of DHEA per day, which I recommended because his blood level was found to be quite low.

After 6 months, he reported his symptoms were gone. He was able to taper off the prednisone and discontinue the sulfasalazine; and, following desensitization, was able to return most of the eliminated foods to his diet over the next few months, although I insisted he stay away from cow's milk and other dairy products. With his wife's help, he's stayed away from sugar, processed food, hydrogenated fats, and food chemicals, with "only an occasional lapse." He has continued the hydrochloric acid-pepsin supplements, the vitamin-mineral supplements, and DHEA. He reduced the amount of vitamin A gradually to 50,000 IU daily, and the zinc to 30 milligrams twice daily, along with an "offsetting" amount of copper (as copper sebacate), 4 milligrams daily. He tapered down, then stopped the butyrate enemas over 9 months' time. Three years after starting the program, he insisted on a complete exam with "the scope thing", and was told he'd had a "spontaneous remission," as there was no sign of ulcerative colitis or other colon disease.

DR. GABY'S COMMENTARY

THERE ARE A number of effective natural remedies for ulcerative colitis. In addition to improving the chances for success, these natural treatments may also reduce the need for dangerous prescription drugs. In our experience, most patients with ulcerative colitis have benefited from the nutritional approach, and many have seen dramatic results. As is often the case with nutritional medicine, many doctors are unaware of—or resistant to—these safe and effective alternatives. Fortunately, this is changing, as more and more physicians are becoming open-minded to new possibilities.

Dietary Considerations
Food Allergies

THE first and most important step in treating ulcerative colitis is to identify food allergies. Numerous medical journal reports over the years have shown that food allergy is a major contributing factor in ulcerative colitis.[1, 2, 3, 4] The most common offending foods are wheat, dairy products, corn products, and eggs. Other foods, including citrus fruits, yeast, coffee, tea, alcohol, sugar, and various food additives may also provoke symptoms. Carrageenan is a compound derived from seaweed and used as a stabilizer in processed foods.

It has been shown to cause ulceration of the colon in animals,[5] but its effect on humans is not known. Until more information becomes available, we advise our patients to avoid carrageenan.

Food allergies can be identified by means of a medically supervised elimination diet. If symptoms improve on the diet (usually in 3 weeks or less, if they are going to improve at all), foods are reintroduced one at a time. Foods that provoke abdominal pain, diarrhea, bleeding, or other symptoms are then removed from the diet. At least half of the patients we have seen with ulcerative colitis report significant improvement with dietary modification alone. In some cases, the colitis just disappears and does not return unless the patient goes off the diet.

One of the elimination diets I have used in my practice is presented in appendix A. Some doctors use other tests for allergy and sensitivity, as well as desensitization techniques. The reliability and effectiveness of some of these methods is controversial (see chapter 3 for additional discussion).

Other Allergies

INHALANT ALLERGIES (particularly to molds) also seem to play an important role in some patients with ulcerative colitis. A few of my patients who failed to respond to the nutritional approach experienced complete resolution after they received desensitization therapy for their mold sensitivity. Some individuals are apparently allergic to *Candida albicans* (the common yeast germ) or to other types of fungi that live in their intestinal tract. Although diagnosing a yeast or fungal infection involves some guesswork, some patients with ulcerative colitis clearly improve after taking anti-yeast medication.

Unfortunately, allergies have been routinely ignored by the average medical doctor, even though reasonable scientific evidence shows that allergies are a factor in many patients with ulcerative colitis. The connection between yeast overgrowth and ulcerative colitis, also ignored by most doctors, is not as well documented scientifically. Neverthe-

less, we have observed that eliminating candida is helpful for some people, and the medications that kill yeast are relatively safe.

Nutritional Deficiencies

INDIVIDUALS WITH ULCERATIVE colitis are often deficient in many different nutrients, including zinc, vitamin C, magnesium, vitamin A, folic acid, and iron. Persistent bleeding and diarrhea contribute to the loss of nutrients, as does chronic inflammation and malabsorption. Nutritional deficiencies impair immune function and decrease the body's ability to heal the inflamed bowel wall. A deficiency of one nutrient (folic acid) might even make diarrhea worse.[6] Nutritional supplements are therefore an important component of a comprehensive treatment program.

While nutritional deficiencies have been well documented in people with ulcerative colitis, the therapeutic effect of nutritional supplements has not been investigated as extensively. In one study, 51 patients with ulcerative colitis were given either zinc or a placebo for 4 weeks. More patients improved in the zinc group than in the placebo group (46% versus 32%).[7] Although this difference was not statistically significant, the results are consistent with the known beneficial effects of zinc. This mineral has an anti-inflammatory activity, promotes tissue healing, and enhances immune function. Each of those actions would be expected to be helpful for someone with ulcerative colitis. In another study, supplementing with fish oil resulted in a small reduction in the severity of ulcerative colitis.[8] Not much other research has been done using nutritional supplements to treat ulcerative colitis. However, common sense dictates that we do our best to correct every known nutritional deficiency, if an ailing person is to have the best chance of getting well. Patients suffering from ulcerative colitis frequently tell us that supplements give them more energy and increase their resistance to infection.

Butyrate

ONE NATURAL TREATMENT that shows great promise in treating ulcerative colitis is butyrate. Butyrate is a short-chain fatty acid that is produced when colonic bacteria break down carbohydrates and protein. In contrast to most cells in the body which depend on glucose and fat for energy, the cells that line the colon use butyrate as a major source of fuel and energy. Decreased levels of butyrate have been found in the stool of individuals with ulcerative colitis. It has therefore been suggested that one of the causes of this disease is a "nutritional deficiency" of butyrate, and that increasing the amount of butyrate in the colon might promote healing. Another reason for increasing butyrate levels is that reduced concentrations are associated with an increased risk of colon cancer, one of the diseases that occurs frequently in individuals with ulcerative colitis.

In one study, 10 patients with ulcerative colitis who had failed to respond to usual treatments were given enemas containing butyrate twice a day for 2 weeks. For comparison, each patient was also given placebo enemas during a separate 2-week period. After butyrate treatment, the average daily number of bowel movements decreased by 55% and rectal bleeding stopped in 9 of 10 cases. In contrast, there was no improvement with the placebo treatment.[9]

Butyrate enemas represent a significant advance in the treatment of ulcerative colitis. It is a promising therapy, even for those who have a severe case of the disease. It should be noted that butyrate enemas have been studied primarily in individuals whose disease was on the left side of the colon— the area that can be reached most easily by the contents of an enema. Although the research on butyrate was published in a major gastroenterology journal more than 7 years ago and confirmed by follow-up studies,[10] few gastroenterologists use butyrate. If your doctor is willing to write a prescription for butyrate enemas, the material can be obtained from a compounding pharmacist.

Butyrate is also available orally as a nutritional supplement, but taking butyrate by mouth is not likely to improve ulcerative colitis very much. It may be possible to increase colonic butyrate levels somewhat by consuming adequate amounts of fiber in the diet.

Hormone Therapy: DHEA

IN A STUDY of 46 individuals with ulcerative colitis, 79% had abnormally low blood levels of the adrenal hormone dehydroepiandrosterone (DHEA).[11] In 1994, this hormone was shown to be effective in treating individuals with lupus,[12] an autoimmune disease. At that time, we considered the possibility that DHEA also might be helpful in treating patients with other autoimmune diseases, including ulcerative colitis. Some of our patients with this disease have improved after taking DHEA. We prefer to use "physiologic" doses of DHEA (i.e., amounts similar to those produced in the body), such as 5 to 15 mg per day for women and 10 to 30 mg per day for men. However, individuals with severe ulcerative colitis may require larger amounts of DHEA. Although this hormone is available over the counter, DHEA therapy should be supervised by a doctor. For additional information on DHEA, please refer to chapter 4.

Summary of Recommendations for Ulcerative Colitis

PRIMARY RECOMMENDATIONS:

- Diet: Eliminate refined sugar, refined carbohydrates. Work with food allergies.

- High-potency multiple vitamin/mineral (adjust doses of other nutrients as needed).

OTHER RECOMMENDATIONS:

(NOTE: under medical supervision)

- Zinc (picolinate or citrate), 30 mg, 1 to 3 times per day.

- Copper (to balance zinc), 2 to 4 mg per day.

- Vitamin A, 25,000 IU per day for maintenance. With active disease, larger amounts of vitamin A have been used for short periods of time.

- Vitamin C (buffered), 1,000 to 3,000 mg per day in divided doses, to promote tissue healing. Watch for diarrhea as a side effect; reduce the dose it this occurs.

- Butyrate enemas (available by prescription), for left-sided (also called "distal") ulcerative colitis. Used mainly for severe or non-responsive cases.

- DHEA, in selected cases.

- Anti-candida medication, in selected cases.

ALLERGY ELIMINATION DIET

by Alan R. Gaby, M.D.

(modified from *Tracking Down Hidden Food Allergies,* by William Crook, M.D.)

THE FOLLOWING IS one of the elimination diets used in Dr. Gaby's medical practice. If not properly supervised, elimination diets can result in nutritional deficiencies. In addition, exaggerated allergic reactions can occur with individual food challenges. For those reasons, allergy elimination diets should be supervised by a doctor.

Purpose

TO IDENTIFY HIDDEN food allergens that may be causing some or all of your symptoms. During the elimination period, all common allergens are completely eliminated from the diet for 2 to 3 weeks. After your symptoms improve, foods are added back, one at a time, to determine which foods provoke symptoms.

Foods You Must Avoid
Dairy Products

MILK, cheese, butter, yogurt, sour cream, cottage cheese, whey, casein, sodium caseinate, calcium caseinate, any food containing these.

Wheat

MOST breads, spaghetti, noodles, pasta, most flour, baked goods, durum semolina, farina, and many gravies.

Corn

INCLUDING any product with corn oil, vegetable oil from an unspecified source, corn syrup, corn sweetener, dextrose, glucose, corn chips, tortillas, popcorn.

Eggs

AVOID whites, yolks, and any product containing eggs.

Citrus Fruits

AVOID oranges, grapefruits, lemons, limes, tangerines and foods containing citrus.

Coffee, Tea, and Alcohol

AVOID both caffeinated and decaffeinated coffee, as well as standard (such as Lipton) tea and decaffeinated tea. Herb teas are OK, except those containing citrus.

Refined Sugars

ELIMINATE table sugar and any foods that contain it, candy, soda, pies, cake, and cookies. Other names for sugar include sucrose, glucose, dextrose, corn syrup, corn sweetener, fructose, maltose, and levulose. These must all be avoided. Some patients (those without suspected "blood sugar problems") are allowed 1 to 3 teaspoons per day of pure, unprocessed honey, maple syrup or barley malt. This is decided on an individual basis. If you are restricted from all sugars, please do not eat dried fruit. Otherwise unsulfured, organically grown dried fruits may be used sparingly.

Honey, Maple, or Barley Syrup, 1 to 3 teaspoons per day

Allowed ❑ Not allowed ❑ (depending on suspected sensitivity to refined sugar)

Food Additives

ELIMINATE artificial colors, flavors, preservatives, texturing agents, and artificial sweeteners. Most diet sodas and other dietetic foods contain artificial ingredients and must be avoided. Grapes, prunes, and raisins that are not organically grown contain sulfites and must be avoided.

Any Other Food You Eat More than 3 Times a Week

ANY food you are now eating more than 3 times a week should be avoided and tested later.

Known Allergens

AVOID any food you know you are allergic to, even if it is allowed on this diet.

Water (includes cooking water)

USE spring or distilled water bottled in glass or heavy plastic. Water bottled in soft (collapsible) plastic containers tends to leach plastic into the water. Some water-filtration systems do not remove all potential allergens. Take your water with you, including to work and restaurants.

Read Labels

HIDDEN ALLERGENS ARE frequently found in packaged foods. "Flour" usually means wheat. "Vegetable oil" may mean corn oil. Casein and whey are dairy products. Make sure your vitamins are free of wheat, corn, sugar, citrus, yeast, and artificial colorings. Vary your diet by choosing from a wide variety of foods. Do not rely on just a few foods, as you may become allergic to foods you eat every day!

Foods You May Eat
Cereals

OATMEAL, oat bran, cream of rye, Rice and Shine, puffed rice, puffed millet, Oatio's (wheat-free), and others. Diluted apple juice with apple slices and nuts go well on cereal. You may use soy milk that has no corn oil added (such as some Eden Soy products; please read the ingredients carefully). You also may use almond nut milk. Most of these foods are available in health-food stores.

Grains and Flour Products

YOU may eat 100% rice cakes, rice crackers, rye crackers; any 100% rye or spelt bread with no wheat; Oriental noodles, such as 100% buckwheat Soba noodles; soy, rice, potato, buckwheat, and bean flours; rice or millet bread (as long as they do not contain dairy, eggs, sugar, or wheat); cooked whole grains including oats, millet, barley, buckwheat groats (kasha), rice macaroni, spelt (flour and pasta), brown rice, amaranth, quinoa. Most of these grains are available at health-food stores.

Legumes (Beans)

THE foods you may eat include: soybeans, tofu, lentils, peas, chickpeas, navy beans, kidney beans, black beans, string beans, and others. Dried beans should be soaked overnight. Pour off the water and rinse before cooking. Canned beans often contain added sugar or other potential allergens. Some cooked beans packaged in glass jars, and sold at health-food stores, contain no sugar. Read labels. You may also use bean dips without sugar, lemon, or additives. Canned soups include split pea and lentil soup (without additives).

Vegetables

USE a wide variety of vegetables. All vegetables except corn are permitted.

Proteins

FOR protein, you may eat poultry, fowl, and fresh fish (such as tuna and salmon, packed in spring water). Shrimp and most canned or packaged shellfish (such as lobster, crab, and oysters) may contain sulfites and should be avoided. Canned tuna, salmon, and other canned fish are OK. Beef and pork may be eaten unless specified otherwise. Lamb rarely causes allergic reactions, and may be used even when other meats are restricted. Also recommended are grain-and-bean casseroles (recipes may be found in vegetarian cookbooks).

Nuts and Seeds

YOU may eat nuts and seeds, either raw or roasted without salt or sugar. To prevent rancidity, nuts and seeds should be kept in an air-tight container in the refrigerator. You may also use nut butters from health-food stores or from fresh ground nuts (this includes peanut butter, almond butter, cashew butter, walnut butter, sesame butter, and sesame tahini). Nut butters go well on celery sticks and crackers.

Oils and Fats

ACCEPTABLE fats and oils include sunflower, safflower, olive, sesame, peanut, flaxseed, canola, and soy. Use cold-pressed or expeller-pressed oils (available from health-food stores), as they are safer for the heart and blood vessels. Do not use corn oil. Vegetable oil from an unspecified source is usually corn oil. Soy, sunflower, and safflower margarines are OK from an allergy standpoint, but we do not consider margarine a desirable food, as there is evidence that it may promote heart disease. It is acceptable to use margarine during the elimination and testing period. However, if you are not allergic to butter, we recommend it instead of margarine, once you have completed food testing. We also suggest vegetable and bean spreads, instead of butter or margarine.

Snacks

ANY food on the allowed-foods list can be eaten as a snack, any time of day. Also suggested are celery, carrot sticks, or other vegetables; fruit in moderation (no citrus); unsalted fresh nuts and seeds; Barbara's Granola Bars (from health-food stores); and wheat-free cookies (check ingredients).

Beverages

HERB teas (with no lemon or orange); spring water in glass bottles or hard plastic, seltzer (salt free); Perrier; pure fruit juices without sugar or additives (dilute 50:50 with water); almond nut milk (Nut Quick); soy milk without corn oil (such as Eden Soy Plain); Cafix, Inka, and Roma may be used as coffee substitutes.

Thickeners

YOU may use rice, oat, millet, barley, soy, or amaranth flours; and arrowroot and agar.

Spices and Condiments

YOU can use salt in moderation, as well as pepper. You can also use herbal spices that do not contain preservatives, citrus, or sugar. Also OK are garlic, ginger, and onions, as well as catsup and mustard from the health-food store (without sugar); wheat-free tamari sauce; and Bragg liquid aminos. Use vitamin C crystals in water as a substitute for lemon juice.

Miscellaneous

YOU can use sugar-free spaghetti sauce; fruit jellies without sugar or citrus; and soups such as split pea, lentil, and turkey/vegetable.

General Suggestions
Do Not Restrict Your Calories

START with a good breakfast, eat frequently throughout the day, and consume at least 4 glasses of water per day. If you do not eat enough, you may experience symptoms of low blood sugar, such as fatigue, irritability, headache, and too-rapid weight loss. To ensure adequate fiber, eat beans, permitted whole grains, whole fruits and vegetables, homemade vegetable soup, and nuts and seeds. Be sure to chew thoroughly, in order to enhance digestion.

Plan Your Meals for the Week and Take a List With You to the Health-Food Store

IF your schedule is very busy, and you have a hard time thinking of what to fix, take some time before starting the diet to make a list of all of your favorite types of foods and possible meal plans. For ideas, look through cookbooks that specialize in hypoallergenic diets. Most meals can be modified easily to meet the requirements of the diet without changing the meal plan for the rest of your family. When you go to the health-food store, ask for assistance in locating "allowed" versions of breads, crackers, cereals, muffins, soups, etc. Some people find it helpful to prepare additional foods on the weekend, in order to cut down on preparation time during the week.

Dining Out

DO not hesitate to ask questions or make requests at restaurants. For example, you could ask for fish topped with slivered almonds and cooked without added seasoning, butter, or lemon. Get a baked potato with a slice of onion on top. Order steak or lamb chops with fresh vegetables, also prepared without added seasonings (with the exception of garlic and plain herbs). Eat only at salad bars that do not use sulfites as a preservative, and bring your own dressing (oil and cider vinegar with chopped nuts, seeds, and fresh herbs). Get into the habit of carrying pure water, snacks, seasonings, etc., wherever you go, to supplement your meals or to have something on hand if you get hungry.

Withdrawal Symptoms

ABOUT 1 in 4 patients develops mild "withdrawal" symptoms within a few days after starting the diet. Withdrawal symptoms may include fatigue, irritability, headaches, malaise, or increased hunger. These symptoms generally disappear within 2 to 5 days, and they are usually followed by an improvement in your original symptoms. If withdrawal symptoms are uncomfortable, take buffered vitamin C (calcium ascorbate, 1,000 mg in tablet form or ¼ teaspoon of the crystals, up to 4 times a day), for several days. Your doctor may also prescribe "alkali salts" for withdrawal symptoms. In most cases, withdrawal symptoms are not severe and do not require treatment. We find it is best to discontinue all the foods abruptly ("cold turkey"), rather than easing into the diet slowly.

Testing Individual Foods

IT MAY TAKE 3 weeks for your symptoms to improve enough to allow you to retest foods. However, you may begin retesting after 2 weeks if you are sure you are feeling better. If you have been on the diet for 4 weeks and feel no better, check with your health-care practitioner for further instructions. Most patients do improve. Some patients feel so well on the diet that they decide not to test the foods. That could be a mistake. If you wait too long to retest foods, your allergies may "settle down," and you will not be able to provoke your symptoms by food testing. Then you will not know which foods you are allergic to. If reintroducing certain foods causes a recurrence of symptoms, you are probably allergic to those foods.

Food Sources for Testing

TEST pure sources of a food. For example, do not use pizza to test cheese, because pizza also contains wheat and corn oil. Do not use bread to test wheat, as it contains other ingredients. Organic sources are the best to use for testing, as you will not experience interference from pesticides, hormones, or other additives that may be used in commercial preparations.

Test One New Food Each Day. If your main symptom is arthritic pain, test one new food every other day. Allergic reactions to test foods usually occur within 10 minutes to 12 hours after ingestion. However, joint pains may be delayed by as much as 48 hours.

Eat a Relatively Large Amount of Each Test Food. For instance, on the day you are testing milk, drink a large glass at breakfast, along with any of the other foods on the "permitted" list. If after one serving, your original symptoms come back, or if you develop a headache, bloating, nausea, dizziness, or fatigue, do not eat that food anymore, and place it on your "allergic" list. If no symptoms occur, eat the food again for lunch and supper and watch for reactions.

How and What to Test

EVEN if the food is well tolerated, do not add it back into your diet until you have finished testing all of the foods. If you do experience a reaction, wait until your symptoms have improved before testing the next food. If you wake up the next morning with head or joint pain, nausea, or any other suspicious symptom, you may be experiencing a delayed reaction to the food you tested the day before. If you are uncertain whether you have reacted to a particular food, remove it from your diet and retest it 4 or 5 days later. You do not have to test foods you never eat. Do not test foods you already know cause symptoms.

Foods May be Tested in Any Order

BEGIN testing on a day you are feeling well (without colds, unusual headaches, or flu). Review the list of symptoms to watch for, and keep a journal of how you feel.

Conducting Specific Tests

Dairy Tests

Test milk and cheese on separate days. You may wish to test several cheeses on different days, since some people are allergic to one cheese but not another. It is usually not necessary to test yogurt, cottage cheese, or butter separately.

Wheat Test

Test Wheatena (with no milk or sugar) or another pure wheat cereal. You may add soy or nut milk.

Corn Test

Use fresh ears of corn or frozen corn (without sauces or preservatives).

Egg Test

Test the whites and yolks on separate days, using hard-boiled eggs.

Citrus Test

Test oranges, grapefruits, lemons, and limes. Test these individually on 4 separate days. The lemon and lime can be squeezed into water. In the case of orange and grapefruit, use the whole fruit.

Frequently Eaten Foods

Test tap water, if you have eliminated it, followed by those foods you have restricted (such as foods you consume more than 3 times a week).

Optional Tests

THE following foods and beverages are considered undesirable, regardless of whether or not you are allergic to them. If any of them are not now a part of your diet, or if you are fully committed to eliminating them from your diet, you don't need to test them. However, if you have been consuming any of them regularly, it is a good idea to test them and find out how they affect you. Reactions to these foods and beverages may be severe in some cases. They should be tested only on days that you can afford to feel bad.

Coffee and Tea Tests (separate days)

Do not add milk, non-dairy creamer, or sugar. You may add soy milk. If you use decaffeinated coffee, test it separately. Coffee, tea, decaffeinated coffee, and decaffeinated tea are separate tests.

Sugar Test

Put 4 teaspoons of sugar in a drink or on cereal, or mix with another food.

Chocolate Test

Use 1 to 2 tablespoons of pure baker's chocolate or Hershey's cocoa powder.

Alcohol Test (test this last)

Beer, wine, and hard liquor may require testing on different days, as the reactions to each may be different. Have 2 drinks per test day, but only if you can afford not to feel well that day and possibly the next day.

Food-Additive Test

Buy a set of McCormick's or French's food dyes and colors. Put ½ teaspoon of each color in a glass. Add 1 teaspoon of the mixture to a glass of water and drink. If you wish, you may test each color separately.

Follow-up Review of Tests

AFTER the testing is finished, please return to the office for a follow-up visit. Bring your journal with you, so that you may review your experiences with the doctor.

Suggestions for Self-Help if You Are Allergic to Foods
Rotation Diets

IF you have an allergic constitution and eat the same foods every day, you may eventually become allergic to them. After you have discovered which foods you can eat safely, make an attempt to rotate your diet. A 4-day schedule is necessary for some severely allergic patients, but most people can tolerate foods more frequently than every 4 days. You may eventually be able to tolerate allergenic foods, after you have avoided them for 6 to 12 months. However, if you continue to eat these foods more frequently than every fourth day, your symptoms may return.

Use common sense, and consume a wide variety of foods. Do not just latch onto a few favorites. If you are rotating foods, be sure to avoid all forms of the food when you are on an "off" day. For instance, if you are rotating corn, be sure to avoid corn chips, corn oil, corn sweeteners, etc., except on the days that you are eating corn and corn products. It is not necessary to do strict food rotation during the elimination and retesting periods.

Watch for Other Allergic Reactions

IF you have an allergic constitution, you may be allergic to foods other than those you have eliminated and tested on this diet. Pay attention to what you are eating. If you develop symptoms, review your recent meals, and try to identify the offending food. You can then eliminate that food for 2 weeks and test it to see if it provokes the same symptoms.

Symptoms that May Be Due to Food Allergy

- GENERAL: Fatigue, anxiety, depression, insomnia, food cravings, obesity.

- INFECTIONS: Recurrent colds, urinary tract infections, sore throats, ear infections, yeast infections.

- EAR, NOSE, AND THROAT: Chronic nasal congestion, postnasal drip, fluid in the ears, Meniere's syndrome.

- GASTROINTESTINAL: Irritable bowel syndrome, constipation, diarrhea, abdominal cramping, ulcerative colitis, Crohn's disease, gallbladder disease.

- CARDIOVASCULAR: High blood pressure, arrhythmia, angina.

- DERMATOLOGIC: Acne, eczema, psoriasis, canker sores (aphthous ulcers), hives.

- RHEUMATOLOGIC: Muscle aches, osteoarthritis, rheumatoid arthritis.

- NEUROLOGIC: Migraines, other headaches, numbness.

- MISCELLANEOUS: Asthma, frequent urination, teeth grinding, bedwetting, infantile colic. (NOTE: *Most of these disorders have more than one cause, but food allergy is a relatively common and frequently overlooked cause.*)

Additional Reading

Allergy Self Help Cookbook (Jones MH, Jones MH)

If It's Tuesday, It Must Be Chicken (a primer on rotation diets)(Golos N, Golbitz FG)

INTRAVENOUS VITAMIN AND MINERAL PROTOCOL

("Myers' Cocktail")

by Alan R. Gaby, M.D.

Materials and Method of Administration

Magnesium chloride hexahydrate (20%)	2 to 5 ml
Calcium gluconate (10%)	2 to 3 ml
Hydroxocobalamin (1,000 mcg/ml)	1 ml
Pyridoxine hydrochloride (100 mg/ml)	1 ml
Dexpanthenol (250 mg/ml)	1 ml
B-complex 100	1 ml
Vitamin C (222 mg/ml)	4 to 20 ml

Draw all of the ingredients into one syringe. Add 6 to 15 ml of sterile water (depending on the dosage of nutrients used), in order to reduce the hypertonicity of the solution. Diluting the solution reduces the incidence of occasional pain at the injection site and the rare incidence of phlebitis. Administer slowly over 5 to 15 minutes (depending on the dosage of minerals used and on individual tolerance), through a 25G butterfly needle.

Precautions

MOST PATIENTS EXPERIENCE warmth during the injection. Too-rapid administration of magnesium can cause hypotension, which can be severe. Patients with low blood pressure tend to tolerate less magnesium. When administering this treatment to a patient for the first time, it is best to give 0.5 to 1.0 ml, then wait 30 seconds or so, before proceeding with the rest of the infusion. For elderly or frail individuals, start with lower doses or consider intramuscular administration of magnesium and B-vitamins as an alternative to intravenous therapy. In patients at risk for hypokalemia (such as those taking certain diuretics, beta-agonists, or glucocorticoids, or patients with diarrhea), measure the serum potassium and correct the hypokalemia before administering this treatment. When in doubt, give 10 to 20 mEq of potassium orally at the time of the infusion, and repeat the oral potassium 4 to 6 hours later.

Indications

- Chronic fatigue, including chronic fatigue syndrome
- Chronic depression (occasionally effective)
- Acute or chronic muscle spasm; fibromyalgia
- Acute or chronic asthma
- Acute or chronic urticaria
- Seasonal allergic rhinitis, chronic sinusitis

- Congestive heart failure
- Angina
- Ischemic vascular disease
- Acute infections
- Senile dementia

Notes

- In patients with heart disease, calcium should not be included.
- For asthma or urticaria, 6 to 30 ml of vitamin C and double doses of pyridoxine, dexpanthenol, and vitamin B$_{12}$ may be necessary.
- For infections and allergic rhinitis, use 10 to 30 ml of vitamin C.

In some patients, the treatment works better if vitamin B$_{12}$ is given intramuscularly in a separate syringe. It is not clear whether this is due to the short half-life of intravenously administered B$_{12}$, or whether vitamin B$_{12}$ interacts with some other component of the injection.

---

*Dexpanthenol is the injectable form of pantothenic acid. B-complex 100 is a commercial product that contains (per ml): 100 mg each of thiamine and niacinamide, and 2 mg each of riboflavin-5'-phosphate, dexpanthenol, and pyridoxine hydrochloride. All of the materials listed above are available from a number of medical suppliers. At the time of this writing, hydroxocobalamin (vitamin B$_{12}$) and B-complex 100 are not available through commercial sources, but can be manufactured by a compounding pharmacist. Cyanocobalamin is an acceptable alternative to hydroxocobalamin, but it may be slightly less effective.

NOTES

Introduction

1. Goodwin JS, Tangum MR. Battling quackery: attitudes about micronutrient supplements in American academic medicine. Arch Intern Med 1998;158: 2187–2191.

Chapter One

1. Wong E, et al. The oestrogenic activity of red clover isoflavones and some of their degradation products. J Endocrinol 1962;24:341–348.

2. Albertazzi P, et al. The effect of dietary soy supplementation on hot flushes. Obstet Gynecol 1998; 91:6–11.

3. Bingham SA, et al. Phyto-oestrogens: where are we now? Br J Nutr 1998;79:393–406.

4. Anthony MS, et al. Soy protein versus soy phytoestrogens in the prevention of diet-induced coronary artery atherosclerosis of male cynomolgus monkeys. Arterioscler Thromb Vasc Biol 1997;17:2524–2531.

5. Wattenberg LW, et al. Dietary constituents altering the responses to chemical carcinogens. Fed Proc 1976;35:1327–1331.

6. Levy J, et al. Lycopene is a more potent inhibitor of human cancer cell proliferation than either alpha-carotene or beta-carotene. Nutr Cancer 1995; 24:257–266.

7. Giovannucci E, et al. Intake of carotenoids and retinol in relation to risk of prostate cancer. J Natl Cancer Inst 1995;87:1767–1776.

8. Seddon JM, et al. Dietary carotenoids, vitamins A, C, and E, and advanced age-related macular degeneration. JAMA 1994;272:1413–1420.

9. Landrum JT, et al. A one year study of the macular pigment: the effect of 140 days of a lutein supplement. Exp Eye Res 1997;65:57–62.

10. Hudspeth WJ, et al. Neurobiology of the hypoglycemia syndrome. J Holistic Med 1981; 3(1):60–71.

11. Hill EG, et al. Intensification of essential fatty acid deficiency in the rat by dietary *trans*-fatty acids. J Nutr 1979;109:1759–1766.

12. Hu FB, et al. Dietary fat intake and the risk of coronary heart disease in women. N Engl J Med 1997; 337:1491–1499.

13. Kummerow FA, et al. The influence of three sources of dietary fats and cholesterol on lipid composition of swine serum lipids and aorta tissue. Artery 1978; 4:360–384.

14. Hubbard RW, et al. Atherogenic effect of oxidized products of cholesterol. Progr Food Nutr Sci 1989; 13:17–44.

15. Karjalainen J, et al. A bovine albumin peptide as a possible trigger of insulin-dependent diabetes mellitus. N Engl J Med 1992;327:302–307.

16. Scott FW, et al. Milk and type I diabetes. Diabetes Care 1996;19:379–383.

17. Oster KA. Plasmalogen diseases: a new concept of the etiology of the atherosclerotic process. AJCR 1971;2(1):30–35.

18. Anonymous. Atherosclerosis. Am Family Physician 1987;36(6):250.

19. Ross DJ, et al. The presence of ectopic xanthine oxidase in atherosclerotic plaques and myocardial tissues. Proc Soc Exp Biol Med 1973;144:523–526.

20. Oster KA, Ross DJ. *The XO Factor*. Park City Press, New York, 1983, pp. 44–45.

21. Walton RG, et al. Adverse reactions to aspartame:

double-blind challenge in patients from a vulnerable population. Biol Psychiatry 1993;34:13–17.

22. Roberts HJ. Reactions attributed to aspartame-containing products: 551 cases. J Appl Nutr 1988; 40(2):85–94.

23. Stanton GA. The cause of arterial disease. Am Heart J 1974;87:796–798.

24. Mughal FH. Chlorination of drinking water and cancer: a review. J Environ Pathol Toxicol Oncol 1992;11:287–292.

25. Danielson C, et al. Hip fractures and fluoridation in Utah's elderly population. JAMA 1992;268:746–748.

26. Gutfeld R. Excessive lead found in water of many cities. Wall Street Journal, October 21, 1992, p. B7.

27. Abou-Donia MB, et al. Neurotoxicity resulting from coexposure to pyridostigmine bromide, DEET, and permethrin: implications of Gulf War chemical exposures. J Toxicol Environ Health 1996;48:35–56.

28. Settle DM, et al. Lead in Albacore: guide to lead pollution in Americans. Science 1980;207: 1167–1176.

29. Gaby AR. *Preventing and Reversing Osteoporosis.* Prima Publishing, Rocklin, CA, 1994, chapter 19.

30. Frustaci A, et al. Myocardial magnesium content, histology, and antiarrhythmic response to magnesium infusion. Lancet 1987;2:1019.

31. van Tiggelen CJM, et al. Vitamin B$_{12}$ levels of cerebrospinal fluid in patients with organic mental disorder. J Orthomolec Psychiatry 1983;12:305–311.

32. Gaby AR. *The Doctor's Guide to Vitamin B$_6$.* Rodale Press, Emmaus, PA, 1984.

33. Ellis JM. Treatment of carpal tunnel syndrome with vitamin B$_6$. South Med J 1987;80:882–884.

34. Phalen GS. Reflections on 21 years' experience with the carpal tunnel syndrome. JAMA 1970;212: 1365–1367.

35. Murata A. Virucidal activity of vitamin C for prevention and treatment of viral diseases. In Hasegawa T (ed.). Proceedings of the First Intersectional Congress of the International Association of Microbiological Societies. Tokyo, September 1–7, 1974.

36. Subramanian N. Histamine degradative potential of ascorbic acid: considerations and evaluations. Agents Actions 1978;8:484–487.

37. Hallson PC, et al. Magnesium reduces calcium oxalate crystal formation in human whole urine. Clin Sci 1982;62:17–19.

38. Anibarro B, et al. Asthma with sulfite intolerance in children: a blocking study with cyanocobalamin. J Allergy Clin Immunol 1992;90:103–109.

Chapter 2

1. Niwa Y, et al. Why are natural plant medicinal products effective in some patients and not in others with the same disease? Planta Med 1991; 57:299–304.

2. Cater RE II. Helicobacter (aka Campylobacter) pylori as the major causal factor in chronic hypochlorhydria. Med Hypotheses 1992; 39:367–374.

3. Kokkonen J, et al. Impaired gastric function in children with cow's milk intolerance. Eur J Pediatr 1979; 132:1–6.

Chapter 3

1. Breneman JC. *Basics of Food Allergy.* Charles C. Thomas, Springfield, IL, 1978, p. 8.

2. Darlington LG, et al. Placebo-controlled, blind study of dietary manipulation therapy in rheumatoid arthritis. Lancet 1986;1:236–238.

3. Egger J, et al. Controlled trial of oligoantigenic treatment in the hyperkinetic syndrome. Lancet 1985; 1:540–545.

4. Jones VA, et al. Food intolerance: a major factor in the pathogenesis of irritable bowel syndrome. Lancet 1982;2:1115–1117.

5. Dickey L (ed.). *Clinical Ecology.* Charles C. Thomas, Springfield, IL, 1976.

6. Breneman JC. *Basics of Food Allergy.* Charles C. Thomas, Springfield, IL, 1978.

7. Gaby AR. The role of hidden food allergy/intolerance in chronic disease. Altern Med Rev 1998; 3:90–100.

8. AAAI Board of Directors. Measurement of specific and nonspecific IgG$_4$ levels as diagnostic and prognostic tests for clinical allergy. J Allergy Clin Immunol 1995;95:652–654.

9. Hoj L. Diagnostic value of ALCAT test in intolerance to food additives compared with double-blind placebo-controlled (DBPC) oral challenges. Presented at the 52nd Annual Meeting of the American Academy of Allergy, Asthma and Immunology, March 15–20, 1996, New Orleans.

10. Fell PJ, et al. ALCAT—"a new test for food induced problems in medicine?" Presented at the Annual Meeting of the American Academy of Otolaryngic Allergy, October 1, 1988, Washington, D.C.

11. Miller JB. A double-blind study of food extract injection therapy: a preliminary report. Ann Allergy 1977;38:185–191.

12. Lehman CW. A double-blind study of sublingual provocative food testing: a study of its efficacy. Ann Allergy 1980;45:144–149.

Chapter 4

1. Gaby AR. Treatment with thyroid hormone. JAMA 1989;262:1774.
2. Bunevicius R, et al. Effects of thyroxine as compared with thyroxine plus triiodothyronine in patients with hypothyroidism. N Engl J Med 1999;340:424–429.
3. Cleare AJ, et al. Low-dose hydrocortisone in chronic fatigue syndrome: a randomised crossover trial. Lancet 1999;353:455–458.
4. Jefferies WM. Safe Uses of Cortisol. Charles C. Thomas, Springfield, IL, 1996.
5. Howlett TA. An assessment of optimal hydrocortisone replacement therapy. Clin Endocrinol 1997; 46:263–268.
6. Anonymous. Antiobesity drug may counter aging. Science News 1981;19(3):39.
7. Yen SSC, et al. Replacement of DHEA in aging men and women. Potential remedial effects. Ann NY Acad Sci 1995;774:128–142.
8. Gaby AR. Dehydroepiandrosterone: biological significance and clinical effects. Altern Med Rev 1996; 1:60–69.
9. Labrie F, et al. Effect of 12-month dehydroepiandrosterone replacement therapy on bone, vagina, and endometrium in postmenopausal women. J Clin Endocrinol Metab 1997;82:3498–3505.
10. Wolkowitz OM, et al. Dehydroepiandrosterone (DHEA) treatment of depression. Biol Psychiatry 1997;41:311–318.
11. Wolkowitz OM, et al. Double-blind treatment of major depression with dehydroepiandrosterone. Am J Psychiatry 1999;156:646–649.
12. van Vollenhoven RF, et al. Dehydroepiandrosterone in systemic lupus erythematosus. Arthritis Rheum 1995;38:1826–1831.
13. Follingstad AH. Estriol, the forgotten estrogen? JAMA 1978;239:29–30.
14. Tzingounis VA, et al. Estriol in the management of the menopause. JAMA 1978;239:1638–1641.
15. Granberg S, et al. Endometrial sonographic and histologic findings in women with and without hormonal replacement therapy suffering from postmenopausal bleeding. Maturitas 1997;27:35–40.
16. Head KA. Estriol: safety and efficacy. Altern Med Rev 1998;3:101–113.
17. Wright JV, Morgenthaler J. Natural Hormone Replacement for Women Over 45. Smart Publications, Petaluma, CA, 1997.
18. Lee JR. Natural Progesterone: the Multiple Roles of a Remarkable Hormone. BLL Publishing (P.O. Box 2068, Sebastopol, CA, 95473), 1993.
19. The Writing Group for the PEPI Trial. Effects of estrogen or estrogen/progestin regimens on heart disease risk factors in postmenopausal women. The Postmenopausal Estrogen/Progestin Interventions (PEPI) Trial. JAMA 1995;273:199–208.
20. Sih R, et al. Testosterone replacement in older hypogonadal men: a 12-month randomized controlled trial. J Clin Endocrinol Metab 1997; 82:1661–1667.
21. Gaby AR. Preventing and Reversing Osteoporosis. Prima Publishing, Rocklin, CA, 1994.
22. Wright JV, Lenard L. Maximize Your Vitality and Potency: for Men Over 40. Smart Publications, Petaluma, CA, 1999.

Acne Rosacea

1. Ryle JA, et al. Gastric analysis in acne rosacea. Lancet 1920;2:1195–1196.
2. Tulipan L. Acne rosacea: a vitamin B complex deficiency. Arch Dermatol Syph 1947;56:589–591.
3. Poole WL. Effect of vitamin B complex and S-factor on acne rosacea. South Med J 1957;50:207–210.
4. Schellenberg D, et al. Treatment of Clostridium difficile diarrhoea with brewer's yeast. Lancet 1994;343: 171–172.
5. Perkins RB. Effect of vitamin B group in rosacea. Aust J Dermatol 1959;5:202–203.
6. Werbach M. Nutritional Influences on Illness, Second Edition. Third Line Press, Tarzana, CA, 1993, p. 3.
7. Graupe K, et al. Efficacy and safety of topical azelaic acid (20 percent cream): an overview of results from European clinical trials and experimental reports. Cutis 1996; 57(Number 1S):20–35.

Acne Vulgaris

1. Schaefer O. When the Eskimo comes to town. Nutr Today, Nov/Dec 1971, pp. 8–16.

2. Hillstrom L, et al. Comparison of oral treatment with zinc sulfate and placebo in acne vulgaris. Br J Dermatol 1977;97:679–684.

3. Michaelsson G, et al. A double-blind study of the effect of zinc and oxytetracycline in acne vulgaris. Br J Dermatol 1977;97:561–566.

4. Gibson JR. Rationale for the development of new topical treatments for acne vulgaris. Cutis 1996; 57(Number 1S):13–19.

5. Graupe K, et al. Efficacy and safety of topical azelaic acid (20 percent cream): an overview of results from European clinical trials and experimental reports. Cutis 1996;57(Number 1S):20–35.

6. Shalita AR, et al. Topical nicotinamide compared with clindamycin gel in the treatment of inflammatory acne vulgaris. Int J Dermatol 1995;34:434–437.

7. Snider B, Dietman DF. Pyridoxine therapy for premenstrual acne flare. Arch Dermatol 1974;110: 130–131.

8. Kligman AM, et al. Oral vitamin A in acne vulgaris. Int J Dermatol 1981;20:278–285.

9. Michaelsson G, Edqvist L-E. Erythrocyte glutathione peroxidase activity in acne vulgaris and the effect of selenium and vitamin E treatment. Acta Derm Venereol 1984;64:9–14.

Alcoholism

1. Anonymous. New alcoholism Rx: hold the coffee and give vitamins. Med Tribune, Sept. 12, 1979, pp. 3, 29.

2. Randolph TG. The role of specific alcoholic beverages. In Dickey L (ed.). *Clinical Ecology.* Charles C. Thomas, Springfield, IL, 1976, chapter 31.

3. Anonymous. High carbohydrate diet affects rat's alcohol intake. JAMA 1970;212:976.

4. Pekkanen L. Effects of thiamine deprivation and antagonism on voluntary ethanol intake in rats. J Nutr 1980;110:937–944.

5. Pekkanen L. Effects of thiamine deprivation and antagonism on voluntary ethanol intake in rats. J Nutr 1980;110:937–944.

6. Brown RV. Vitamin deficiency and voluntary alcohol consumption in mice. Q J Stud Alcohol 1969; 30:592–597.

7. Williams RJ, et al. Dietary deficiencies in animals in relation to voluntary alcohol and sugar consumption. Q J Stud Alcohol 1955;16:234–244.

8. Smith JA, et al. The treatment of alcoholism by nutritional supplement. Q J Stud Alcohol 1951; 12:381–385.

9. Trulson MF, et al. Vitamin medication in alcoholism. JAMA 1954;155:114–119.

10. Smith RF. A five-year field trial of massive nicotinic acid therapy of alcoholics in Michigan. J Orthomolec Psychiatry 1974;3:327–331.

11. Rogers LL, Pelton RB. Glutamine in the treatment of alcoholism. Q J Stud Alcohol 1957;18:581–587.

12. Horrobin DF. A biochemical basis for alcoholism and alcohol-induced damage including the fetal alcohol syndrome and cirrhosis: interference with essential fatty acid and prostaglandin metabolism. Med Hypotheses 1980;6:929–942.

13. Horrobin DF. Essential fatty acids, prostaglandins, and alcoholism: an overview. Alcoholism: Clin Exp Res 1987;11:2–9.

14. Branchey L, et al. Ethanol impairs tryptophan transport into the brain and depresses serotonin. Life Sci 1981;29:2751–2755.

15. Anonymous. Tryptophan may relieve insomnia of hospitalized mental patients. Clin Psychiatry News, March, 1983, p. 7.

16. Asheychik R, et al. The efficacy of L-tryptophan in the reduction of sleep disturbance and depressive state in alcoholic patients. J Stud Alcohol 1989; 50:525–532.

17. Kline NS, et al. Evaluation of lithium therapy in chronic and periodic alcoholism. Am J Med Sci 1974;268:15–22.

18. Dorus W, et al. Lithium treatment of depressed and nondepressed alcoholics. JAMA 1989;262: 1646–1652.

19. Gallimberti L, et al. Gamma-hydroxybutyric acid in the treatment of alcohol dependence: a double-blind study. Alcoholism: Clin Exp Res 1992;16:673–676.

20. Addolorato G, et al. Maintaining abstinence from alcohol with gamma-hydroxybutyrate. Lancet 1998;351:38.

Angina

1. Roberts HJ. The role of diabetogenic hyperinsulinism in nocturnal angina pectoris, with special reference to the etiology of ischemic heart disease. J Am Geriatr Soc 1967;15:545–555.

2. Rea WJ. Environmentally triggered cardiac disease. Ann Allergy 1978;40:243–251.

3. Ornish D, et al. Can lifestyle changes reverse coronary heart disease? Lancet 1990;336:129–133.

4. Ouchi Y, et al. Effect of dietary magnesium on development of atherosclerosis in cholesterol-fed rabbits. Arteriosclerosis 1990;10:732–737.

5. Malkiel-Shapiro B. Further observations on parenteral magnesium sulfate therapy in coronary heart disease: a clinical appraisal. S Afr Med J 1958; 32:1211–1215.

6. Kamikawa T, et al. Effects of L-carnitine on exercise tolerance in patients with stable angina pectoris. Jpn Heart J 1984;25:587–597.

7. Cherchi A, et al. Effects of L-carnitine on exercise tolerance in chronic stable angina: a multicenter, double-blind, randomized, placebo controlled crossover study. Int J Clin Pharm Ther Toxicol 1985;23:569–572.

8. Kamikawa T, et al. Effects of coenzyme Q10 on exercise tolerance in chronic stable angina pectoris. Am J Cardiol 1985;56:247–251.

9. Anderson TW, et al. A double-blind trial of vitamin E in angina pectoris. Am J Clin Nutr 1974;27: 1174–1178.

10. Hodis HN, et al. Serial coronary angiographic evidence that antioxidant vitamin intake reduces progression of coronary artery atherosclerosis. JAMA 1995;273:1849–1854.

11. Stephens NG, et al. Randomised controlled trial of vitamin E in patients with coronary disease: Cambridge Heart Antioxidant Study (CHAOS). Lancet 1996;347:781–786.

12. Willis GC, et al. Serial arteriography in atherosclerosis. Can Med Assoc J 1954;71:562–568.

13. Chappell LT, Stahl JP. The correlation between EDTA chelation therapy and improvement in cardiovascular function: a meta-analysis. J Advancement Med 1993;6:139–160.

14. Moller J, Einfeldt H. *Testosterone Treatment of Cardiovascular Diseases.* Springer-Verlag, Berlin, 1984.

15. Wright JV, Lenard L. *Maximize Your Vitality and Potency: for Men Over 40.* Smart Publications, Petulama, CA, 1999.

16. Lesser MA. Testosterone propionate therapy in one hundred cases of angina pectoris. J Clin Endocrinol 1946;6:549–557.

17. Wu SZ, Weng XZ. Therapeutic effects of an androgenic preparation on myocardial ischemia and cardiac function in 62 elderly male coronary heart disease patients. Chin Med J 1993;106:415–418

18. Rosano GM, et al. 17-beta-Estradiol therapy lessens angina in postmenopausal women with syndrome X. J Am Coll Cardiol 1996;28:1500–1505.

Anxiety

1. Salzer HM. Relative hypoglycemia as a cause of neuro-psychiatric illness. J Natl Med Assoc 1966; 58:12–17.

2. Hoffmann RH, et al. Hyperinsulinism: a factor in the neuroses. Am J Dig Dis 1949;16:242–247.

3. Kalow W. Variability of caffeine metabolism in humans. Arzneimittelforschung 1985;35:319–324.

4. Bruce M, et al. Anxiogenic effects of caffeine in patients with anxiety disorders. Arch Gen Psychiatry 1992;49:867–869.

5. Boulenger JP, et al. Increased sensitivity to caffeine in patients with panic disorders. Arch Gen Psychiatry 1984;41:1067–1071.

6. Alvarez WC. Puzzling "nervous storms" due to food allergy. Gastroenterology 1946;7:241–242.

7. Mohler H, et al. Nicotinamide is a brain constituent with benzodiazepine-like actions. Nature 1979;278: 563–565.

8. Gaby. *Magnesium.* Keats Publishing, Inc., New Canaan, 1994.

9. Weston PG, et al. Magnesium sulphate as a sedative. Am J Med Sci 1923;165:431–433.

10. Ellis FR, Nasser S. A pilot study of vitamin B_{12} in the treatment of tiredness. Br J Nutr 1973;30: 277–283.

11. Bhattacharya SK, et al. Anxiolytic activity of *Panax ginseng* roots: an experimental study. J Ethnopharmacology 1991;34:87–92.

12. Kinzler E, et al. Effect of a special kava extract in patients with anxiety-, tension-, and excitation states of non-psychotic genesis. Double-blind study with placebos over 4 weeks. Arzneimittelforschung 1991;41:584–588 (cited in Werbach MR, Murray, MT. *Botanical Influences on Illness.* Third Line Press, Tarzana, CA, 1994, p. 51).

13. Almeida JC. Coma from the health food store: interaction between kava and alprazolam. Ann Intern Med 1996;125:940–941.

Asthma

1. Rowe AH, Young EJ. Bronchial asthma due to food allergy alone in ninety-five patients. JAMA 1959; 169:1158–1162.

2. Ogle KA, Bullock JD. Children with allergic rhinitis and/or bronchial asthma treated with elimination diet. Ann Allergy 1977;39:8–11.

3. Collipp PJ, et al. Tryptophane metabolism in bronchial asthma. Ann Allergy 1975;35:153–158.

4. Weir MR, et al. Depression of vitamin B6 levels due to theophylline. Ann Allergy 1990;65:59–62.

5. Collipp PJ, et al. Pyridoxine treatment of childhood bronchial asthma. Ann Allergy 1975;35:93–97.

6. Reynolds RD, Natta CL. Depressed plasma pyridoxal phosphate concentrations in adult asthmatics. Am J Clin Nutr 1985;41:684–688.

7. Haury VG. Blood serum magnesium in bronchial asthma and its treatment by the administration of magnesium sulfate. J Lab Clin Med 1940;26:340–344.

8. Rayssiguier Y. Hypomagnesemia resulting from adrenaline infusion in ewes: its relation to lipolysis. Horm Metab Res 1977;9:309–314.

9. Phillips PJ, et al. Metabolic and cardiovascular side effects of the beta-2-adrenoceptor agonists salbutamol and rimiterol. Br J Clin Pharmacol 1980 9:483–491.

10. Durlach J. Magnesium and allergy: experimental and clinical relationships between magnesium and hypersensitivity. Rev Franc Allergol 1975;15:133–146.

11. Skobeloff EM, et al. Intravenous magnesium sulfate for the treatment of acute asthma in the emergency department. JAMA 1989;262:1210–1213.

12. Ciarallo L, et al. Intravenous magnesium therapy for moderate to severe pediatric asthma: results of a randomized, placebo-controlled trial. J Pediatr 1996; 129:809–814.

13. Wright JV. Treatment of childhood asthma with parenteral vitamin B12, gastric re-acidification, and attention to food allergy, magnesium and pyridoxine: three case reports with background and an integrated hypothesis. J Nutr Med 1990;1:277–282.

14. Anibarro B, et al. Asthma with sulfite intolerance in children: a blocking study with cyanocobalamin. J Allergy Clin Immunol 1992;90:103–109.

15. Johnson JL, et al. Molybdenum cofactor deficiency in a patient previously characterized as deficient in sulfite oxidase. Biochem Med Metab Biol 1988; 40:86–93.

16. Malamud D, Kroll Y. Ascorbic acid inhibition of cyclic nucleotide phosphodiesterase activity. Proc Soc Exp Biol Med 1980;164:534–536.

17. Anah CO, et al. High dose ascorbic acid in Nigerian asthmatics. Trop Geogr Med 1980;32:132–137.

18. Hawthorne AB, et al. High dose eicosapentaenoic acid ethyl ester: effects on lipids and neutrophil leukotriene production in normal volunteers. Br J Clin Pharmacol 1990;30:187–194.

19. Dry J, Vincent D. Effect of a fish oil diet on asthma: results of a 1-year double-blind study. Int Arch Allergy Appl Immunol 1991;95:156–157.

20. Bray GW. The hypochlorhydria of asthma in childhood. Q J Med 1931(January):181–197.

Atherosclerosis (prevention)

1. Kummerow FA, et al. Swine as an animal model in studies on atherosclerosis. Fed Proc 1975;33:235.

2. Willett WC, et al. Intake of *trans*-fatty acids and risk of coronary heart disease among women. Lancet 1993;341:581–585.

3. Taylor CB, et al. Spontaneously occurring angiotoxic derivatives of cholesterol. Am J Clin Nutr 1979; 32:40–57.

4. Yudkin J, Morland J. Sugar intake and myocardial infarction. Am J Clin Nutr 1967;20:503–506.

5. Gaby AR. Nutritional factors in cardiovascular disease. J Holistic Med 1983;5(2):107–120.

6. Stanton GA. The cause of arterial disease. Am Heart J 1974;87:796–798.

7. Hu FB, et al. Frequent nut consumption and risk of coronary heart disease in women: prospective cohort study. BMJ 1998;317:1341–1345.

8. Fraser GE, et al. A possible protective effect of nut consumption on risk of coronary heart disease. Arch Intern Med 1992;152:1416–1424.

9. Oster KA. Plasmalogen diseases: a new concept of the etiology of the atherosclerotic process. AJCR 1971;2(1):30–35.

10. Oster KA, Ross DJ. *The XO Factor*. Park City Press, New York, 1983, pp. 44–45.

11. Verhoef P, et al. Homocysteine metabolism and risk of myocardial infarction: relation with vitamins B6, B12, and folate. Am J Epidemiol 1996;143:845–859.

12. Stampfer MJ, et al. A prospective study of plasma homocysteine and risk of myocardial infarction in US physicians. JAMA 1992;268:877–881.

13. Glueck CJ, et al. Evidence that homocysteine is an independent risk factor for atherosclerosis in hyperlipidemic patients. Am J Cardiol 1995;75:132–36.

14. Ubbink JB,.et al. Vitamin B$_{12}$, vitamin B$_6$, and folate nutritional status in men with hyperhomocysteinemia. Am J Clin Nutr 1993;57:47–53.

15. Ubbink JB, et al. Vitamin requirements for the treatment of hyperhomocysteinemia in humans. J Nutr 1994;124:1927–33.

16. Boers GHJ, et al. Heterozygosity for homocystinuria in premature peripheral and cerebral occlusive arterial disease. N Engl J Med 1985;313:709–715.

17. Vitale JJ, et al. Interrelationships between experimental hypercholesterolemia, magnesium requirement and experimental atherosclerosis. J Exp Med 1957;106:757–767.

18. Gaby AR. *Magnesium.* Keats Publishing, New Canaan, CT, 1994.

19. Stampfer MJ, et al. Vitamin E consumption and the risk of coronary disease in women. N Engl J Med 1993;328:1444–1449.

20. Rimm EB, et al. Vitamin E consumption and the risk of coronary heart disease in men. N Engl J Med 1993;328:1450–1456.

21. Takamatsu S, et al "Effects on health of dietary supplementation with 100 mg d-alpha-tocopheryl acetate, daily for 6 years. J Int Med Res 1995;23:342–357.

22. *Nutritional Therapy in Medical Practice,* by Drs. Gaby and Wright, is a 309-page annotated bibliography of more than 3,500 medical-journal articles. It provides an extensive review of atherosclerosis and of many other nutritional topics. For information on obtaining this manual, send an email to gaby@halcyon.com.

23. Salonen JT, et al. High stored iron levels are associated with excess risk of myocardial infarction in eastern Finnish men. Circulation 1992;86:803–811.

Atherosclerosis (treatment)

1. Moller J, Einfeldt H. *Testosterone Treatment of Cardiovascular Diseases.* Springer-Verlag, Berlin, 1984, and Moller J. C*holesterol: Interactions with Testosterone and Cortisol in Cardiovascular Diseases.* Springer-Verlag, Berlin, 1987.

2. Pritikin N, McGrady PM Jr. *The Pritikin Program for Diet and Exercise.* Bantam Books, New York, 1979.

3. Ornish D. Can lifestyle changes reverse coronary heart disease? Lancet 1990;336:129–133.

4. Willis GC, et al. Serial arteriography in atherosclerosis. Can Med Assoc J 1954;71:562–568.

5. Neglen P, et al. Peroral magnesium hydroxide therapy and intermittent claudication. Vasa 1985;14:285–288.

6. Browne SE. Parenteral magnesium sulphate in arterial disease. Practitioner 1964;192:791.

7. Haeger K. Long-time treatment of intermittent claudication with vitamin E. Am J Clin Nutr 1974;27:1179–1181.

8. Hove EL, et al. The effect of tocopherol and of fat on the resistance of rats to anoxic anoxia. Arch Biochem 1945;8:395–404.

9. Tyson VCH. Treatment of intermittent claudication. Practitioner 1979;223:121–126.

10. Brevetti G, et al. Increases in walking distance in patients with peripheral vascular disease treated with L-carnitine: a double-blind, cross-over study. Circulation 1988;77:767–773.

11. Clarke NE, et al. Treatment of angina pectoris with disodium ethylene diamine tetraacetic acid. Am J Med Sci 1956;232:654–666.

12. Lamar CP. Chelation endarterectomy for occlusive atherosclerosis. J Am Geriatr Soc 1966;14:272–294.

13. Rudolph CJ, et al. A nonsurgical approach to obstructive carotid stenosis using EDTA chelation. J Advancement Med 1991;4:157–166.

14. Olszewer E, et al. A pilot double-blind study of sodium-magnesium EDTA in peripheral vascular disease. J Natl Med Assoc 1990;82:173–177.

15. Sehnert KW, et al. The improvement in renal function following EDTA chelation and multi-vitamin-trace mineral therapy: a study in creatinine clearance. Med Hypotheses 1984;15:301–304.

Attention Deficit-Hyperactivity Disorder

1. Ott JN. *Health and Light.* Pocket Books, New York, 1973, pp. 127–128.

2. Swain A, et al. Salicylates, oligoantigenic diets, and behaviour. Lancet 1985;2:41–42.

3. Wolraich ML, et al. Effects of diets high in sucrose or aspartame on the behavior and cognitive performance of children. N Engl J Med 1994;330:301–307.

4. Rippere V. Placebo-controlled tests of chemical food additives: are they valid? Med Hypotheses 1981;7:819–823.

5. Boris M, et al. Foods and additives are common causes of the attention deficit hyperactive disorder in children. Ann Allergy 1994;72:462–468.

6. Egger J, et al. Controlled trial of oligoantigenic treatment in the hyperkinetic syndrome. Lancet 1985; 1:540–545.

7. Coleman M, et al. A preliminary study of the effect of pyridoxine administration in a subgroup of hyperkinetic children: a double-blind crossover comparison with methylphenidate. Biol Psychiatry 1979; 14:741–751.

8. Brenner A. The effects of megadoses of selected B complex vitamins on children with hyperkinesis: controlled studies with long term followup. J Learn Disabil 1982;15:258–264.

Benign Prostatic Hyperplasia (enlarged prostate)

1. McConnell JD, et al. The effect of finasteride on the risk of acute urinary retention and the need for surgical treatment among men with benign prostatic hyperplasia. N Engl J Med 1998;338:557–563.

2. Hart JP, Cooper WL. Vitamin F in the treatment of prostatic hypertrophy. Report #1, Lee Foundation for Nutritional Research, November, 1941, Milwaukee, Wisconsin.

3. Bush IM, et. al. Zinc and the prostate. (Presented at the annual meeting of the American Medical Association, Chicago, 1974.)

4. Klein LA, Stoff JS. Prostaglandins and the prostate: an hypothesis on the etiology of benign prostatic hyperplasia. Prostate 1983;4:247–251.

5. Hill EG, et al. Intensification of essential fatty acid deficiency in the rat by dietary trans-fatty acids. J Nutr 1979;109:1759–1766.

6. Holman RT, Peifer JJ. Acceleration of essential fatty acid deficiency by dietary cholesterol. J Nutr 1960; 70:411–417.

7. Damrau F. Benign prostatic hypertrophy: amino acid therapy for symptomatic relief. J Am Geriatr Soc 1962;10:426–430.

8. Champault G, et al. A double-blind trial of an extract of the plant Serenoa repens in benign prostatic hyperplasia. Br J Clin Pharmacol 1984;18:461–462.

9. Wilt TJ, et al. Saw palmetto extracts for treatment of benign prostatic hyperplasia: a systematic review. JAMA 1998;280:1604–1609.

10. Breza J, et al. Efficacy and acceptability of Tadenan (Pygeum africanum extract) in the treatment of benign prostatic hyperplasia (BPH): a multicentre trial in central Europe. Curr Med Res Opin 1998; 14:127–139.

11. Andro MC, Riffaud JP. Pygeum africanum extract for the treatment of patients with benign prostatic hyperplasia: a review of 25 years of published experience. Curr Ther Res 1995;56:796–817.

12. Klippel KF, et al. A multicentric, placebo-controlled, double-blind clinical trial of beta-sitosterol (phytosterol) for the treatment of benign prostatic hyperplasia. Br J Urol 1997;80:427–432.

13. Berges RR, et al. Randomised, placebo-controlled, double-blind clinical trial of beta-sitosterol in patients with benign prostatic hyperplasia. Lancet 1995;345:1529–1532.

14. Wagner H, et al. Search for the antiprostatic principle of stinging nettle (Urtica dioica) roots. Phytomedicine 1994;1:213–224.

Birth Defects

1. Davis SD, et al. Teratogenicity of vitamin B6 deficiency: omphalocele, skeletal and neural defects, and splenic hypoplasia. Science 1970;169:1329–1330.

2. McGuire R. Lack of magnesium in pregnancy eyed. Med Tribune, April 17, 1985, p. 10.

3. Warkany J, et al. Congenital malformations of the central nervous system in rats produced by maternal zinc deficiency. Teratology 1972;5:319–334.

4. Nelson MM, et al. Pantothenic acid deficiency and reproduction in the rat. J Nutr 1946;31:497–507.

5. Peer LA, et al. Induction of cleft palate in mice by cortisone and its reduction by vitamins. J Int Coll Surg 1958;30:249–253.

6. Laurence KM, et al. Double-blind randomised controlled trial of folate treatment before conception to prevent recurrence of neural-tube defects. Br Med J 1981;282:1509.

7. Czeizel AE, Dudas I. Prevention of the first occurrence of neural-tube defects by periconceptional vitamin supplementation. N Engl J Med 1992;327: 1832–1835.

8. Kirke PN, et al. Maternal plasma folate and vitamin B12 are independent risk factors for neural tube defects. Q J Med 1993;86:703–708.

9. Cavdar AO, et al. Zinc deficiency and anencephaly in Turkey. Teratology 1980;22:141.

10. Rothman KJ, et al. Teratogenicity of high vitamin A intake. N Engl J Med 1995;333:1369–1373.

11. Shaw GM, et al. High maternal vitamin A intake and risk of anomalies of structure with a cranial neural crest cell contribution. Lancet 1996;347:899–900.

12. Mills JL, et al. Vitamin A and birth defects. Am J Obstet Gynecol 1997;177:31–36.

13. Phuapradit W, et al. Serum vitamin A and beta-carotene levels in pregnant women infected with human immunodeficiency virus-1. Obstet Gynecol 1996;87:564–567.

14. Semba RD, et al. Maternal vitamin A deficiency and mother-to-child transmission of HIV-1. Lancet 1994;343:1593–1597.

15. Millen JW, et al. Effect of vitamin B complex on the teratogenic activity of hypervitaminosis A. Nature 1958;182:940.

Bursitis

1. Klemes IS. Vitamin B_{12} in acute subdeltoid bursitis. Indust Med Surg 1957;26:290–292.

Canker Sores

1. Hay KD, Reade PC. The use of an elimination diet in the treatment of recurrent aphthous ulceration of the oral cavity. Oral Surg 1984;57:504–507.

2. Wray D. Gluten-sensitive recurrent aphthous stomatitis. Dig Dis Sci 1981;26:737–740.

3. Merchant HW, et al. Zinc sulfate supplementation for treatment of recurring oral ulcers. South Med J 1977;70:559–561.

4. Nolan A, et al. Recurrent aphthous ulceration: vitamin B_1, B_2 and B_6 status and response to replacement therapy. J Oral Pathol Med 1991;20:389–391.

5. Wray D, et al. Nutritional deficiencies in recurrent aphthae. J Oral Pathol 1978;7:418–423.

6. Nally FF, Blake GC. Recurrent aphthae: treatment with vitamin B_{12}, folic acid, and iron. Br Med J 1975;3:308.

7. Rapoport L, Levine WI. Treatment of oral ulceration with lactobacillus tablets. Report of forty cases. Oral Surg Oral Med Oral Pathol 1965;20:591–593.

8. Das SK, et al. Deglycyrrhizinated liquorice in aphthous ulcers. J Assoc Physicians India 1989;37:647.

9. Herlofson BB, Barkvoll P. Sodium lauryl sulfate and recurrent aphthous ulcers. Acta Odontol Scand 1994;52:257–259.

Cholesterol

1. Taylor CB, et al. Spontaneously occurring angiotoxic derivatives of cholesterol. Am J Clin Nutr 1979; 32:40–57.

2. Gey KF, et al. Inverse correlation between plasma vitamin E and mortality from ischemic heart disease in cross-cultural epidemiology. Am J Clin Nutr 1991;53:326S–334S.

3. Rose GA, et al. Corn oil in treatment of ischemic heart disease. Br Med J 1965;1:1531–1533.

4. Newman TB, Hulley SB. Carcinogenicity of lipid-lowering drugs. JAMA 1996;275:55–60.

5. Yudkin J, et al. Effects of high dietary sugar. Br Med J 1980;281:1396.

6. Jenkins DJ, et al. Effect of a diet high in vegetables, fruit, and nuts on serum lipids. Metabolism 1997; 46:530–537.

7. Morgan JM, et al. Effect of dietary (egg) cholesterol on serum cholesterol in free-living adults. J Appl Nutr 1993;45(3,4):73–84.

8. Newbold HL. Reducing the serum cholesterol level with a diet high in animal fat. South Med J 1988; 81:61–63.

9. Maggi GC, et al. Pantethine: a physiological lipo-modulating agent, in the treatment of hyperlipid-emias. Curr Ther Res 1982;32:380–386.

10. Galeone F, et al. The lipid-lowering effect of pan-tethine in hyperlipidemic patients: a clinical investi-gation. Curr Ther Res 1983;34:383–390.

11. Gaddi A, et al. Controlled evaluation of pantethine, a natural hypolipidemic compound, in patients with different forms of hyperlipoproteinemia. Atherosclerosis 1984;50:73–83.

12. Arsenio L, et al. Effectiveness of long-term treatment with pantethine in patients with dyslipidemia. Clin Ther 1986;8:537–545.

13. Horwitz N. Cut cholesterol for $5 a month? Med Tribune, February 19, 1986, p. 7.

14. Urberg M, et al. Hypocholesterolemic effects of nicotinic acid and chromium supplementation. J Family Pract 1988;27:603–606.

15. Bell L, et al. Cholesterol-lowering effects of calcium carbonate in patients with mild to moderate hyper-cholesterolemia. Arch Intern Med 1992;152: 2441–2444.

16. Hermann WJ. The failure of alpha-tocopherol sup-plementation to alter the distribution of lipoprotein cholesterol in normal and hyperlipoproteinemic per-sons. Am J Clin Pathol 1981;76:124–126.

17. Horsey J, et al. Ischaemic heart disease and aged patients: effects of ascorbic acid on lipoproteins. J Hum Nutr 1981;35:53–58.

18. Davis WH, et al. Monotherapy with magnesium increases abnormally low high-density lipoprotein cholesterol: a clinical assay. Curr Ther Res 1984;36:341–346.

19. Nityanand S, et al. Clinical trials with gugulipid: a new hypolipidaemic agent. J Assoc Physicians India 1989;37:323–328.

Chronic Fatigue Syndrome

1. Demitrack MA, et al. Evidence for impaired activation of the hypothalamic-pituitary-adrenal axis in patients with chronic fatigue syndrome. J Clin Endocrinol Metab 1991;73:1224–1234.

2. Cox IM, et al. Red blood cell magnesium and chronic fatigue syndrome. Lancet 1991;337:757–760.

3. Bralley JA, Lord RS. Treatment of chronic fatigue syndrome with specific amino acid supplementation. J Appl Nutr 1994;46(3):74–78.

4. Jefferies WM. *Safe Uses of Cortisol.* Charles C. Thomas, Springfield, IL, 1996.

5. Cleare AJ, et al. Low-dose hydrocortisone in chronic fatigue syndrome: a randomised crossover trial. Lancet 1999;353:455–458.

6. McKenzie R, et al. Low-dose hydrocortisone for treatment of chronic fatigue syndrome: a randomized controlled trial. JAMA 1998;280:1061–1066.

7. Barnes BO, Galton L. *Hypothyroidism: the Unsuspected Illness,* Crowell, New York, 1976.

8. Sklar SH. CFS Forum, April 15, 1989.

Congestive Heart Failure

1. Frustaci A, et al. Myocardial magnesium content, histology, and antiarrhythmic response to magnesium infusion. Lancet 1987;2:1019.

2. Wener J, et al. The effects of prolonged hypomagnesemia on the cardiovascular system in young dogs. Am Heart J 1964;67:221–231.

3. Dyckner T, Wester PO. Ventricular extrasystoles and intracellular electrolytes before and after potassium and magnesium infusions in patients on diuretic treatment. Am Heart J 1979;97:12–18.

4. Iseri LT, et al. Magnesium and potassium therapy in multifocal atrial tachycardia. Am Heart J 1985;110:789–794.

5. Ishiyama T, et al. A clinical study of the effect of coenzyme Q on congestive heart failure. Jpn Heart J 1976;17:32–42.

6. Morisco C, et al. Effect of coenzyme Q10 in patients with congestive heart failure: a long-term multicenter randomized study. Clin Invest 1993;71:S134–S136.

7. Langsjoen PH, et al. Long-term efficacy and safety of coenzyme Q10 therapy for idiopathic dilated cardiomyopathy. Am J Cardiol 1990;65:521–523.

8. Azuma J, et al. Taurine for treatment of congestive heart failure. Int J Cardiol 1982;2:303.

9. Azuma J, et al. Double-blind randomized crossover trial of taurine in congestive heart failure. Curr Ther Res 1983;34:543.

10. Seligmann H, et al. Thiamine deficiency in patients with congestive heart failure receiving long-term furosemide therapy: a pilot study. Am J Med 1991;91:151–155.

11. Rector TS, et al. Randomized, double-blind, placebo-controlled study of supplemental oral L-arginine in patients with heart failure. Circulation 1996;93:2135–2141.

12. Berkowitz D, et al. Malabsorption as a complication of congestive heart failure. Am J Cardiol 1963;11:43–47.

13. Moller J, Einfeldt H. *Testosterone Treatment of Cardiovascular Diseases.* Springer-Verlag, Berlin, 1984.

14. Wright JV, Lenard L. *Maximize Your Vitality and Potency: for Men Over 40.* Smart Publications, Petuluma, CA, 1999.

15. Blesken R. Crataegus in cardiology. Fortschr Med 1992;110:290–292. [article in German]

16. Leuchtgens H. Crataegus Special Extract WS 1442 in NYHA II heart failure. A placebo controlled randomized double-blind study. Fortschr Med 1993;111:352–354. [article in German]

Crohn's Disease

1. Rowe AH, et al. Regional enteritis: its allergic aspects. Gastroenterology 1953;23:554–571.

2. Riordan AM, et al. Treatment of active Crohn's disease by exclusion diet: East Anglian Multicentre Controlled Trial. Lancet 1993;342:1131–1134.

3. Jones VA, et al. Crohn's disease: maintenance of remission by diet. Lancet 1985;2:177–180.

4. Gottschall E. *Breaking the Vicious Cycle.* Kirkton Press, Ontario, 1994.

5. Skogh M, et al. Vitamin A in Crohn's disease. Lancet 1980;1:766.

6. Wright JP, et al. Vitamin A therapy in patients with Crohn's disease. Gastroenterology 1985;88:512–514.

7. Belluzzi A, et al. Effect of an enteric-coated fish-oil preparation on relapses in Crohn's disease. N Engl J Med 1996;334:1557–1560.

Diabetes

1. Jenkins DJA, et al. Slow release dietary carbohydrate improves second meal tolerance. Am J Clin Nutr 1982;35:1339–1346.

2. Gutierrez M, et al. Utility of a short-term 25% carbohydrate diet on improving glycemic control in type 2 diabetes mellitus. J Am Coll Nutr 1998;17:595–600.

3. Schroeder HA. Chromium deficiency in rats: a syndrome simulating diabetes mellitus with retarded growth. J Nutr 1966;88:439–445.

4. Toepfer EW, et al. Preparation of chromium-containing material of glucose tolerance factor activity from brewer's yeast extracts and by synthesis. J Agric Food Chem 1977;25:162–166.

5. Anderson RA, Kozlovsky AS. Chromium intake, absorption and excretion of subjects consuming self-selected diets. Am J Clin Nutr 1985;41:1177–1183.

6. Martinez OB, et al. Dietary chromium and effect of chromium supplementation on glucose tolerance of elderly Canadian women. Nutr Res 1985;5:609–620.

7. Anderson RA, et al. Elevated intakes of supplemental chromium improve glucose and insulin variables in individuals with type 2 diabetes. Diabetes 1997;46:1786–1791.

8. Urberg M, Zemel MB. Evidence for synergism between chromium and nicotinic acid in the control of glucose tolerance in elderly humans. Metabolism 1987;36:896–899.

9. Reddi A, et al. Biotin supplementation improves glucose and insulin tolerances in genetically diabetic KK mice. Life Sci 1988;42:1323–1330.

10. Coggeshall JC, et al. Biotin status and plasma glucose in diabetics. Ann NY Acad Sci 1985;447:389–393.

11. Maebashi M, et al. Therapeutic evaluation of the effect of biotin on hyperglycemia in patients with non-insulin dependent diabetes mellitus. J Clin Biochem Nutr 1993;14:211–218.

12. Paolisso G, et al. Pharmacologic doses of vitamin E improve insulin action in healthy subjects and non-insulin-dependent diabetic patients. Am J Clin Nutr 1993;57:650–656.

13. Gaby AR, Wright JV. Nutritional regulation of blood glucose. J Advancement Med 1991;4(1):57–71.

14. Shanmugasundaram ERB, et al. Possible regeneration of the islets of Langerhans in streptozotocin-diabetic rats given *Gymnema sylvestre* leaf extracts. J Ethnopharmacol 1990;3:265–279.

15. Shanmugasundaram ERB, et al. Use of *Gymnema sylvestre* leaf extract in the control of blood glucose in insulin-dependent diabetes mellitus. J Ethnopharmacol 1990;30:281–294.

16. Baskaran K, et al. Antidiabetic effect of a leaf extract from *Gymnema sylvestre* in non-insulin-dependent diabetes mellitus patients. J Ethnopharmacol 1990;30:295–305.

Diabetes (preventing complications)

1. Bates CJ, et al. Effect of vitamin C on sorbitol in the lens of guinea-pigs made diabetic with streptozotocin. Br J Nutr 1992;67:445–456.

2. Vinson JA, et al. In vitro and in vivo reduction of erythrocyte sorbitol by ascorbic acid. Diabetes 1989;38:1036–1041.

3. Cunningham JJ, et al. Reduced mononuclear leukocyte ascorbic acid content in adults with insulin-dependent diabetes mellitus consuming adequate dietary vitamin C. Metabolism 1991;40:146–149.

4. Solomon LR, Cohen K. Erythrocyte O_2 transport and metabolism and effects of vitamin B_6 therapy in type II diabetes mellitus. Diabetes 1989;38:881–886.

5. Ceriello A, et al. Vitamin E reduction of protein glycosylation in diabetes. Diabetes Care 1991;14:68–72.

6. Davie SJ, et al. Effect of vitamin C on glycosylation of proteins. Diabetes 1992;41:167–173.

7. Lagrue G, et al. Pathology of the microcirculation in diabetes and alterations of the biosynthesis of intracellular matrix molecules. Front Matrix Biol S Karger 1979;7:324–335.

8 Scharrer A, Ober M. Anthocyanosides in the treat-

ment of retinopathies. Klin Mbl Augenheilk 1981; 178:386–389.

9. Griffith JQ Jr. Clinical application of quercetin: preliminary report. J Am Pharm Assoc 1953;42:68–69.

10. Koutsikos D, et al. Biotin for diabetic peripheral neuropathy. Biomed Pharmacother 1990;44:511–514.

11. Sancetta SM, et al. The use of vitamin B_{12} in the management of the neurologic manifestations of diabetes mellitus, with notes on the administration of massive doses. Ann Intern Med 1951;35: 1028–1048.

12. Keen H, et al. Treatment of diabetic neuropathy with gamma-linolenic acid. Diabetes Care 1993;16:8–15.

13. Jamal GA, et al. Treatment of diabetic neuropathy with gamma-linolenic acid (GLA) as evening primrose oil (Efamol). J Am Coll Nutr 1987;6:86.

14. Jones CL, Gonzalez V. Pyridoxine deficiency: a new factor in diabetic neuropathy. J Am Podiatry Assoc 1978;68:646–653.

15. Levin ER, et al. The influence of pyridoxine in diabetic peripheral neuropathy. Diabetes Care 1981; 4:606–609.

16. McNair P, et al. Hypomagnesemia, a risk factor in diabetic retinopathy. Diabetes 1978;27:1075–1077.

17. Kornerup T, Strom L. Vitamin B_{12} and retinopathy in juvenile diabetics. Acta Paediatr 1958;47:646–651.

18. Cameron AJ, Ahern GJ. Diabetic retinopathy and cyancobalamin (vitamin B_{12}). A preliminary report. Br J Ophthalmal 1958;42:686–693.

19. Franconi F, et al. Plasma and platelet taurine are reduced in subjects with insulin-dependent diabetes mellitus: effects of taurine supplementation. Am J Clin Nutr 1995;61:1115–1119.

Ear Infections

1. Williams RL, et al. Use of antibiotics in preventing recurrent acute otitis media and in treating otitis media with effusion. JAMA 1993;270:1344–1351.

2. Scheck A. Tympanostomy tubes may cause hearing loss. Family Pract News, March 15, 1993, pp. 3, 24.

3. Berg AO. Middle ear effusion guideline: the co-chair's thoughts. Am Family Physician 1994;50(5): 897–898.

4. Otitis Media Guideline Panel. Managing otitis media with effusion in young children. Am Family Physician 1994;50(5):1003–1010.

5. Ringsdorf WM Jr, et al. Sucrose, neutrophilic phago-

cytosis and resistance to disease. Dent Survey 1976; 52(12):46–48.

6. Sanchez A, et al. Role of sugars in human neutrophilic phagocytosis. Am J Clin Nutr 1973;26: 1180–1184.

7. Nalder BN, et al. Sensitivity of the immunological response to the nutritional status of rats. J Nutr 1972;102:535–542.

8. Noun LJ. Chronic otorrhea due to food sensitivity. J Allergy 1942;14:82–86.

9. Bellioni P, et al. Allergy: a leading role in otitis media with effusion. Allergol Immunopathol 1987;15: 205–208.

10. Nsouli TM, et al. Role of food allergy in serous otitis media. Ann Allergy 1994;73:215–219.

11. Chandra RK. Effect of vitamin and trace–element supplementation on immune responses and infection in elderly subjects. Lancet 1992;340:1124–1127.

Eczema

1. Atherton DJ, et al. A double-blind controlled cross-over trial of an antigen avoidance diet in atopic eczema. Lancet 1978;1:401–403.

2. Sampson HA, McCaskill CC. Food hypersensitivity and atopic dermatitis: evaluation of 113 patients. J Pediatr 1985;107:669–675.

3. Hansen AE. Serum lipid changes and therapeutic effects of various oils in infantile eczema. Proc Soc Exp Biol Med 1933;31:160–161.

4. Wright S, Burton JL. Oral evening primrose seed oil improves atopic eczema. Lancet 1982;2:1120–1122.

5. Schalin-Karrila M, et al. Evening primrose oil in the treatment of atopic eczema: effect on clinical status, plasma phospholipid fatty acids and circulating blood prostaglandins. Br J Dermatol 1987;117:11–19.

6. Bjorneboe A, et al. Effect of dietary supplementation with eicosapentaenoic acid in the treatment of atopic dermatitis. Br J Dermatol 1987;117:463–469.

7. Gross P. Nummular eczema: its clinical picture and successful therapy. Arch Dermatol Syph 1941; 44:1060–1077.

8. Stoesser AV, Nelson LS. Synthetic vitamin A in treatment of eczema in children. Ann Allergy 1952;10: 703–704.

Emphysema and Chronic Bronchitis (chronic obstructive lung disease)

1. Rowe AH, et al. Food allergy: its role in the symptoms of obstructive emphysema and chronic bronchitis. J Asthma Res 1967;5:11–20.

2. Tattersall AB, et al. Acetylcysteine (Fabrol) in chronic bronchitis—a study in general practice. J Int Med Res 1983;11:279–284.

3. British Thoracic Society Research Committee. Oral N-acetylcysteine and exacerbation rates in patients with chronic bronchitis and severe airways obstruction. Thorax 1985;40:832–835.

4. Fiaccadori E, et al. Muscle and serum magnesium in pulmonary intensive care unit patients. Crit Care Med 1988;16:751–760.

5. Okayama H, et al. Bronchodilating effect of intravenous magnesium sulfate in bronchial asthma. JAMA 1987;257:1076–1078.

6. Molloy DW, et al. Hypomagnesemia and respiratory muscle power. Am Rev Respir Dis 1984;129: 497–498.

7. Dal Negro R, et al. L-carnitine and physiokinesiotherapy in chronic respiratory insufficiency. Clin Trials J 1985;22:353–360.

8. Fujimoto S, et al. Effects of coenzyme Q10 administration on pulmonary function and exercise performance in patients with chronic lung diseases. Clin Investig 1993;71:S162–S166.

9. Soskel NT, et al. A copper-deficient, zinc-supplemented diet produces emphysema in pigs. Am Rev Respir Dis 1982;126:316–325.

10. Sparrow D, et al. The relationship of pulmonary function to copper concentrations in drinking water. Am Rev Respir Dis 1982;126:312–315.

11. Buhl R, et al. Oxidant-protease interactions in the lung. Prospects for antioxidant therapy. Chest 1996;110:267S–272S.

12. Lamson D. Personal communication. Seattle, WA, 1998.

Epilepsy

1. Fabrykant M, et al. The association of spontaneous hypoglycemia with hypocalcemia and electro-cerebral dysfunction. Proc Am Diabetes Assoc 1947;7: 233–242.

2. Egger J, et al. Oligoantigenic diet treatment of children with epilepsy and migraine. J Pediatr 1989; 114:51–58.

3. Gasch AT. Use of the traditional ketogenic diet for treatment of intractable epilepsy. J Am Diet Assoc 1990;90:1433–1434.

4. Gordon N. Medium-chain triglycerides in a ketogenic diet. Develop Med Child Neurol 1977;19: 535–544.

5. Coursin DB. Convulsive seizures in infants with pyridoxine-deficient diet. JAMA 1954;154:406–408.

6. Crowell GF, et al. Pyridoxine-dependent seizures. Am Family Physician 1983;27(3):183–187.

7. Hagberg B, et al. Tryptophan load tests and pyridoxal-5-phosphate levels in epileptic children. II. Cryptogenic epilepsy. Acta Paediatr Scand 1966;55:371–384.

8. Ogunmekan AO, et al. A randomized, double-blind, placebo-controlled, clinical trial of d-alpha-tocopheryl acetate (vitamin E), as add-on therapy, for epilepsy in children. Epilepsia 1989;30:84–89.

9. Carl GF, et al. Association of low blood manganese concentrations with epilepsy. Neurology 1986;36: 1584–1587.

10. Papavasiliou PS, et al. Seizure disorders and trace metals: manganese tissue levels in treated epileptics. Neurology 1979;29:1466–1473.

11. Sampson P. Low manganese level may trigger epilepsy. JAMA 1977;238:1805.

12. Goldman RS, Finkbeiner SM. Therapeutic use of magnesium sulfate in selected cases of cerebral ischemia. N Engl J Med 1988;319:1224–1225.

13. Barbeau A, et al. Zinc, taurine, and epilepsy. Arch Neurol 1974;30:52–58.

14. Roach ES, et al. N,N-dimethylglycine for epilepsy. N Engl J Med 1982;307:1081–1082.

15. Backman N, et al. Folate treatment of diphenylhydantoin-induced gingival hyperplasia. Scand J Dent Res 1989;97:222–232.

16. Drew HJ, et al. Effect of folate on phenytoin hyperplasia. J Clin Periodontol 1987;14:350–356.

17. Callaghan N, et al. The correction of defective vitamin B_{12} absorption due to anti-convulsant drugs by folic acid. Ir J Med Sci 1970;3:401–405.

18. Fischer MH, et al. Bone status in nonambulant, epileptic, institutionalized youth. Improvement with vitamin D therapy. Clin Pediatr 1988;27:499–505.

19. van Wouwe JP. Carnitine deficiency during valproic acid treatment. Int J Vitam Nutr Res 1995;65: 211–214.

Fibrocystic Breast Disease

1. Minton JP, et al. Clinical and biochemical studies on methylxanthine-related fibrocystic breast disease. Surgery 1981;90:299–304.
2. Ernster VL, et al. Effects of a caffeine-free diet on benign breast disease: a randomized trial. Surgery 1982;91:263–267.
3. Abrams AA. Use of vitamin E in chronic cystic mastitis. N Engl J Med 1965;272:1080.
4. London RS, et al. Mammary dysplasia: clinical response and urinary excretion of 11-deoxy-17-ketosteroids and pregnanediol following alpha-tocopherol therapy. Breast 1978;4(2):19–22.
5. Ernster VL, et al. Vitamin E and benign breast "disease": a double-blind, randomized clinical trial. Surgery 1985;97:490–494.
6. Krouse TB, et al. Age-related changes resembling fibrocystic disease in iodine-blocked rat breasts. Arch Pathol Lab Med 1979;103:631–634.
7. Eskin BA, et al. Mammary gland dysplasia in iodine deficiency. JAMA 1967;200:691–695.
8. Anonymous. Iodine supplements relieve painful, swollen breasts. Family Pract News, Dec 1, 1986.
9. Ghent WR, et al. Iodine replacement in fibrocystic disease of the breast. Can J Surg 1993;36:453–460.
10. Estes NC. Mastodynia due to fibrocystic disease of the breast controlled with thyroid hormone. Am J Surg 1981;142:764–766.
11. Gateley CA, et al. Plasma fatty acid profiles in benign breast disorders. Br J Surg 1992;79:407–409.

Gallstones (avoiding gallbladder sugery)

1. Breneman JC. Allergy elimination diet as the most effective gallbladder diet. Ann Allergy 1968;26:83–87.
2. Walzer M. The allergic reaction in the gallbladder. Experimental studies in the rhesus monkey. Gastroenterology 1943;1:565–572.
3. Thornton JR, et al. Diet and gallstones: effects of refined carbohydrate diets on bile cholesterol saturation and bile acid metabolism. Gut 1983;24:2–6.
4. Capper WM, et al. Gallstones, gastric secretion and flatulent dyspepsia. Lancet 1967;1:413–415.
5. Jenkins SA. Biliary lipids, bile acids and gallstone formation in hypovitaminotic C guinea-pigs. Br J Nutr 1978;40:317–322.
6. Gustafsson U, et al. The effect of vitamin C in high doses on plasma and biliary lipid composition in patients with cholesterol gallstones: prolongation of the nucleation time. Eur J Clin Invest 1997;27:387–391.
7. Robins SJ, Fasulo J. Mechanism of lithogenic bile production: studies in the hamster fed an essential fatty acid-deficient diet. Gastroenterology 1973;65:104–114.
8. Tuzhilin SA, et al. The treatment of patients with gallstones by lecithin. Am J Gastroenterol 1976;65:231–235.
9. Bell GD, Doran J. Gall stone dissolution in man using an essential oil preparation. Br Med J 1979;1:24.
10. Ellis WR, et al. Pilot study of combination treatment for gallstones with medium dose chenodeoxycholic acid and a terpene preparation. Br Med J 1984;289:153–156.

Gout

1. Israel KD, et al. Serum uric acid, inorganic phosphorus, and glutamic-oxalacetic transaminase and blood pressure in carbohydrate-sensitive adults consuming three different levels of sucrose. Ann Nutr Metab 1983;27:425–435.
2. Emmerson BT. Effect of oral fructose on urate production. Ann Rheum Dis 1974;33:276–280.
3. Harkavy J. Allergic factors in gout. JAMA 1949;139:75–80.
4. Blau LW. Cherry diet control for gout and arthritis. Tex Rep Biol Med 1950;8:309–311.
5. Oster KA. Evaluation of serum cholesterol reduction and xanthine oxidase inhibition in the treatment of atherosclerosis. In Dhalla NS (ed.). *Recent Advances in Studies on Cardiac Structure,* vol. 3, University Press, Baltimore, 1973, pp. 73–80.
6. Oster KA. Xanthine oxidase and folic acid. Ann Intern Med 1977;87:252–253.
7. Stein HB, et al. Ascorbic acid-induced uricosuria: a consequence of megavitamin therapy. Ann Intern Med 1976;84:385–388.
8. Garrod AB. Uric acid: its physiology and its relation to renal calculi and gravel. Lancet 1883;1:669–673.
9. Lieb J. Linoleic acid in the treatment of lithium toxicity and familial tremor. Prostaglandins Med 1980;4:275–279.

10. Klevay LM. Hyperuricemia in rats due to copper deficiency. Nutr Rep Int 1980;22:617–621.
11. Garg A, et al. Nicotinic acid as therapy for dyslipidemia in non-insulin-dependent diabetes mellitus. JAMA 1990;264:723–726.

Hepatitis (acute and chronic)

1. Beyer KH. Protective action of vitamin C against experimental hepatic damage. Arch Intern Med 1943;71:315–324.
2. Murata A. Virucidal activity of vitamin C for prevention and treatment of viral diseases. In Proc First Int Congr IAMS, Takezi Hasegawa (ed.), Science Council of Japan, 1975.
3. Baur H, Staub H. Treatment of hepatitis with infusions of ascorbic acid: comparison with other therapies. JAMA 1954;156:565(Abstract).
4. Calleja HB, Brooks RH. Acute hepatitis treated with high doses of vitamin C. Ohio State Med J 1960;56:821–823.
5. Campbell RE, Pruitt FW. The effect of vitamin B_{12} and folic acid in the treatment of viral hepatitis. Am J Med Sci 1955;229:8–15.
6. Andreone P, et al. Vitamin E for chronic hepatitis B. Ann Intern Med 1998;128:156–157.
7. Houglum K, et al. A pilot study of the effects of d-alpha-tocopherol on hepatic stellate cell activation in chronic hepatitis C. Gastroenterology 1997;113:1069–1073.
8. Fujisawa K, et al. Therapeutic approach to chronic active hepatitis with glycyrrhizin. Asian Med J 1980;23:745–756.
9. Xianshi S, et al. Clinical and laboratory observation on the effect of glycyrrhizin in acute and chronic viral hepatitis. J Traditional Chin Med 1984;4:127–132.
10. Acharya SK, et al. A preliminary open trial on interferon stimulator (SNMC) derived from *Glycyrrhiza glabra* in the treatment of subacute hepatic failure. Indian J Med Res 1993;98:69–74.
11. Thyagarajan SP, et al. Effect of Phyllanthus amarus on chronic carriers of hepatitis B virus. Lancet 1988;2:764–766.
12. Yu SY, et al. Protective role of selenium against hepatitis B virus and primary liver cancer in Qidong. Biol Trace Elem Res 1997;56:117–124.

Herpes Simplex

1. Murata A. Virucidal activity of vitamin C for prevention and treatment of viral diseases. In Proc First Int Congr IAMS, Takezi Hasegawa (ed.), Science Council of Japan, 1975.
2. Holden M, et al. Further experiments on the inactivation of herpes virus by vitamin C (l-ascorbic acid). J Immunol 1937;33:251–257.
3. Terezhalmy GT, et al. The use of water-soluble bioflavonoid-ascorbic acid complex in the treatment of recurrent herpes labialis. Oral Surg 1978;45:56–62.
4. Griffith RS, et al. A multicentered study of lysine therapy in herpes simplex infection. Dermatologica 1978;156:257–267.
5. McCune MA, et al. Treatment of recurrent herpes simplex infections with L-lysine hydrochloride. Cutis 1984;34:366–373.
6. Nead DE. Effective vitamin E treatment for ulcerative herpetic lesions. Dent Survey 1976;52(7):50–51.
7. Fink M, et al. Treatment of herpes simplex by alpha-tocopherol (vitamin E). Br Dent J 1980;148:246.
8. Sklar SH, et al. Adenosine in the treatment of recurrent herpes labialis. Oral Surg 1979;48:416–417.
9. Skinner GRB, et al. The effect of lithium chloride on the replication of herpes simplex virus. Med Microbiol Immunol 1980;168:139–148.
10. Amsterdam JD, et al. A possible antiviral action of lithium carbonate in herpes simplex virus infections. Biol Psychiatry 1990;27:447–453.
11. Skinner GRB. Lithium ointment for genital herpes. Lancet 1983;2:288.

Hypertension

1. el Zein M, et al. Long-term effects of excess sucrose ingestion on three strains of rats. Am J Hypertens 1990;3:560–562.
2. Abraira C, et al. Systolic blood pressure (B.P.) enhancing effect of dietary sucrose (S) in humans. J Am Coll Nutr 1987;6:79.
3. Silagy CA, et al. A meta-analysis of the effect of garlic on blood pressure. J Hypertens 1994;12:463–468.
4. Louria DB, et al. Onion extract in treatment of hypertension and hyperlipidemia: a preliminary communication. Curr Ther Res 1985;37:127–131.
5. Lang T, et al. Relation between coffee drinking and

blood pressure: analysis of 6,321 subjects in the Paris region. Am J Cardiol 1983;52:1238–1242.

6. Robertson D, et al. Caffeine and hypertension. Am J Med 1984;77:54–60.

7. Puddey IB, et al. Regular alcohol use raises blood pressure in treated hypertensive subjects. Lancet 1987;1:647–651.

8. Gay LP. Nonreaginic food allergy in the management of essential hypertension. J Appl Nutr 1959;12:71–74.

9. Grant ECG. Food allergies and migraine. Lancet 1979;1:966–969.

10. Cappuccio FP, et al. Does potassium supplementation lower blood pressure? A meta-analysis of published trials. J Hypertens 1991;9:465–473.

11. Resnick LM, et al. Calcium metabolism in essential hypertension: relationship to altered renin system activity. Fed Proc 1986;45:2739–2745.

12. Dyckner T, Wester PO. Effect of magnesium on blood pressure. Br Med J 1983;286:1847–1849.

13. Cappuccio FP, et al. Lack of effect of oral magnesium on high blood pressure: a double blind study. Br Med J 1985;291:235–238.

14. Rao RH, et al. Effect of polyunsaturate-rich vegetable oils on blood pressure in essential hypertension. Clin Exp Hypertension 1981;3:27–38.

15. Lungershausen YK, et al. Reduction of blood pressure and plasma triglycerides by omega-3 fatty acids in treated hypertensives. J Hypertens 1994;12:1041–1045.

16. Digiesi V, et al. Coenzyme Q10 in essential hypertension. Molec Aspects Med 1994;15(Suppl):S257–S263.

17. Digiesi V, et al. Effect of coenzyme Q10 on essential hypertension. Curr Ther Res 1990;47:841–845.

18. Saito I, et al. Hypothyroidism as a cause of hypertension. Hypertension 1983;5:112–115.

Infertility (male and female)

1. Hurley D. Pollutants blamed for steady decline in sperm counts, ejaculate volume. Med Tribune, October 8, 1992, p. 14.

2. Comhaire F, et al. Declining sperm quality in European men. Andrologia 1996;28:300–301.

3. Danzo BJ. Environmental xenobiotics may disrupt normal endocrine function by interfering with the binding of physiological ligands to steroid receptors and binding proteins. Environ Health Perspect 1997;105:294–301.

4. Gilfillan SC. Lead poisoning and the fall of Rome. J Occup Med 1965;7(2):53–60.

5. Bolumar F, et al. Caffeine intake and delayed conception: a European multicenter study on infertility and subfecundity. Am J Epidemiol 1997;145:324–334.

6. Holt LE Jr, et al. Studies of experimental amino acid deficiency in man. I. Nitrogen balance. Fed Proc 1942;1:116–117.

7. Schacter A, et al. Treatment of oligospermia with the amino acid arginine. J Urol 1973;110:311–313.

8. Anonymous. Sperm swim singly after vitamin C therapy. JAMA 1983;249:2747–2751.

9. Igarashi M. Augmentative effect of ascorbic acid upon induction of human ovulation in clomiphene-ineffective anovulatory women. Int J Fertil 1977;22:168–173.

10. Hargrove JT, Abraham GE. Effect of vitamin B6 on infertility in women with the premenstrual tension syndrome. Infertility 1979;2:315–322.

11. Vitali G, et al. Carnitine supplementation in human idiopathic asthenospermia: clinical results. Drugs Exp Clin Res 1995;21:157–159.

12. Marmar JL, et al. Semen zinc levels in infertile and postvasectomy patients and patients with prostatitis. Fertil Steril 1975;26:1057–1063.

13. Netter A, et al. Effect of zinc administration on plasma testosterone, dihydrotestosterone, and sperm count. Arch Androl 1981;7:69–73.

14. Rushton DH, et al. Ferritin and fertility. Lancet 1991;337:1554.

15. Sieve BF. The clinical effects of a new B complex factor, para-aminobenzoic acid, on pigmentation and fertility. South Med Surg 1942(March);104:135–139.

16. Buxton CL, Herrmann WL. Effect of thyroid therapy on menstrual disorders and sterility. JAMA 1954;155:1035–1039.

17. Reed DC, et al. Male subfertility: treatment with liothyronine (Cytomel). J Urol 1958;79:868–872.

Irritable Bowel Syndrome

1. Jones VA, et al. Food intolerance: a major factor in the pathogenesis of irritable bowel syndrome. Lancet 1982;2:1115–1117.

2. Nanda R, et al. Food intolerance and the irritable bowel syndrome. Gut 1989;30:1099–1104.

3. Bentley SJ, et al. Food hypersensitivity in irritable bowel syndrome. Lancet 1983;2:295–297.

4. Zwetchkenbaum J, Burakoff R. The irritable bowel syndrome and food hypersensitivity. Ann Allergy 1988;61:47–49.

5. Rees WDW, et al. Treating irritable bowel syndrome with peppermint oil. Br Med J 1979;2:835–836.

Kidney Stones

1. Lemann J, et al. Possible role of carboydrate-induced calciuria in calcium oxalate kidney-stone formation. N Engl J Med 1969;280:232–237.

2. Robertson WG, et al. The effect of high animal protein intake on the risk of calcium stone-formation in the urinary tract. Clin Sci 1979;57:285–288.

3. Coe FL, et al. The contribution of dietary purine over-consumption to hyperuricosuria in calcium oxalate stone formers. J Chronic Dis 1976;29: 793–800.

4. Burtis WJ, et al. Dietary hypercalciuria in patients with calcium oxalate kidney stones. Am J Clin Nutr 1994;60:424–429.

5. Hollingbery PW, et al. Effect of dietary caffeine and aspirin on urinary calcium and hydroxyproline excretion in pre- and postmenopausal women. Fed Proc 1985;44:1149.

6. Shah PJR, et al. Idiopathic hypercalciuria: its control with unprocessed bran. Br J Urol 1980;52:426–429.

7. Ebisuno S, et al. Rice-bran treatment for calcium stone formers with idiopathic hypercalciuria. Br J Urol 1986;58:592–595.

8. Shuster J, et al. Soft drink consumption and urinary stone recurrence: a randomized prevention trial. J Clin Epidemiol 1992;45:911–916.

9. Ettinger B, et al. Potassium-magnesium citrate is an effective prophylaxis against recurrent calcium oxalate nephrolithiasis. J Urol 1997;158:2069–2073.

10. Seltzer MA, et al. Dietary manipulation with lemonade to treat hypocitraturic calcium nephrolithiasis. J Urol 1996;156:907–909.

11. Wabner CL, Pak CYC. Effect of orange juice consumption on urinary stone risk factors. J Urol 1993; 149:1405–1408.

12. Johansson G, et al. Effects of magnesium hydroxide in renal stone disease. J Am Coll Nutr 1982;1: 179–185.

13. Thind SK, et al. Role of vitamin B6 in oxalate metabolism in urolithiasis. Am J Clin Nutr 1979;32(6):xx (Abstract).

14. Rattan V, et al. Effect of combined supplementation of magnesium oxide and pyridoxine in calcium-oxalate stone formers. Urol Res 1994;22:161–165.

15. Prien EL, Gershoff SN. Magnesium oxide-pyridoxine therapy for recurrent calcium oxalate calculi. J Urol 1974;112:509–512.

16. Will EJ, et al. Primary oxalosis: clinical and biochemical response to high-dose pyridoxine therapy. Metabolism 1979;28:542–548.

17. Kancha RK, Anasuya A. Contribution of vitamin A deficiency to calculogenic risk factors of urine: studies in children. Biochem Med Metabol Biol 1992; 47:1–9.

18. Robertson WG, Peacock M. The cause of idiopathic calcium stone disease: hypercalciuria or hyperoxaluria? Nephron 1980;26:105–110.

19. Curhan GC, et al. A prospective study of dietary calcium and other nutrients and the risk of symptomatic kidney stones. N Engl J Med 1993;328: 833–838.

20. Curhan GC, et al. Comparison of dietary calcium with supplemental calcium and other nutrients as factors affecting the risk of kidney stones in women. Ann Intern Med 1997;126:497–504.

21. Ringsdorf WM Jr, Cheraskin E. Nutritional aspects of urolithiasis, South Med J 1981;74:41–44.

22. Curhan GC, et al. A prospective study of the intake of vitamins C and B6, and the risk of kidney stones in men. J Urol 1996;155:1847–1851.

23. Wright JV. High-dose vitamin C and kidney stones. In *Dr. Wright's Book of Nutritional Therapy*. Rodale Press, 1979, pp. 272–277.

Lupus

1. Anderson JA, et al. Hyperreactivity to cow's milk in an infant with LE and tart cell phenomenon. J Pediatr 1974;84:59–67.

2. Cooke HM, Reading CM. Dietary intervention in systemic lupus erythematosis: 4 cases of clinical remission and reversal of abnormal pathology. Int Clin Nutr Rev 1985;5(4):166–176.

3 Crook W. *The Yeast Connection and the Woman*. Professional Books, Jackson TN, 1995.

4 Lahita RG, et al. Low plasma androgens in women with systemic lupus erythematosus. Arthritis Rheum 1987;30:241–247.

5. Lucas JA, et al. Prevention of autoantibody formation and prolonged survival in New Zealand Black/New Zealand White mice fed dehydroisoandrosterone. J Clin Invest 1985;75:2091–2093.

6. Van Vollenhoven RF, et al. An open study of dehydroepiandrosterone in systemic lupus erythematosus. Arthritis Rheum 1994;37:1305–1310.

7. van Vollenhoven RF, et al. Dehydroepiandrosterone in systemic lupus erythematosus. Arthritis Rheum 1995;38:1826–1831.

8. Lahita RG, et al. Increased oxidation of testosterone in systemic lupus erythematosus. Arthritis Rheum 1983;26:1517–1521.

9. Olsen NJ, Kovacs WJ. Case report: testosterone treatment of systemic lupus erythematosus in a patient with Klinefelter's syndrome. Am J Med Sci 1995;310:158–160.

10. Ayres S Jr, Mihan R. Is vitamin E involved in the autoimmune mechanism? Cutis 1978;21:321–325.

11. Gaby AR. *B6: the Natural Healer.* Keats, New Canaan, CT, 1987.

Macular Degeneration

1. Mobarhan S, et al. Dietary zinc deficiency produces electroretinogram (ERG) abnormalities without depleting total ocular zinc. Fed Proc 1984;43:685.

2. Wyszynski RE, et al. A donor-age-dependent change in the activity of alpha-mannosidase in human cultured RPE cells. Invest Ophthalmol Vis Sci 1989;30:2341–2347.

3. Newsome DA, et al. Oral zinc in macular degeneration. Arch Ophthalmol 1988;106:192–198.

4. Fosmire GJ, et al. Dietary intakes and zinc status of an elderly rural population. J Nutr Elderly 1984;4(1):19–30.

5. Jacobsen JG. Possible physiological functions of taurine in mammalian systems. In Cavallini D, et al. (eds.). Proc 2nd Int Meeting on Low Molecular Weight Sulfur-Containing Natural Products. Rome, June 18–21, 1979, pp. 163–172.

6. Geggel HS, et al. Nutritional requirement for taurine in patients receiving long-term parenteral nutrition. N Engl J Med 1985;312:142–146.

7. Franconi F, et al. Plasma and platelet taurine are reduced in subjects with insulin-dependent diabetes mellitus: effects of taurine supplementation. Am J Clin Nutr 1995;61:1115–1119.

8. Li Z-Y, et al. Amelioration of photic injury in rat retina by ascorbic acid: a histopathologic study. Invest Ophthalmol Vis Sci 1985;26:1589–1598.

9. Hayes KC. Pathophysiology of vitamin E deficiency in monkeys. Am J Clin Nutr 1974;27:1130–1140.

10. Adayeva Y, et al. Vitamin E treatment in dystrophy of the macula lutea. Am J Ophthalmol 1963;56:498 (Abstract).

11. Wright JV, et al. Improvement of vision in macular degeneration associated with intravenous zinc and selenium therapy: two cases. J Nutr Med 1990;1:133–138.

12. Goldberg J, et al. Factors associated with age-related macular degeneration. An analysis of data from the First National Health and Nutrition Examination Survey. Am J Epidemiol 1988;128:700–710.

13. Seddon JM, et al. Dietary carotenoids, vitamins A, C, and E, and advanced age-related macular degeneration. JAMA 1994;272:1413–1420.

14. Landrum JT, et al. A one year study of the macular pigment: the effect of 140 days of a lutein supplement. Exp Eye Res 1997;65:57–62.

15. Lebuisson DA, et al. Treatment of senile macular degeneration with Ginkgo biloba extract. A preliminary double-blind, drug versus placebo study. Presse Med 1986;15:1556–1558.

16. Gloria E. Perla A. Effect of anthocyanosides on the absolute visual threshold. Ann Ottalmol Clin Ocul 1966;92:595–607.

17. Jayle G-E, Aubert L. Action des glucosides d'anthocyanes sur la vision scotopique et mesopique du sujet normal. Therapie 1964;19:171–185.

Memory Loss and Depression (age-related)

1. Joosten E, et al. Metabolic evidence that deficiencies of vitamin B12 (cobalamin), folate, and vitamin B6 occur commonly in elderly people. Am J Clin Nutr 1993;58:458–476.

2. van Tiggelen CJM, et al. Assessment of vitamin B12 status in CSF. Am J Psychiatry 1984;141:136.

3. Frank O, et al. Superiority of periodic intramuscular vitamin injections over daily oral vitamins in maintaining normal vitamin titers in a geriatric population. Am J Clin Nutr 1977;30:630.

4. Anonymous. Antiobesity drug may counter aging. Science News 1981;19(3):39.

5. Flood JF, et al. Memory-enhancing effects in male mice

of pregnenolone and steroids metabolically derived from it. Proc Natl Acad Sci 1992;89:1567–1571.

6. Boschert S. Testosterone loss linked with memory dysfunction. Family Pract News, October 1, 1994, p. 5.

7. Paganini-Hill A, et al. Estrogen replacement therapy and risk of Alzheimer's disease. Arch Intern Med 1996;156:2213–2217.

8. Ohkura T, et al. Evaluation of estrogen treatment in female patients with dementia of the Alzheimer type. Endocrine J 1994;41:361–371.

9. Honjo H, et al. Senile dementia-Alzheimer's type and estrogen. Horm Metab Res 1995;27:204–207.

10. Vorberg G. Ginkgo biloba extract (GBE): a long-term study of chronic cerebral insufficiency in geriatric patients. Clin Trials J 1985;22:149–157.

11. Taillandier J, et al. Ginkgo biloba extract in the treatment of cerebral disorders due to ageing. Presse Med 1986;15:1583–1587.

12. Kleijnen J, Knipschild P. Ginkgo biloba for cerebral insufficiency. Br J Clin Pharmacol 1992;34:352–358.

13. Hopfenmuller W. Proof of the therapeutic effectiveness of a Ginkgo biloba special extract. Meta-analysis of 11 clinical trials in aged patients with cerebral insufficiency. Arzneimittelforschung 1994;44:1005–1013.

14. Le Bars PL, et al. A placebo-controlled, double-blind, randomized trial of an extract of Ginkgo biloba for dementia. JAMA 1997;278:1327–1332.

15. Nunzi MG, et al. Dendritic spine loss in hippocampus of aged rats. Effect of brain phosphatidylserine administration. Neurobiol Aging 1987;8:501–510.

16. Lombardi GF. Terapia farmacologica con fosfatidil serina in 40 patzienti ambulatoriali con sindrome demenziale senile. Minerva Med 1989;80:599–602.

17. Kidd PM. Phosphatidylserine: membrane nutrient for memory. A clinical and mechanistic assessment. Altern Med Rev 1996;1:70–84.

18. Gaby AR. Don't believe everything you read. Townsend Letter for Doctors and Patients, July 1997, pp. 125–126.

19. Vecchi GP, et al. Acetyl-l-carnitine treatment of mental impairment in the elderly: evidence from a multicentre study. Arch Gerontol Geriatr 1991;Suppl 2:159–168.

20. Thal LJ, et al. A 1-year multicenter placebo-controlled study of acetyl-L-carnitine in patients with Alzheimer's disease. Neurology 1996;47:705–711.

Menopause

1. Felson DT, et al. The effect of postmenopausal estrogen therapy on bone density in elderly women. N Engl J Med 1993;329:1141–1146.

2. Gaby AR. *Preventing and Reversing Osteoporosis.* Prima Publ., Rocklin, CA, 1994.

3 . Hulley S, et al. Randomized trial of estrogen plus progestin for secondary prevention of coronary heart disease in postmenopausal women. JAMA 1998;280:605–613.

4. The Writing Group for the PEPI Trial. Effects of estrogen or estrogen/progestin regimens on heart disease risk factors in postmenopausal women. The Postmenopausal Estrogen/Progestin Interventions (PEPI) Trial. JAMA 1995;273:199–208.

5. Rubenstein BB. Vitamin E diminishes the vasomotor symptoms of menopause. Fed Proc 1948;7:106.

6. Perloff WH. Treatment of the menopause. Am J Obstet Gynecol 1949;58:684–694.

7. McLaren HC. Vitamin E in the menopause. Br Med J 1949;2:1378–1382.

8. Blatt MHG, et al. Vitamin E and climacteric syndrome. Failure of effective control as measured by menpausal index. Arch Intern Med 1953;91:792–799.

9. Smith CJ. Non-hormonal control of vaso-motor flushing in menopausal patients. Chicago Med 1964(March 7);67:193–195.

10. Adlercreutz H, et al. Dietary phyto-oestrogens and the menopause in Japan. Lancet 1992;339:1233.

11. Albertazzi P, et al. The effect of dietary soy supplementation on hot flushes. Obstet Gynecol 1998;91:6–11.

12. Erdman JW Jr. Control of serum lipids with soy protein. N Engl J Med 1995;333:313–315.

13. Ziegler J. Soybeans show promise in cancer prevention. J Natl Cancer Inst 1994;86:1666–1667.

14. Lehmann-Willenbrock E, Riedel HH. Clinical and endocrinologic examinations concerning therapy of climacteric symptoms following hysterectomy and remaining ovaries. Zent Bl Gynakol 1988;110:611–618.

15. Zhy DPQ. Dong quai. Am J Chin Med 1987;15(3–4):117–125.

16. Mehta AI. The liquorice story. Lancet 1951;1:113.

17. Elakovich SD, Hampton JM. Analysis of coumestrol, a phytoestrogen, in alfalfa tablets sold for human consumption. J Agric Food Chem 1984;32:173–175.

18. Punnonen R, Lukola A. Oestrogen-like effect of ginseng. Br Med J 1980;281:1110.

19. Hirata JD, et al. Does dong quai have estrogenic effects in postmenopausal women? A double-blind, placebo-controlled trial. Fertil Steril 1997;68:981–986.

20. Follingstad AH. Estriol, the forgotten estrogen? JAMA 1978;239:29–30.

21. Head KA. Estriol: safety and efficacy. Altern Med Rev 1998;3:101–113.

22. Tzingounis VA, et al. Estriol in the management of the menopause. JAMA 1978;239:1638–1641.

23. Granberg S, et al. Endometrial sonographic and histologic findings in women with and without hormonal replacement therapy suffering from postmenopausal bleeding. Maturitas 1997;27:35–40.

24. Wright JV, Morgenthaler J. *Natural Hormone Replacement for Women Over 45.* Smart Publications, Petaluma, CA, 1997.

Menorrhagia and Cervical Dysplasia

1. Lithgow DM, Politzer WM. Vitamin A in the treatment of menorrhagia. S Afr Med J 1977;51:191–193.

2. Taymor ML, et al. The etiological role of chronic iron deficiency in production of menorrhagia. JAMA 1964;187:323–327.

3. Samuels AJ. Studies in patients with functional menorrhagia: the antihemorrhagic effect of the adequate repletion of iron stores. Isr J Med Sci 1965;1:851–853.

4. Cohen JD, Rubin HW. Functional menorrhagia: treatment with bioflavonoids and vitamin C. Curr Ther Res 1960;2:539–542.

5. Barnes BO, Galton L. *Hypothyroidism: the Unsuspected Illness.* Crowell, New York, 1976.

6. Stoffer SS. Menstrual disorders and mild thyroid insufficiency: intriguing cases suggesting an association. Postgrad Med 1982;72(2):75–82.

7. Palan PR, et al. Plasma levels of antioxidant beta-carotene and alpha-tocopherol in uterine cervix dysplasias and cancer. Nutr Cancer 1991;15:13–20.

8. Dawson EB, et al. Serum vitamin and selenium changes in cervical dysplasia. Fed Proc 1984;43:612.

9. Wassertheil-Smoller S, et al. Dietary vitamin C and uterine cervical dysplasia. Am J Epidemiol 1981;114:714–724.

10. Romney SL, et al. Retinoids and the prevention of cervical dysplasias. Am J Obstet Gynecol 1981;141:890–894.

11. Butterworth CE, et al. Improvement in cervical dysplasia associated with folic acid therapy in users of oral contraceptives. Am J Clin Nutr 1982;35:73–82.

12. Butterworth CE Jr, et al. Folate deficiency and cervical dysplasia. JAMA 1992;267:528–533.

Migraine Headache

1. Wilkinson CF Jr. Recurrent migrainoid headaches associated with spontaneous hypoglycemia. Am J Med Sci 1949;218:209–212.

2. Stoll W. Teen headaches disappear. Med Tribune, March 31, 1982, p. 23.

3. DeGowin EL. Allergic migraine: a review of sixty cases. J Allergy 1932;3:557–566.

4. Grant ECG. Food allergies and migraine. Lancet 1979;1:966–969.

5. Baker B. New research approach helps clarify magnesium/migraine link. Family Pract News, August 15, 1993, p. 16.

6. Weaver K. Magnesium and migraine. Headache 1990;30:168.

7. Faccinetti F, et al. Magnesium prophylaxis of menstrual migraine: effects on intracellular magnesium. Headache 1991;31:298–304.

8. Peikert A, et al. Prophylaxis of migraine with oral magnesium: results from a prospective, multi-center, placebo-controlled and double-blind randomized study. Cephalalgia 1996;16:257–263.

9. Pfaffenrath V, et al. Magnesium in the prophylaxis of migraine—a double-blind, placebo-controlled study. Cephalalgia 1996;16:436–440.

10. Mauskop A, et al. Intravenous magnesium sulphate relieves migraine attacks in patients with low serum ionized magnesium levels: a pilot study. Clin Sci 1995;89:633–636.

11. Schoenen J, et al. High-dose riboflavin as a prophylactic treatment of migraine: results of an open pilot study. Cephalalgia 1994;14:328–329.

12. Schoenen J, et al. High-dose riboflavin as a novel prophylactic antimigraine therapy: results from a double blind, randomized, placebo-controlled trial. Cephalalgia 1997;17:244.

13 Johnson ES, et al. Efficacy of feverfew as prophylactic treatment of migraine. Br Med J 1985;291:569–573.

14. Murphy JJ, et al. Randomised double-blind placebo-controlled trial of feverfew in migraine prevention. Lancet 1988;2:189–192.

Multiple Sclerosis

1. Meyer MG, et al. Is multiple sclerosis a manifestation of idioblaptic allergy? Psychiatr Q 1954(January); 28:57–71.
2. Ehrentheil OF, et al. Role of food allergy in multiple sclerosis. Neurology 1952;2:412–426.
3. Crook WG. *The Yeast Connection Handbook.* Professional Books, Jackson, TN, 1996.
4. Swank RL, et al. Effect of low saturated fat diet in early and late cases of multiple sclerosis. Lancet 1990;336:37–39.
5. Swank RL. Multiple sclerosis: fat-oil relationship. Nutrition 1991;7:368–376.
6. Dworkin RH, et al. Linoleic acid and multiple sclerosis: a reanalysis of three double-blind trials. Neurology 1984;34:1441–1445.
7. Clark WF, Parbtani A. Omega-3 fatty acid supplementation in clinical and experimental lupus nephritis. Am J Kidney Dis 1994;23:644–647.
8. Horrobin DF, et al. Polyunsaturated fatty acids and colchicine in multiple sclerosis. Br Med J 1979; 1:199–200.
9. Bates D, et al. Polyunsaturated fatty acids in treatment of acute remitting multiple sclerosis. Br Med J 1978;2:1390–1391.
10. Anonymous. Vitamin B_{12} in multiple sclerosis. JAMA 1950;143:1272.
11. Korwin-Piotrowska T, et al. Experience of Padma 28 in multiple sclerosis. Phytother Res 1992;6:133–136.
12. Adaptrin may be obtained by prescription from Pacific Biologic: 1-800-869-8783.
13. Lowry ML, et al. Adenosine-5-monophosphate in the treatment of multiple sclerosis. Am J Med Sci 1953;226:73–83.

Osteoarthritis

1. Rashad S, et al. Effect of non-steroidal anti-inflammatory drugs on the course of osteoarthritis. Lancet 1989;2:519–522.
2. Childers NF, Russo GM. *The Nightshades and Health.* Horticultural Publications, Somerset Press, Inc., Somerville, NJ, 1973.
3. Kaufman W. *The Common Form of Joint Dysfunction: its Incidence and Treatment.* E.L. Hildreth Co., Brattleboro, VT, 1949.
4. Jonas WB, et al. The effect of niacinamide on osteoarthritis: a pilot study. Inflamm Res 1996; 45:330–334.
5. Kaufman W. Niacinamide: a most neglected vitamin. J Int Acad Prev Med 1983(Winter):5–25.
6. Pujalte JM, et al. Double-blind clinical evaluation of oral glucosamine sulphate in the basic treatment of osteoarthritis. Curr Med Res Opin 1980;7:110–114.
7. Noack W, et al. Glucosamine sulfate in osteoarthritis of the knee. Osteoarthritis Cartilage 1994;2:51–59.
8. Vaz AL. Double-blind clinical evaluation of the relative efficacy of glucosamine sulphate in the management of osteoarthritis of the knee in out-patients. Curr Med Res Opin 1982;8:145–149.
9. Drovanti A, et al. Therapeutic activity of oral glucosamine sulfate in osteoarthrosis: a placebo-controlled double-blind investigation. Clin Ther 1980;3:260–272.
10. Morreale P, et al. Comparison of the antiinflammatory efficacy of chondroitin sulfate and diclofenac sodium in patients with knee osteoarthritis. J Rheumatol 1996;23:1385–1391.
11. Uebelhart D, et al. Effects of oral chondroitin sulfate on the progression of knee osteoarthritis: a pilot study. Osteoarthritis Cartilage 1998;6(Suppl A): 39–46.
12. Verbruggen G, et al. Chondroitin sulfate: S/DMOAD (structure/disease modifying anti-osteoarthritis drug) in the treatment of finger joint OA. Osteoarthritis Cartilage 1998;6(Suppl A):37–38.
13. Conte A, et al. Biochemical and pharmacokinetic aspects of oral treatment with chondroitin sulfate. Arzneimittelforschung 1995;45:918–925.
14. Machtey I, Ouaknine L. Tocopherol in osteoarthritis: a controlled pilot study. J Am Geriatr Soc 1978; 26:328–330.
15. Peretz A, et al. Adjuvant treatment of recent onset rheumatoid arthritis by selenium supplementation: preliminary observations. Br J Rheumatol 1992; 31:281–286.
16. Tarp U, et al. Selenium treatment in rheumatoid arthritis. Scand J Rheumatol 1985;14: 364–368.
17. Caruso I, Pietrogrande V. Italian double-blind multicenter study comparing S-adenosylmethionine, naproxen, and placebo in the treatment of degenerative joint disease. Am J Med 1987;83(Suppl 5A): 66–71.

18. Montrone F, et al. Double-blind study of S-adenosyl-methionine versus placebo in hip and knee arthrosis. Clin Rheumatol 1985;4:484–485.

19. Vetter G. Double-blind comparative clinical trial with S-adenosylmethionine and indomethacin in the treatment of osteoarthritis. Am J Med 1987;83 (Suppl 5A):78–80.

20. Czap A. Beware the son of SAMe. Altern Med Rev 1999;4(2):Editorial preceding page 74.

Osteoporosis

1. Chiu J-F, et al. Long-term vegetarian diet and bone mineral density in postmenopausal Taiwanese women. Calcif Tissue Int 1997;60:245–249.

2. Feskanich D, et al. Milk, dietary calcium, and bone fractures in women: a 12-year prospective study. Am J Public Health 1997;87:992–997.

3. Ishida H, et al. Preventive effects of the plant isoflavones, daidzin and genistin, on bone loss in ovariectomized rats fed a calcium-deficient diet. Biol Pharm Bull 1998;21:62–66.

4. Harrison E, et al. The effect of soybean protein on bone loss in a rat model of postmenopausal osteoporosis. J Nutr Sci Vitaminol 1998;44:257–268.

5. Knight DC, et al. A review of the clinical effects of phytoestrogens. Obstet Gynecol 1996;87:897–904.

6. Hart JP, et al. Electrochemical detection of depressed circulating levels of vitamin K_1 in osteoporosis. J Clin Endocrinol Metab 1985;60:1268–1269.

7. Tomita A. Postmenopausal osteoporosis [47]Ca kinetic study with vitamin K_2. Clin Endocrinol (Jpn) 1971;19:731–736. Article in Japanese (summary taken from review by Gallop PM. N Engl J Med 1980;302:1460–1466).

8. Feskanich D, et al. Vitamin K intake and hip fractures in women: a prospective study. Am J Clin Nutr 1999;69:74–79.

9. Cohen L, Kitzes R. Infrared spectroscopy and magnesium content of bone mineral in osteoporotic women. Isr J Med Sci 1981;17:1123–1125.

10. Vikhanski L. Magnesium may slow bone loss. Med Tribune July 22, 1993.

11. Gold M. Basketball bones. Science 80, May/June 1980, pp. 101–102.

12. Brattstrom LE, et al. Folic acid responsive postmenopausal homocysteinemia. Metabolism 1985; 34:1073–1077.

13. Nielsen FH. Boron—an overlooked element of potential nutritional importance. Nutr Today 1988 (Jan/Feb):4–7.

14. Lee JR. Is natural progesterone the missing link in osteoporosis prevention and treatment? Med Hypotheses 1991;35:316–318.

15. Leonetti HB, etal. Transdermal progesterone cream for vasomotor symptoms and postmenopausal bone loss. Obstet Gynecol 1999;94:225–228.

16. Labrie F, et al. Effect of 12-month dehydroepiandrosterone replacement therapy on bone, vagina, and endometrium in postmenopausal women. J Clin Endocrinol Metab 1997;82:3498–3505.

17. Katznelson L, et al. Increase in bone density and lean body mass during testosterone administration in men with acquired hypogonadism. J Clin Endocrinol Metab 1996;81:4358–4365.

18. Wright JV, Lenard L. *Maximize Your Vitality and Potency: for Men Over 40.* Smart Publications, Petaluma, CA, 1999.

19. de Aloysio D, et al. Bone density changes in postmenopausal women with the administration of ipriflavone alone or in association with low-dose ERT. Gynecol Endocrinol 1997;11:289–293.

20. Adami S, et al. Ipriflavone prevents radial bone loss in postmenopausal women with low bone mass over 2 years. Osteoporos Int 1997;7:119–125.

21. Mazzuoli GF. Inhibitory effect of ipriflavone on vertebral bone mass loss in postmenopausal women with low bone mass. Osteoporos Int 1996;6(Suppl 1):93.

22. Monostory K, et al. Ipriflavone as an inhibitor of human cytochrome P450 enzymes. Br J Pharmacol 1998;123:605–610.

23. Gutfeld R. Excessive lead found in water of many cities. Wall Street Journal, October 21, 1992, p. B7.

Peptic Ulcer

1. Anonymous. Aluminum in antacids shown to accumulate in brain and bone tissue. Gastroenterol Observer 1986;5(6):1–2.

2. Gaby AR. *Preventing and Reversing Osteoporosis.* Prima Publishing, Rocklin, CA, 1994.

3. Siegel J. Gastrointestinal ulcer: Arthus reaction. Ann Allergy 1974;32:127–130.

4. Siegel J. Immunologic approach to the treatment and prevention of gastrointestinal ulcers. Ann Allergy 1977;38:27–41.

5 Turpie AGG, et al. Clinical trial of deglycyrrhizinized liquorice in gastric ulcer. Gut 1969;10:299–302.

6. Kassir ZA. Endoscopic controlled trial of four drug regimens in the treatment of chronic duodenal ulceration. Ir Med J 1985;78:153–156.

7. Glick L. Deglycyrrhizinated liquorice for peptic ulcer. Lancet 1982;2:817.

8. Takeuchi K, et al. Effect of L-glutamine on acetylsalicylic acid-induced gastric lesions in pregnant and non-pregnant rats. Jpn J Pharmacol 1976; 26:267.

9. Shive W, et al. Glutamine in treatment of peptic ulcer. Texas State J Med 1957;53:840–843.

10. Cho CH, et al. A correlative study of the antiulcer effects of zinc sulphate in stressed rats. Eur J Pharmacol 1978;48:97–105.

11. Ogle CW, et al. Protection by zinc sulphate against reserpine-induced ulceration and other gastric effects in the rat. Pharmacology 1978;17:254–261.

12. Frommer DJ. The healing of gastric ulcers by zinc sulphate. Med J Aust 1975;2:793–796.

13. Sorenson JRJ. Copper chelates as possible active forms of antiarthritic agents. J Medicinal Chem 1976;19:135–148.

14. Schumpelick VV, Farthmann E. Study on the protective effect of vitamin A on stress ulcer of the rat. Arzneimittelforschung 1976;26:386–388.

15. Chernov MS, et al. Stress ulcer: a preventable disease. J Trauma 1972;12:831–846.

16. Huwez FU, et al. Mastic gum kills *Helicobacter pylori*. N Engl J Med 1998;339:1946.

17. Al-Habbal MJ, et al. A double-blind controlled clinical trial of mastic and placebo in the treatment of duodenal ulcer. Clin Exp Pharmacol Physiol 1984; 11:541–544.

18. Huwez FU, Al-Habbal MJ. Mastic in the treatment of benign gastric ulcers. Gastroenterol Jpn 1986; 21:273–274.

19. Jorosz M, et al. Effects of high dose vitamin C treatment on *Helicobacter pylori* infection and total vitamin C concentration in gastric juice. Eur J Cancer Prev 1998;7:449–454.

Pregnancy (preventing and treating toxemia)

1. Brewer T. Metabolic toxemia: the mysterious affliction. J Appl Nutr 1972;24:56–63.

2. Conradt A, et al. Magnesium deficiency, a possible cause of pre-eclampsia: reduction of frequency of premature rupture of membranes and premature or small-for-date deliveries after magnesium supplementation. J Am Coll Nutr 1985;4:321.

3. Bucher HC, et al. Effect of calcium supplementation on pregnancy-induced hypertension and preeclampsia. A meta-analysis of randomized controlled trials. JAMA 1996;275:1113–1117.

4. Wachstein M, et al. Influence of vitamin B$_6$ on the incidence of preeclampsia. Obstet Gynecol 1956; 8:177–180.

5. Hillman RW, et al. Pyridoxine supplementation during pregnancy. Clinical and laboratory observations. Am J Clin Nutr 1963;12:427–430.

6. Shute E. The effect of vitamin E upon impaired kidney function. Can Med Assoc J 1945;52:151–153.

7. Hipsley EH. Dietary "fibre" and pregnancy toxaemia. Br Med J 1953;2:420–422.

8. Burger H. Modification by rutin of capillary resistance and capillary permeability during pregnancy. JAMA 1952;148:586(Abstract).

9. Ellis JM, Presley J. *Vitamin B$_6$: the Doctor's Report.* Harper and Row, New York, 1973.

Premenstrual Syndrome

1. Rossignol AM. Caffeine-containing beverages and premenstrual syndrome in young women. Am J Public Health 1985;75:1335–1337.

2. Prior JC, et al. Conditioning exercise decreases premenstrual symptoms: a prospective, controlled 6-month trial. Fertil Steril 1987;47:402–408.

3. Gaby AR. *The Doctor's Guide to Vitamin B$_6$.* Rodale Press, Emmaus, PA, 1984, chapter 2.

4. Abraham GE, Hargrove JT. Effect of vitamin B$_6$ on premenstrual symptomatology in women with premenstrual tension syndrome: a double-blind crossover study. Infertility 1980;3:155–165.

5. Kerr GD. The management of premenstrual syndrome. Curr Med Res Opin 1977;4(Suppl 4): 29–34).

6. Snider B, et al. Pyridoxine therapy for premenstrual acne flare. Arch Dermatol 1974;110:130–131.

7. Sherwood RA, et al. Magnesium and the premenstrual syndrome. Ann Clin Biochem 1986;23: 667–670.

8. Facchinetti F, et al. Oral magnesium successfully relieves premenstrual mood changes. Obstet Gynecol 1991;78:177–181.

9. Walker AF, et al. Magnesium supplementation

alleviates premenstrual symptoms of fluid retention. J Womens Health 1998;7:1157–1165.

10. Thys-Jacobs S, et al. Calcium carbonate and the premenstrual syndrome: effects on premenstrual and menstrual symptoms. Am J Obstet Gynecol 1998; 179:444–452.

11. London RS, et al. The effect of alpha-tocopherol on premenstrual symptomatology: a double-blind study. J Am Coll Nutr 1983;2:115–122.

12. Larsson B, et al. Evening primrose oil in the treatment of premenstrual syndrome: a pilot study. Curr Ther Res 1989;46:58–63.

13. Khoo SK, et al. Evening primrose oil and treatment of premenstrual syndrome. Med J Aust 1990;153: 189–192.

14. Brayshaw ND, Brayshaw DD. Thyroid hypofunction in premenstrual syndrome. N Engl J Med 1986; 315:1486–1487.

15. Roy-Byrne PP, et al. TSH and prolactin responses to TRH in patients with premenstrual syndrome. Am J Psychiatry 1987;144:480–484.

16. Dalton K. *The Premenstrual Syndrome and Progesterone Therapy.* Yearbook Medical Publishers, Inc., Chicago, 1984.

17. Wahlen T. Endocrine allergy. A study in 35 cases with premenstrual symptoms of allergic-type. Acta Obstet Gynaecol Scand 1955;34:161–170.

Psoriasis

1. Bazex A, et al. Diet without gluten and psoriasis. Ann Dermatol Syph 1976;103:648–650.

2. Michaelsson G, Gerden B. How common is gluten intolerance among patients with psoriasis? Acta Derm Venereol 1991;71:90.

3. Bittiner SB, et al. A double-blind, randomised placebo-controlled trial of fish oil in psoriasis. Lancet 1988;1:378–380.

4. Perez A, et al. Efficacy and safety of topical calcitriol (1,25-dihydroxyvitamin D_3) for the treatment of psoriasis. Br J Dermatol 1996;134:238–246.

5. Morimoto S, et al. Topical administration of 1,25-dihydroxyvitamin D_3 for psoriasis: report of five cases. Calcif Tissue Int 1986;38:119–122.

6. Morimoto S, et al. Treatment of psoriasis vulgaris by oral administration of 1alpha-hydroxyvitamin D_3— open design study. Calcif Tissue Int 1986;39: 209–212.

7. Oster KA. A cardiologist considers psoriasis. Cutis 1977;20:39–41.

8. Ruedemann R Jr. Treatment of psoriasis with large doses of vitamin B_{12}; 1,100 micrograms per cubic centimeter. Arch Dermatol 1954;69:738–739.

9. Cohen EL. Vitamin B_{12} in psoriasis. Br Med J 1963;1:125.

10. Altmeyer PJ, et al. Antipsoriatic effect of fumaric acid derivatives. Results of a multicenter double-blind study in 100 patients. J Am Acad Dermatol 1994;30:977–981.

11. Nieboer C, et al. Systemic therapy with fumaric acid derivates: new possibilities in the treatment of psoriasis. J Am Acad Dermatol 1989;20:601–608.

12. Pelkowitz D. A new treatment for psoriasis. S Afr Med J 1981;60:804.

Recurrent Infections

1. Ringsdorf WM Jr, et al. Sucrose, neutrophilic phagocytosis and resistance to disease. Dent Survey 1976; 52(12):46–48.

2. Sanchez A, et al. Role of sugars in human neutrophilic phagocytosis. Am J Clin Nutr 1973;26: 1180–1184.

3. Nalder BN, et al. Sensitivity of the immunological response to the nutritional status of rats. J Nutr 1972;102:535–542.

4. Samaranayake LP, MacFarlane TW. On the role of dietary carbohydrates in the pathogenesis of oral candidosis. FEMS Microbiol Lett 1985;27:1–5.

5. Nsouli TM, et al. Role of food allergy in serous otitis media. Ann Allergy 1994;73:215–219.

6. Sommer A. Vitamin A, infectious disease, and childhood mortality: a 2¢ solution? J Infect Dis 1993; 167:1003–1007.

7. Pinnock CB, et al. Vitamin A status in children who are prone to respiratory tract infections. Aust Paediatr J 1986;22:95–99.

8. Ritzel G. Kritische beurteilung des vitamins C als prophylacticum und therapeuticum der erkaltungskrankheiten. Helvetia Med Acta 1961;28:63–68.

9. Anderson TW, et al. Vitamin C and the common cold: a double-blind trial. Can Med Assoc J 1972; 107:503–508.

10. Cathcart RF III. Vitamin C in the treatment of acquired immune deficiency syndrome (AIDS). Med Hypotheses 1984;14:423–433.

11. Brody I. Treatment of recurrent furunculosis with oral zinc. Lancet 1977;2:1358.

12. Mocchegiani E, et al. Benefit of oral zinc supplementation as an adjunct to zidovudine (AZT) therapy against opportunistic infections in AIDS. Int J Immunopharmacol 1995;17:719–727.

13. Sazawal S, et al. Zinc supplementation reduces the incidence of acute lower respiratory infections in infants and preschool children: a double-blind, controlled trial. Pediatrics 1998;102:1–5.

14. Wolf WR, et al. Daily intake of zinc and copper from self selected diets. Fed Proc 1977;36:1175.

15. Chandra RK. Effect of vitamin and trace-element supplementation on immune responses and infection in elderly subjects. Lancet 1992;340:1124–1127.

16. Palmblad J, et al. Neutrophil function in hypothyroid patients. Acta Med Scand 1981;210:287–291.

Rheumatoid Arthritis

1. Hicklin JA, et al. The effect of diet in rheumatoid arthritis. Clin Allergy 1980;10:463.

2. Anonymous. Environmental factors in arthritis: certain foods deemed reactive. American Rheumatism Association, Convention Reporter 1980, vol 10, No. 28.

3. Darlington LG, et al. Placebo-controlled, blind study of dietary manipulation therapy in rheumatoid arthritis. Lancet 1986;1:236–238.

4. Simkin PA. Oral zinc sulfate in rheumatoid arthritis. Lancet 1976;2:539–542.

5. Rasker JJ, Kardaun SH. Lack of beneficial effect of zinc sulphate in rheumatoid arthritis. Scand J Rheumatol 1982;11:168–170.

6. Walker WR, Keats DM. An investigation of the therapeutic value of the "copper bracelet": dermal assimilation of copper in arthritic/rheumatoid conditions. Agents Actions 1976;6:454–459.

7. Sorenson JRJ. Copper chelates as possible active forms of the antiarthritic agents. J Medicinal Chem 1976;19:135–148.

8. Tarp U, et al. Low selenium level in severe rheumatoid arthritis. Scand J Rheumatol 1985;14:97–101.

9. Peretz A, et al. Adjuvant treatment of recent onset rheumatoid arthritis by selenium supplementation: preliminary observations. Br J Rheumatol 1992; 31:281–286.

10. Tarp U, et al. Selenium treatment in rheumatoid arthritis. Scand J Rheumatol 1985;14:364–368.

11. Leventhal LJ, et al. Treatment of rheumatoid arthritis with gammalinolenic acid. Ann Intern Med 1993; 119:867–873.

12. van der Tempel H, et al. Effects of fish oil supplementation in rheumatoid arthritis. Ann Rheum Dis 1990;49:76–80.

13. Leventhal LJ, et al. Treatment of rheumatoid arthritis with blackcurrant seed oil. Br J Rheumatol 1994; 33:847–852.

14. Kaufman W. *The Common Form of Joint Dysfunction: its Incidence and Treatment.* E.L. Hildreth Co., Brattleboro, VT., 1949.

15. Jonas WB, et al. The effect of niacinamide on osteoarthritis: a pilot study. Inflamm Res 1996; 45:330–334.

16. Srivastava KC, Mustafa T. Ginger (Zingiber officinale) and rheumatic disorders. Med Hypotheses 1989;29:25–28.

Shingles (herpes zoster)

1. Murata A. Virucidal activity of vitamin C for prevention and treatment of viral diseases. In Proc First Int Congr IAMS, Takezi Hasegawa (ed.), Science Council of Japan, 1975.

2. Brody I. Topical treatment of recurrent herpes simplex and post-herpetic erythema multiforme with low concentrations of zinc sulphate solution. Br J Dermatol 1981;104:191–194.

3. Pompei JR, et al. Glycyrrhizic acid inhibits virus growth and inactivates virus particles. Nature 1979; 281:689–690.

4. Yu S-Y, et al. Chemoprevention trial of human hepatitis with selenium supplementation in China. Biol Trace Elem Res 1989;20:15–22.

5. Ayres S Jr, et al. Post-herpes zoster neuralgia: response to vitamin E therapy. Arch Dermatol 1973; 108:855–866.

6. Heyblon R. Vitamin B_{12} in herpes zoster. JAMA 1951;146:1338(Abstract).

7. Sklar SH, et al. Herpes zoster. Br J Dermatol 1981; 104:351–352.

8. Sklar SH, et al. Herpes zoster: the treatment and prevention of neuralgia with adenosine monophosphate. JAMA 1985;253:1427–1430.

9. Bernstein JE, et al. Treatment of chronic postherpetic neuralgia with topical capsaicin. J Am Acad Dermatol 1987;17:93–96.

Ulcerative Colitis

1. Andresen AFR. Ulcerative colitis: an allergic phenomenon. Am J Dig Dis 1942;9:91–98.

2. Siegel J. Inflammatory bowel disease: another possible facet of the allergic diathesis. Ann Allergy 1981; 47:92–94.

3. Rider JA, Moeller HC. Food hypersensitivity in ulcerative colitis: further experience with an intramucosal test. Am J Gastroenterol 1962;37:497–507.

4. Rowe AH, Rowe A Jr. Chronic ulcerative colitis: atopic allergy in its etiology. Am J Gastroenterol 1960;34:49–60.

5. Grasso P, et al. Studies on carrageenan and large-bowel ulceration in mammals. Food Cosmet Toxicol 1973;11:555–564.

6. Carruthers LB. Chronic diarrhea treated with folic acid. Lancet 1946;1:849.

7. Dronfield MW, et al. Zinc in ulcerative colitis: a therapeutic trial and report on plasma levels. Gut 1977;18:33–36.

8. Stenson WF, et al. Dietary supplementation with fish oil in ulcerative colitis. Ann Intern Med 1992;116: 609–614.

9. Scheppach W, et al. Effect of butyrate enemas on the colonic mucosa in distal ulcerative colitis. Gastroenterology 1992;103:51–56.

10. Steinhart AH, et al. Treatment of refractory ulcerative proctosigmoiditis with butyrate enemas. Am J Gastroenterol 1994;89:179–183.

11. de la Torre B, et al. Blood and tissue dehydroepiandrosterone sulphate levels and their relationship to chronic inflammatory bowel disease. Clin Exp Rheumatol 1998;16:579–582.

12. Van Vollenhoven RF, et al. An open study of dehydroepiandrosterone in systemic lupus erythematosus. Arthritis Rheum 1994;37:1305–1310.

INDEX